A Consumer's Guide to the Pill and other Drugs.

Second Edition.

FULLY REVISED AND UPDATED.

John Wilks B.Pharm M.P.S.

"In an age in which preventative medicine has high priority, it is distressing to have women exploited as guinea pigs in order to establish with absolute certainty the causal relationship of the Pill to cancer and other complications."

Dr Margaret White [1]

Publishing Details.
First published in Australia in October, 1996, by TGB Books, a
part of Freedom Publishing Company Pty Ltd.
582 Queensberry St.
North Melbourne, Victoria 3051 Australia
Telephone: +61 3 93265757
Fax: +61 3 93282877
ISBN 0 646 29226 9
Cover Design by Clare Cannon, Portico Books, Pennant Hills,
NSW, Australia.

This edition published in America in October, 1997, by ALL Inc.,
Stafford, Virginia 22555.
Telephone: 540 659 4171
Fax: 540 659 2586
ISBN 1-890712-25-6
Cover Design by Clare Cannon, Portico Books, Pennant Hills,
NSW, Australia.

Table of Contents

vi

FOREWORD TO THE SECOND EDITION.

The Wilks book is a remarkable piece of work, especially strong on the physiology and pharmacologic endocrinology relating to oral contraception. This tome is encyclopedic in its range. It is must reading for all who are interested in the broad subject of oral contraception: morally, ethically and/or scientifically. I recommend it enthusiastically and without reservation.

Bernard N. Nathanson, M.D., P.C.
Clinical Associate Professor of Obstetrics and Gynaecology
New York Medical College,
Visiting Scholar at Vanderbilt University.
July, 1997.

FOREWORD TO THE FIRST EDITION.

We all have the right to make informed choices about our health and about the chemicals we put inside our bodies. Making such choices is not helped by the manner in which much relevant information is available; either as over-simplified summaries in short booklets, or spread across hundreds of journals in thousands of research papers and scholarly reviews. Mr Wilks provides a critical review of the literature relating to the safety, effectiveness and mode-of-action of drugs developed to manipulate female hormonal physiology. Although not everyone may agree with his conclusions, he raises important questions about the ways in which what is known through research is packaged and presented to prescribers and consumers.

Prof. Tim Usherwood
Professor of General Practice
University of Sydney
N.S.W.   Australia.
1996

PREFACE.

In the past 30 years, hormonal drugs of various types have become common place in the lives of women, from the time of their first menstruation to well into the menopause. There are drugs to suppress or stimulate fertility, drugs to suppress or replicate the effects of a monthly period and drugs to end or maintain a pregnancy. In fact, there is a drug to match almost all the variables in women's health.

Accompanying this variety is an enormous volume of consumption, with the oral 'contraceptive' alone accounting for over 3.9 million scripts per annum in Australia. Yet it has been my experience for fifteen years as a community pharmacist that the average woman knows very little about these drugs and the long-term effects they will have. This book has been written to help the average woman get the answers she needs to these important questions.

Of particular concern with many of these drugs is the substantial body of research which leads to the conclusion that they are associated with a variety of illnesses in women, most notably breast cancer.

There are two methods which I have used in arranging the order of the chapters in this book.

First, I have sought to follow a woman's reproductive and sexual life as closely as possible. The first nine chapters discuss drugs or devices which are used by women during their reproductive years: the pill, Depo-Provera, Norplant, barrier contraceptives, chemical abortifacients and fertility drugs. Chapter Ten deals with hormone replacement therapy (HRT).

Second, I have grouped topics according to similarity of drug use and drug design. It is easier to read material on drugs with a common *modus operandi* than it is to move from one drug delivery system to another because of some lesser similarities such as side-effects or mortality rate. Accordingly, the pill, Norplant, and Depo-Provera are discussed in separate chapters. Whilst they all contain a synthetic version of progesterone, the drug is administered to the patient via different drug delivery systems which have different developmental histories. The pill receives four chapters because of the vast amount of medical literature related to this drug treatment, the on-going controversy surrounding it and the sheer number of women who daily ingest it.

Barrier methods of contraception such as spermicides and condoms are grouped together for obvious reasons. Post-coital 'contraceptives' such as RU-486 and methotrexate are grouped together because they are all chemical abortifacients and they are used post-intercourse. HRT and fertility drugs are dealt with individually, since they are neither 'contraceptive' nor abortifacient.

The final chapter, Chapter Eleven, presents examples of how material in the preceding ten chapters is criticised without foundation, and minimized or ignored to varying degrees by government health agencies, pharmaceutical manufacturers and the media so as to present a particular drug or device in a way which falsifies or ignores published research. Here lies the source of much community ignorance of these drugs and the reason for this book.

CHAPTER ONE.

1.   THE PILL: HOW IT WORKS AND FAILS.

"... suppression of follicular development is incomplete with the
contemporary low-dose pill.".[2]

1.1   INTRODUCTION.

An understanding of the pill's biological action is central to the relevance of the
research I wish to discuss. Without this, the significance of what is to follow
may be missed. The pharmacology of the pill, both of its successes and failures,
is as relevant to Depo-Provera® as it is to Norplant®, post-coital 'contraception'
and RU-486. To understand the pill is to understand these other drug delivery
systems.

1.2   WORDS AND MEANINGS.

Over the years there has been an intemperate degree of word manipulation,
which has had the effect of altering the semantic significance of many
fundamental definitions in embryology. Arguably the three most commonly
misused terms in female reproductive health, and therefore deserving of
particular attention, are conception,[3] pregnancy[4][5][6] and contraception.[7][8][9]

'Conception' refers to the moment at which the sperm penetrates and fertilises
the ovum to form a viable zygote.[10] It does not refer to the process of implantation
which is a separate event, occurring over a few days, beginning on the 7th or
8th day after conception.[11] A woman is pregnant because conception has
occurred, not because implantation has occurred. This distinction is important.
It is upon the correct definition of this term that many of the medical and ethical
issues to be canvassed in this book will depend.

At the precise and unique moment of conception, a woman is *'pregnant'* with **"a new individual".**[12] This is an accurate and informed medical description. It is the same terminology used by Prof. John Dwyer, pre-eminent Australian AIDS expert and researcher, who has described the moment that the sperm enters the ovum as the creation of a **"new and unique individual".**[13] Well known medical writer, Professor Derek Llewellyn-Jones, also has written that when the male genetic material from the sperm joins with the female genetic material in the ovum, **" a new individual is formed".**[14]

To stop conception occurring, that is, to stop sperm and ovum joining, is *contraception.* Condoms, diaphragms, spermicides, vasectomy and tubal ligation are accurately described as methods of contraception (Latin -L- *Contra* against). Any action due to a drug or device used *after* conception has occurred cannot be termed a contraceptive action[15] (also, see glossary). 'Abortifacient' is the precise biological description for any drug or device which employs a post-conception action.[16]

The weight of medical opinion supports the above definitions of 'conception', 'pregnancy' and 'contraception'. In fact, a substantial range of the world's most respected medical text books use definitions which are almost *verbatim* copies when it comes to defining the above.[17][18][19][20][21][22][23] To break from these definitions is to move outside the accepted linguistic norms of embryology and gynaecology.

Now, with these early tasks accomplished, it is appropriate to review the *modus operandi* of the pill.

1.2.1 HOW THE PILL WORKS.

1. To varying degrees the various formulations of the pill act by a *suppression of ovulation*, but neither the progesterone-only pill[24] nor the combined progesterone-oestrogen formulations always inhibits ovulation.[25][26][27]

(N.B. The American and English/Australian spelling of estrogen differ. The former spell it as estrogen, whereas the latter place an 'o' before the 'e'. I shall adopt the English convention in the general text, but employ the same as that used in a reference if I quote from it).

2. All formulations of the pill cause varying degrees of *alterations to cervical mucus.* The cervical mucus may become thicker and hence make it more difficult for sperm to move through the neck of the cervix.[28]

3. Both the progesterone-only and the oestrogen-progesterone formulations act to cause alterations to the *lining of the womb,* converting the proliferative nature of the endometrium, which is naturally designed to accept and sustain a fertilised ovum, to a secretory endometrium,[29] [30] which is a thin, devasculating lining,[31] physiologically unreceptive to receiving and sustaining a zygote.[32]   In many medical text books, this action of the pill is referred to as 'the inhibition of nidation' (Latin *nidus* nest) .

4. The pill causes changes to the *movement of the Fallopian tubes,* which may alter the time taken for the passage of the ovum and hence reduce the possibility of the ovum's being fertilised.[33] [34] [35]

1.2.2 THE PILL: WHAT'S IN A NAME?

It is relevant to note that none of these mechanisms of action of either the mini-pill or combined pill is absolute.[36] Ovulation is not always stopped,[37] [38] [39] [40] cervical mucus is not always made impenetrable,[41] [42] the lining of the womb is not always rendered unreceptive to a fertilised ovum every cycle,[43] [44] and Fallopian tube activity does not always inhibit sperm and ovum unification.[45] Therefore, it is incorrect to describe the mini-pill[46] or the combined pill[47] as an oral 'contraceptive', since these pills have a mechanism of action which goes beyond mere 'contra-ception'. The adjective 'contraceptive' should not be used in conjunction with the noun 'pill'. Henceforth, I will refer to this drug as simply the pill; however, readers will note that most researchers quoted in this book use the term oral contraceptive, usually abbreviated as OC.

1.2.3 PILL FAILURE RATES AND INDUCED ABORTION.

What proof exists to indicate that these inter-connected mechanisms of action do not always operate 'successfully' in every woman? *First,* there is the simplest evidence that women *do* become pregnant whilst on the pill (cf.,p.24). There are two accepted measures of this evident pill failure.

The first measurement of the rate of pill failure, and hence pregnancy, is known as the *theoretical efficacy rate*.

> **"The theoretical-effectiveness of any birth control method is 'the maximum effectiveness of that method, i.e., its effectiveness when used without error, when used perfectly, when used exactly according to instructions'."**[48]

The word 'theoretical' refers to the rate of pregnancy which *should* occur under perfect conditions of pill use.

The second measurement of pregnancy whilst on the pill is the *use-effectiveness rate*. This rate is taken as the measure of what *does* happen in real life. It takes into account many aspects of the 'human factor': i.e., those who use the pill correctly and those who don't.[49]

For the progesterone-only (or mini-pill) the theoretical-effectiveness is 98.5-99%, meaning that only 1- 1.5 women per 100 should become pregnant. The use-effectiveness is lower at 90-95%, meaning that between 5-10% of women do become pregnant .[50]

For the combined pill the theoretical-effectiveness is 99.66%, meaning that only 0.34% or 34 women in 10,000 should become pregnant. The use-effectiveness of the combined pill is 90-96%, that is, within the general population 4-10% of women do become pregnant.[51] Australian medical and science journalist Melissa Sweet has published use-effectiveness figures in the same range.[52]

Instead of indicating the theoretical or use-effectiveness of the pill formulations merely as a percentage of the total number of women using them, there is a more meaningful method of expressing these figures. It is known as the Pearl Index. This index measures how many of every 100 women making use of a particular 'contraceptive' are likely to become pregnant if the method is used for one year.[53] As the reader will notice, the Pearl Index takes into account both the number of women taking the pill (as does a percentage calculation) and *the amount of time* a woman used the pill.

Using the Pearl Index, the theoretical-effectiveness rates for the *mini-pill* has been quoted as 0.3 pregnancies per 100 women years,[54] whereas the use-effectiveness varies between **"1 and 4 pregnancies/100 women years.".** [55] Other researchers confirm these figures.[56]

The Pearl Index of theoretical-effectiveness for the *combined pill* is varyingly quoted in the range of 0.2 to 0.34 pregnancies per 100 women years,[57] [58] whereas the use-effectiveness of the combined pill has been suggested by Khoo as being in the range of 0.5 to 3 pregnancies per 100 women years.[59] Others have place this figure in the range of 3 pregnancies per 100 women years for married women and up to 6 pregnancies per 100 women years for single women.[60]

The explanation given for the substantial gap between the theoretical-effectiveness and use-effectiveness rates for the different rates of the pill is patient compliance. 'Patient compliance' means that the patient must take the drug on a continued and correct basis.

Factors which may interfere with proper patient compliance include forgetting to take a tablet, nausea and vomiting leading to a reduction in the absorption of a daily dose[61] or a drug interaction with antibiotics (such as amoxycillin, co-trimoxazole, tetracycline, erythromycin and amphotericin), large doses of vitamin C, anti-epileptic medication, barbiturates and rifampicin (used for T.B.).[62] [63] [64]

Whilst imperfect patient compliance can validly lead to pill failure, and hence pregnancy, another physiological phenomena also exists which may more adequately explain an unexpected pregnancy for women who otherwise show a high level of patient compliance. This event is known as *'break-through ovulation'*, which, as the name suggests, means that a woman ovulates despite the regular taking of her daily pill.

This brings us to the *second* proof that the inter-connected mechanisms of the pill do not always 'work' and that consequently 'break-through' ovulation occurs. The pioneering research in this area was done by Dr. Nine Van der Vange, State University of Utrecht, Dept. of Obstetrics. & Gynaecology.[65] The results of her studies have been reported at a Contraceptive Promotion Forum in Jakarta (1984) and published in London in 1988 by Butterworths.

Dr Van der Vange's research used high resolution ultra-sound which visually demonstrated that: **"ovariaň suppression is far from complete with the low dose OC".**[66] This visual proof was further supported by the back-up evidence of blood oestradiol levels (E2) and serum progesterone (P) levels. E2 and P are hormones which are released by the body just before and after ovulation. The presence of these "ovulation" hormones confirmed what the ultra-sound showed: that ovarian activity to the stage of maturation and follicular rupture - the release of a *mature* egg - had occurred.[67] Her research found that amongst the women involved in the study, break-through ovulation occurred in 6 of 420 cycles. By the application of some mathematical formulae to these figures (see appendix 6 for a variation of the Pearl Index computation) it can be demonstrated that even within the environment of a strictly regulated study, with women exhibiting a high level of patient compliance, the pill can have an break-through ovulation rate which can be as high as 17 ovulations per 100 women years.

The validity of this ultrasound research and the authenticity of its findings have received endorsement at the highest level:

> **"The advent of ultrasound technology allowed for careful monitoring of ovarian function in women using OC's. In contrast to earlier assumptions, women were found to have varying degrees of residual ovarian activity, which is characterised by follicular development and concurrent plasma** (blood) **oestradiol levels.".**[68] (Corson, 1993).

Other researchers using this same combined ultrasound/E2/P approach have also reported 'break-through ovulation'. Grimes and co-workers (1994) stated that **"suppression of follicular development is incomplete with the contemporary low-dose pill.".**[69] In fact this study reported a rate of break-through ovulation higher than that of Van der Vange; Grimes' results showed that break-through ovulation occurred at a rate of 26.7 ovulations per 100 women years.[70] Importantly, **"the ovulations that occurred did not appear to be due to noncompliance** (by the women), **based on our review of patient pill diaries and returned pill packages.".**[71] This means that patient compliance was high, and the ovulations detected where attributable to a 'failure' of the pill to completely suppress ovulation.

For many people, the occurrence of ovulation whilst on the combined pill may come as something of a surprise, since for many years medical opinion stated that ovulation did not occur when taking the pill (OCs). For example, Dr. Llewellyn-Jones offered this very view in 1978.

> **"At the dose chosen, the** (contraceptive-hormones)**...prevent the release of follicle-stimulating hormone and of leutenising hormone, so ovulation is prevented."**.[72]

The results of Dr. Van der Vange generated an interesting question. If the observed break-though ovulation rate for a group of dedicated and motivated women involved in a scientific research project can be as much as 17 per 100 women-years, how is it that this high ovulation rate results in a low confirmed pregnancy rate of 0.5 per 100 women-years? Both figures were arrived at within the context of clinical trials involving motivated women exhibiting a high level of patient compliance. What events were taking place which could account for the substantial difference between the ovulation rate of 17 per 100 women-years and a *detected* pregnancy rate of just 0.5 per 100-women years?

Much of the answer to this question has recently been supplied by Dr. Ralf G. Rahwan, Prof. of Pharmacology & Toxicology, Ohio State University. He outlined a convincing case for the pill's substantial abortifacient capacity:

> **"It is important to realise that ovulation is** *not* **always suppressed by oral contraceptives** (combined oestrogen and progestin) **containing 50mcg or less of oestrogen... their close to 100% effectiveness in** *interfering with pregnancy* **is due to the effects of the progestin component on the cervix and uterine endometrium in addition to the oestrogenic effects. This hostile environment results in interception."**[73] (original emphasis).

Interception is that part of a pharmaceutical abortion which occurs prior to implantation. In practise, 'interception' means that the fertilized egg, a new individual, is prevented from implanting in the endometrium. Major international pharmacology texts, such as *Goodman & Gilman's The Pharmacological Basis of Therapeutics* (1990), support the view of Prof. Rahwan.[74]

Lest anyone decide to brusquely set aside this claim by Prof. Rahwan on the pretext that there is some unstated 'pro-life' philosophy that may be operative, it should be noted that Prof. Rahwan advocated **"induced abortion"** if a woman became pregnant whilst using an IUD which cannot be removed.[75] Clearly Prof. Rahwan was setting out the medical facts and not a personal ideological view when he made the above statement.

The U.S. Department of Health defined abortifacient procedures in the same way as Prof. Rahwan:

"All the measures which impair the viability of the zygote at any time between the instant of fertilization and the completion of labour constitute, in the strict sense, procedures for inducing abortion.".[76]

Are there any other factors which may interfere with fertilization (conception) and thereby reduce the abortifacient dimension of the pill? The answer is 'yes'. The pill could stop conception by (1) alterations to cervical mucus status, thereby preventing fertilization, or (2) by influencing Fallopian tube movement such that the sperm and ovum could not fuse. A number of scientific publications indicate that in reality these two possibilities have diminished importance.

Taking the first point, it can be stated that the effect of the pill on sperm mobility through cervical mucous is minimal with both the mini-pill (progesterone only) and the combined pill. This is because **"the effect of the progestogen on sperm penetration of the cervical mucus is maximum after 4 hours and remains at that level for the next 16-20 hours"**[77] but **"by 24 hours after ingestion, normal sperm penetration is likely to occur"**.[78]

Thus there is a time-gap in the 'protection' conferred by the mini-pill via the barrier of cervical mucus of 4-8 hours; the first four hour 'gap' exists from the time the pill is ingested until maximum effect is achieved four hours later. The second possible four hour 'gap' is towards the end of the 24 hour day during which the previous pill was taken. Clearly if a woman takes her mini-pill at night just prior to going to bed and having intercourse, the effect of the progestagen will be minimal. The tablet taken the previous night will have little or no remaining effect on cervical mucous, and the new tablet just ingested will not yet have had time to exert its effect. This scenario is a most reasonable one. A New Zealand report stated that 10 out of 19 women in fact *did* take the mini-pill just prior to bedtime near the time of having sexual intercourse. Hence, fertilization would not be impaired, and the abortifacient aspect of the mini-pill , or the combined pill could predominate.[79] (The nature of the cervical mucus which regulates sperm movement towards the ovum is predominantly related to the progestogen hormone in the pill formulations).[80]

On the second point, the magnitude of the pill's effect on ovum movement down the Fallopian tubes is also debatable. Oestrogen and progestins have opposing effects on ovum transport time. Oestrogen speeds up ovum transport and progestins slow ovum transport down.[81] In effect, the actions of the two hormones may neutralise each other, permitting the released ovum to move through the Fallopian tube at an unaffected rate.

Thus we are left with an explanation for the gap between the ovulation rate and *detected* pregnancy rate which in the past has had a diminished, even marginalised importance: the abortifacient impact of both the mini-pill and the commonly prescribed low-dose combined pill.

The abortifacient impact of both formulations of the pill, which is measured as the difference between the ovulation rate and the pregnancy rate, could be termed the 'abortion of undetected pregnancy' rate (AUP rate). This calculation yields the *maximum* possible A.U.P. rate - it will be diminished to some degree because every ovulation does not result in conception, the beginning of the pregnancy.

There is clear corroborate evidence for the suggestion that the pill has an A.U.P. rate. Looking first at the mini-pill , Dr. Edith Weisberg, Medical superintendent of the Family Planning Association of N.S.W.(Aust) , said that: **" in 40%** (of cases) **ovarian cycles are totally normal with normal ovulation and normal hormone production.".**[82]

Based on this figure from Dr Weisberg, 40 out of 100 women taking the mini-pill ovulate. But do 40 out of 100 women on the mini-pill become pregnant? According to research done by Prof. Rahwan, the actual efficacy (success) rate of the mini pill is 90-95%. That is, of the 40% of women who ovulate whilst on the mini-pill, only 5-10% report a detected and confirmed pregnancy. Thus there is a substantial gap between the percentage of women who ovulate (40%), and the percentage who are confirmed pregnant (5-10%).

To calculate a theoretical *maximum* value for the interceptive/early abortifacient capacity of the mini-pill (its AUP rate), we subtract the number of women who have a confirmed pregnancy whilst taking the mini-pill (5-10 per 100 women) from the number who may have ovulated (40 per 100 women). This yields a total number of pharmaceutically induced abortions of undetected pregnancies for the mini-pill of up to 30 and 35 per 100 women.[83] Aside from the evidence presented by these calculations, the fact that fewer women present with a pregnancy than the total who may ovulate argues strongly in favour of the mini-pill having a substantial AUP rate.

Some indication of the AUP rate for the combined pill can be obtained by subtracting the number of women who have a confirmed pregnancy whilst on the combined pill (0.5 per 100 woman-years) from the number of women who have breakthrough ovulation (17 per 100 woman-years). This yields a total maximum number of pharmaceutically induced abortions of undetected pregnancies of just less than 17 per women-years.

The AUP rate for the combined pill is less than that for the mini-pill, a result which is not surprising given that the combined pill contains two hormones which would more fully suppress ovulation than does a formulation of progesterone alone. Nonetheless, the AUP rate is substantial.

1.2.4 CASE STUDY.

The case of Kathyryn Martin, 22, mother of a one year old child, highlighted the tragic consequences of assuming that the pill will always prevent pregnancy. On July 3, 1995, she presented at the Shoalhaven District Memorial Hospital, New South Wales (Australia) with abdominal pains. She was treated for gastro-enteritis and discharged late in the evening. Two days later her husband found her dead on the bedroom floor.

A coronial inquest, as reported in the *Sydney Morning Herald* on September 16, 1997, established that despite taking the low-dose pill and breast feeding, Mrs. Martin had died of an undiagnosed ectopic pregnancy. The treating doctor admitted to the court that he discounted the possibility of pregnancy as the cause of her symptoms because she was on the low-dose pill and breast feeding.

Had the possibility of pregnancy been considered her condition would have been treated appropriately and her life saved. The attending physician remarked that he now does a pregnancy test on any woman presenting with abdominal pain.

1.3   KEY POINTS.

Why is an emphasis on the abortifacient impact of the pill necessary?

The simple answer is that in a pluralistic society many women, notably but not exclusively those of a Judeo-Christian and Islamic heritage, consider it important to be aware of the full range of actions of the pill. It is *their* right to make a family planning decision which is in accordance with the morals and principles of their ethical, religious and cultural milieu. It is not for others, who may have a different set of lifestyle values, to decide what is or isn't important ethical information for a woman to be aware of.

I have set out the facts as they are because this type of information is not readily available elsewhere, unless hidden in the coy vagueness of medical jargon. Let every woman exercise her right to decide for herself.

CHAPTER TWO.

2. THE PILL AND CANCER OF THE CERVIX..

"When we say the pill is safe, we don't mean it is risk free".
Prof. Guillebaud[84] (1995)

2.1 EARLY CONFLICTING DATA.

The issue of whether the pill is linked to cervical cancer has been under active investigation by medical researchers for more than 30 years. Some of the earliest studies go as far back as 1964, only a few years after the pill became commercially available. But rather than clarify the health implications of the pill, many of these initial studies generated conflicting data.

Those who have reviewed the early medical literature have reported that many researchers, such as Tyler (1964), Pincus (1965), Wied (1966), Miller (1973)[85] Worth and Boyes (1972),[86] as well as Thomas (1972), Melamed and Flehinger (1973),[87] and Boyce and Lu (1977),[88] found no link between the disease and the drug.

Contrary to these findings, four studies around the same time by Attwood (1966), Liu (1967), Kline (1970) & Dougherty (1970) did find that pill users had atypia (not standard) cervical cancer rates nearly double that of non-pill users.[89]

Because of the lack of any definitive results, some researchers such as Thomas (1972) suggested that there was a **"danger of reaching premature conclusions due to the long latent period of cervical carcinoma,** (and) **prudently suggested that studies be continued".**[90]

This cautious approach was vindicated in 1977 when Ory[91] reported on a study involving 854 cases of cervical cancer and 147 cases of carcinoma-in-situ (see glossary). The elevated risk of developing these two diseases when compared to the 8553 control subjects was 60% (RR 1.6) and 370 % (RR 4.7) respectively.

13

These results, whilst substantial in their magnitude, have been criticised as misrepresenting the "true" risk of the pill. The critics have suggested that the researcher failed to take into account other factors which might have had some contributory bearing on the results. For example, statistical confounders such as patient age, race, socio-economic status, number of sexual partners, age at first intercourse, genital infection, Pap screening history, age at menarche, reproductive behaviour, smoking and marital status had not been "allowed" for in this statistical analysis.

Another work published in 1977, this time by Peritz[92] and co-workers, which reported a 310% increase in risk (RR 4.10) with 4 years of pill use was also criticised by other researchers as inaccurate because of the failure to allow adequately for the influence of the sexual behaviour of the study subjects.[93] In this study, even the author was aware of certain methodological deficiencies, mentioning that certain estimates **"have a large sampling error and should be regarded with caution."**.[94]

From this early work the worst that could be said against the pill was that the health issue was undecided. There was no clear result, so no firm conclusions could be drawn. Since science is based on demonstrable fact and not supposition or presumption, it was reasonable at this point to give the pill an unsullied report card.

Shortly thereafter this would change.

2.2   IMPORTANT NEW DATA IN THE 80's.

During the early 80's a number of damaging studies, unequivocal in their conclusions, were published. They should have been instrumental in casting a new and more critical light on the safety of the pill. Significantly, these papers bestowed some belated credence on the studies mentioned earlier which in hindsight could have been the victims of a hastier-than-warranted censure.

One of these key studies (Vessey 1983), compared 6838 women who had given birth (parous women) and were now on the pill with 3154 parous women using an IUD. It reported that:

"the overall incidence (of all forms of cervical neoplasia) was

> **nearly 75% higher in the pill group than in the IUD group... we regard our finds, especially those for invasive cancer of the cervix, as disturbing (although not, of course, conclusive).".**[95]

Vessey's study also highlighted a disturbing demographic trend:

> **"... death rates from cancer of the cervix and incidences for invasive cervical cancer and for carcinoma-in-situ have been rising steadily in women up to 34 years of age in England and Wales during the past decade."**[96] (see appendix 3 for stages of cervical cancer development).

It should be noted that this increased mortality rate observed by Vessey had its origins during the very same years when some of the earlier cervical cancer reports, such as those from Ory (1977) and Peritz (1977), were published and strongly criticised.

Dr Vessey, commenting on some of the initial pill studies by Thomas, Worth & Boyce and other researchers who had failed to find a link between the pill and cervical cancer, noted that:

> **"The** (earlier) **negative studies included very few long-term users of oral contraceptives; no association between exposure to the pill and the risk of cervical neoplasia would have been apparent in our study if the data had been restricted to women with up to 48 months' (or even up to 72 months) use of oral contraceptives.".**[97]

Here Dr Vessey is suggesting that a considerable amount of time must transpire before a drug-induced cancer is evident. This is known as the latent period, a concept which I will elaborate in the following chapter. It is sufficient at this stage to note the research significance of this term and the relevance it has to women's health that is highlighted by Dr Vessey's statement that **"our data offer considerable support to the view that long-term contraceptive use may increase the risk of cervical neoplasia"**.[98]

Some five years later, Valerie Beral & Phillip Hannaford (*Lancet* 1988) published one of the most comprehensive studies on the link between the pill and cervical cancer. Their work looked at the medical histories of 47,000 women and concluded that **"those who used oral contraceptives** (ever-users) **had a significantly higher incidence of cervical cancer than never users"**.[99] The researchers found that:

> **"after more than 10 years of use, the incidence is more than four times that in never-users"**[100] (a 300% increase).

It is interesting to note that Valerie Beral addressed, in a frank manner, the pivotal question about the pill:

> **"Are the associations between oral contraceptives and genital cancer causal, or secondary to other factors? It has been argued that the raised incidence of cervical cancer in oral contraceptive users is not a direct effect of the hormonal agents, but secondary to different sexual practices between oral contraceptive users and non-users ... However, in this and other studies, the associations with oral contraceptive use persist after adjustment for other known risk factors.".**[101]

The last sentence of this quote is, from a research perspective, groundbreaking. Beral & Hannaford stated that they took into account statistical confounders such as age, parity (see glossary), smoking, social class, number of previously normal smears and history of STD's, and the substantial residual cancer risk detected by them was *entirely* attributable to the pill. In their mind there was no doubt that a **"direct effect"** existed between the drug and the disease.

2.3   THE PILL: INITIATOR OR PROMOTOR OF CANCER ?

The question which arises is this: is the "direct effect" of the hormonal agents (the pill) such that it is impacting upon pre-existing cervical cancer which begins to grow more aggressively under its influence, or is the "direct effect" of the pill impacting upon normal cervical tissue which then mutates and becomes cancerous? If the former is the case, then the pill would be acting as a 'promotor'. If the latter is the case, then the pill would be acting as an 'initiator'. This is a significant point which I will address as the research unfolds. For the moment it is sufficient to continue to follow that research.

Very soon after Beral's work, Schlesselman (1988) published a review paper on the findings of 135 scientific papers. It reported that:

> **"studies of cervical dysplasia and carcinoma in situ suggest elevated risks with 2 or more years of OC use". It further reported that " there is evidence suggesting an elevated risk which approaches a 2- fold increase at 10 years"**[102] (a 100% increase).

In the same year, a community-based case-control study of women with carcinoma-in-situ of the uterine cervix was conducted by Brock and co-workers in Sydney and published in *The Medical Journal of Australia.* It reported a 130% increased risk of cancer:

> **"the long-term use of oral contraceptive agents was associated with an elevated risk (relative risk 2.3 for more than 6 years of use)"** .[103]

Whilst this study did not produce results identical to those of Beral, it nonetheless pointed in the same direction. Of some sociological interest were a variety of other issues which this research uncovered.

For example, promiscuity was shown to be a major contributing factor in cervical cancer:

> **"...women who had had seven or more sexual partners in a lifetime had a six-fold (500%) increased risk compared with those with one or no partner. Early age at first sexual intercourse was also a risk factor...".** [104]

This latter aspect was associated with a 2-fold increase in cervical cancer if intercourse took place before age 16.

On a positive note this paper also reported that:

> **"A protective effect was found for women who ... practised the rhythm method of birth control, and for women who breast-fed (for more than 7 months) .".**[105]

Also of interest was the postulated mechanism by which the pill may alter normal cervical tissue growth to cancerous tissue growth:

"The mechanism whereby oral contraceptive use might alter the risk of developing cervical cancer remains unknown, although some evidence exists that cervical tissue has hormonal receptor sites and the administration of hormones causes histological alterations in the cervix.".[106]

Receptors are specific cellular proteins onto which a hormone attaches, thereby causing a cellular response to be elicited.[107] The receptor site of a cell could be compared to the ignition key-hole of a car. When the car key is inserted into the key -hole and turned, the car starts. When a hormone 'attaches' to a receptor, that particular cell is 'started', or activated. This concept of drug/receptor interaction is important to the overall understanding of drug-induced action and disease, and therefore a purposeful digression. Now I return to the body of the research.

With ever-mounting pressure, more substantiating material on the pill's relation to cervical cancer began to emerge in 1990. Brinton and Reeves, writing in the *International Journal of Epidemiology*, reported that they had observed an almost doubling of the risk for cervical cancer for women on the pill for 5 years or more.[108] (RR 1.7, 95% CI 1.1-2.6)

Support for this research was also forthcoming in 1991 from the University of Granada, which issued a review of the 53 existing published works on the pill and cancer of the cervix. The authors of this report concluded that there was "**a significant relationship, with the existence of a significant relative risk of the oral contraceptive for cervical cancer**".[109]

A second paper of note from 1991 was by Louise Brinton, a key international researcher of many years standing, who made observations similar to those of Vessey (1983) concerning the inadequacy of earlier, short-term studies which had reported no link between the pill and cervical cancer:

"**Although initial studies examining the relationship of oral contraceptives to risk of cervical neoplasia were reassuring** (i.e. no risk), **more recent studies provide some evidence of a positive**

relationship, particularly for long-term users.".[110]

Given the conservative nature of research papers, this is a refreshingly candid statement. It formally opened the door for serious questioning of the oft-touted view, heard even today, that the pill is safe. Brinton went on to point out **"in several well-controlled studies, residual excess risk** (the true risk when confounders had been taken into account) **of nearly 2-fold persist for users of 5 years or more years"** (my clarification).[111]

Further, Brinton suggested that the pill may have a promotional effect upon cervical cancer. She reported **" a possible promotional effect of oral contraceptives is suggested by higher risks associated with recent usage".**[112] Dr Brinton noted that there was considerable biological plausibility for the pill's role in cervical cancer.

> **"Hormonal steroids are capable of promoting the development of cervical cancer in animals. In humans, cervical tissue has been found to have hormone receptor sites, and, as previously described, histological** (micro tissue) **changes in cervical epithelium** (tissue which covers a surface) **have been demonstrated to result from the administration of contraceptive steroids.".**[113]

Brinton's view of the pill as a promotor of cervical cancer differed from that of Beral & Hannaford (1988), who had postulated an initiator role. These two views contain scientific differences and implications which I shall address later. For the moment we will continue the review of the medical literature which testifies to the carcinogenicity of the pill.

2.4   CERVICAL CANCER AND EARLY AGE PILL USE.

To that end, research by Inger Gram and co-workers (1992), published in the *American Journal of Obstetrics and Gynaecology* is relevant. These researchers reported the results of a 10-year study involving 6,622 Norwegian women on the pill. They found that after allowing for many other issues that could have influenced the results, such as age, smoking, marital status and alcohol consumption, the risk of cervical cancer was 50% greater for pill users compared to non-pill users.[114] (RR 1.5, 95% CI 1.0-1.8)

Gram and co-workers commented that:

> **"... the results of this follow-up study suggest that both current and past oral contraceptive users experience a higher incidence of cervical intra-epithelial neoplasia (CIN) than do those who never used contraceptives. This finding is similar to those of four out of five previous follow-up studies that evaluated oral contraceptive-cervical intra-epithelial neoplasia hypothesis.".**[115]

Despite protestations to the contrary, still being heard, these researchers stated with great certainty that **"these findings support the hypothesis that the occurrence of cervical intra-epithelial neoplasia is increased by oral contraceptive use"**[116] (See appendix 3 for CIN).

Significantly, this paper drew attention to the inherent dangers for women initiated onto the pill at an early age.

> **"Women starting at an earlier age were at an increased risk as compared with those starting later.".**[117]

It should be noted that 'age' at first use of the pill is to become a critical new dimension in pill research. The following chapter on breast cancer devotes considerable space to this issue.

To further support the case against the pill, Delgado-Rodriquez of Spain presented a review of all papers published until 1992 for the 3 progressive stages of cervical intra-epithelial neoplasia (CIN): i.e., dysplasia (any abnormal development of tissues or organs), carcinoma-in-situ (curable, pre-malignant) and invasive cervical cancer. Whilst acknowledging certain limitations of their research, they nonetheless concluded that **"Oral contraceptive use may be a risk factor for *all* stages of the natural history of cervical cancer, which may imply an initiator effect"** (my emphasis).[118]

There are a number of salient issues raised by this particular study. First, its findings are consistent with many earlier studies. This is a simple observation, but one that should not be undervalued. Consistency in research of any type is paramount. Second, and more importantly, this study contained a decided alteration to the terminology used by earlier researchers.

In the past, it was suggested that the pill acts merely as a 'promoter' of cervical cancer. This term presupposed that the 'cause' of the cancer was *another* agent, with the pill having a diminished level of culpability. Now, with the use of the term 'initiator', the pill acquired full responsibility for cervical cancer. There has been more than just a change in the degree of responsibility. There has been a change in the *kind* of responsibility which is attributed to the pill.

In 1993, Kjaer and co-workers reported on a study involving 586 women from Copenhagen with proven cervical carcinoma-in-situ (CIS). This particular study showed that pill users of six to nine years had an associated elevated risk for CIS of 90% when compared to pill non-users.[119] (RR 1.9, CI 1.1-3.1)

It is relevant to observe that not only is there a large measure of consistency in these findings, but they are emanating from different cultural sites (Norway, Spain, England, America). This diversity would seem to argue *against* a strong environmental, dietary or genetic influence as a causative factor.

As we move closer to the present: a study, from Leipzig University detailed one of the highest risk rates so far reported. Kohler and Wuttke stated that after reviewing the medical history of 309 patients with cervical intra-epithelial neoplasia (CIN) or invasive cervical carcinoma, the relative risk was 250% higher for women using hormonal contraception than for never-users (RR 3.5, p=0.006). Other pertinent points made by this research team were **"*easy use* of oral contraceptives and *prolonged use* of oral contraceptives were associated with a significant increase in the relative risk"** (my emphasis.[120]

This last quote, as my emphasis is designed to show, contains a subtle criticism not usually found in the dry, clinical reporting of medical research, though it begs the question of what is 'easy use' and why easy access *is* a problem.

2.5   THE INCIDENCE OF CERVICAL CANCER IN AMERICA AND AUSTRALIA.

More recently, a report by Dr. Ursin from the Department of Preventative Medicine, University of Southern California, provided a revealing historical perspective on the amount of time (the latent period) which might need to transpire before adenocarcinoma, which comprises 10-15 % of all cervical tumors,[121] physiologically manifests itself:

"The incidence of adenocarcinoma of the cervix in the USA more than doubled between the early 1970's and the mid 1980's among women under 35 years of age. It was suggested that this increase was due to the introduction of oral contraceptives in the early 1960's...".[122]

(N.B., The other type of cervical cancer is known as squamous cell carcinoma and accounts for approximately 85% of cases). Graph 1 illustrates the rapid increase in cervical cancer in American women, notably during the ages 20-35, which is further demographic support for the validity of Dr Ursin's findings.

A similar trend exists within the Australian context. Graph 2 shows that there has been an increase in the age- specific incidence rates per 100,000 population for adenocarcinoma of the cervix. Of particular concern is the occurrence of adenocarcinoma in the 15-19 year age bracket during the time period 1988-1992. Prior to 1988 there were no reported cases of adenocarcinoma in the state of New South Wales for this very young age group. Is it beyond the bounds of reasonable deduction to suggest that **"easy use of oral contraceptives ..."** [123] at an early age might be in part responsible for this medical event ?

GRAPH 1: Invasive Cervical Cancer. Annual Age-Specific Rates per 100,000 U.S. Women, 1981-85 (Schlesselman JJ.)[124]

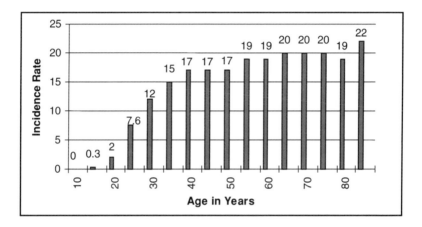

GRAPH 2: Age specific incidence (Adenocarcinoma of cervix) rates per 100,000 population.[125] **(NSW, Australia).**

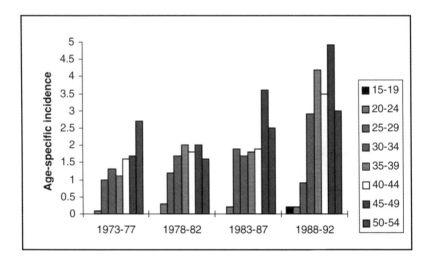

Source: Department of Epidemiology, N.S.W. Cancer Council. (1996).
(Right legend is age range of women, in years.)

Dr Ursin's finding were consistent with those from many other researchers previously quoted. Dr Ursin reported that:

> **"Compared with never use, ever use of oral contraceptives was associated with twice as a great a risk of Adenocarcinoma of the cervix. The highest risk** (a 340% increase) **was observed for oral contraceptive use of more than 12 years."**[126]

Drs' Ursin and Peters also reported that **"the increase was particularly in women aged 20-35 years in the upper socioeconomic strata".**[127] Note that, once again, the susceptibility of young women is a key finding in the medical research. Another salient point and one of much concern was the researchers' observation that **"women who had used oral contraceptives for 1-6 months had an OR of 2.9".**[128] An OR - odds ratio - of 2.9 means that the risk of developing adenocarcinoma was 190% higher (nearly 2 fold greater) for pill users *of only 1-6 months*, compared with non-pill users.

It is important to recall that this high odds-ratio (OR) - a measure of risk - for short term use of the pill is different from some earlier findings which suggested that only longer term use was a risk factor (Beral and Hannaford, 1988, and Brinton, 1991). This research may suggest that there is a certain sub-group of women who are more susceptible to the effects of the pill hormones than others, and who present with clinical symptoms of cervical cellular damage far more quickly than the general population.

Another important paper in 1994 was that of Brisson and co-workers. These Canadian researchers recruited 2,168 women for their study and reported results that bore a striking resemblance to work done in many other parts of the world.

> **"The risk of late-stage** (cervical) **lesions also increased with duration of oral contraceptive use: Those who had used the pill for six or more years, for example, were twice as likely as non-users [of the pill] to have late-stage CIN."** (A two-fold increase in risk is a 100 % increase).[129]

A paper published by the *WHO Collaborative Study of Neoplasia and Steroid Contraceptives* (1995), reported on investigations of 10,979 women who had been recruited from Chile, Thailand and Mexico between 1979 and 1988. The WHO study found that when all other factors had been taken into account (age, condom use, marital history, contraceptive use, abortion history, number of pregnancies and Pap smears), **"ever users of oral contraceptives were 30% more likely to have carcinoma-in-situ than were never-users".**[130]

A second *WHO Collaborative Study of Neoplasia and Steroid Contraceptives* (Jan 6, 1996) reported that the risk of adenocarcinoma of the cervix was 280% greater in women under 20 if they took the pill. Once again, the vulnerability of young women's bodies to the ubiquitous effects of artificial hormones is manifested. Women aged 20-24 years had a 70% increased, and women aged 25-

29 had a 40% greater risk when compared to non-users in the same age range.[131] Further important findings were that the risk of cervical cancer increased with duration of pill use, and the risk declined as time since last use increased. These two findings do, in my view, support the view that there is a pivotal role played by the pill in cervical cancer.

In the same year the *British Journal of Cancer* (1996) reported on a 12 year extension to the 1983 Oxford Family Planning Association contraceptive study. The researchers noted that among current or recent users of the pill, the risk of developing all types of cervical neoplasia (see glossary) was 234% greater than for non-users if the pill had been taken for 49-72 months.[132] This risk decreased over time but was still high, at 104% increased risk for pill use longer than 97 months.

In this study the role of HPV may be considered **"relatively low"** since **"all women who entered the study were married, and the majority (69%) reported having only one sexual partner... It should be noted, however, that we have no data at all on number of sexual partners of the husband that may have influenced the risk of HPV infection for the women in this study.".**[133]

Finally, in the context of the ongoing debate concerning the role of abortion in the etiology of breast cancer, Zondervan noted an increased incidence of cervical cancer in women who had an induced abortion. These women **"were at significantly higher overall risk of developing cervical neoplasia than those not having an induced abortion (OR=1.78, p<0.04).".**[134] An OR of 1.78 means an increased risk of cervical cancer from induced abortion of 78%.

After consideration of the above studies, one important issue still remains to be addressed: what impact does the widespread use of the pill, and its associated increased relative risk, have at a population level? Are these statistical risks merely theoretical probabilities? The answers to these important questions have been supplied by Schlesselman (1995), who conducted a review of all the published research on pill use and cancer between 1980 and July 1994 and listed on the MEDLINE data base. He estimated that for every 100,000 women aged 20-54 who had not taken the pill, the incidence of cervical cancer was 425 cases. For women using the pill for 8 years, there were an additional 125 cases of cervical cancer per 100,000 women.[135]

Oddly, Schlesselman took the view that **"from a population perspective, there are only small cancer-related risks and benefits associated with OC use and, on balance, the net effect is negligible.".**[136] I disagree. The increased incidence of 125 cases of pill-induced cervical cancer, over the non-pill using baseline measure of 425 cases per 100,000 women is an increase of approximately 30%. Given that cervical cancer is the second most common malignancy of the female reproductive tract,[137] it is tragic that in at least 30% of the cases, an avoidable disease was not avoided.

2.6   THE PILL, HUMAN PAPILLOMAVIRUS (HPV) AND CERVICAL CANCER.

Thusfar the focus of this chapter has been on the link between the pill and cervical cancer. There is, however, another issue related to cervical cancer which also deserves attention. The earlier medical literature referred to the possible role of a sexually transmitted 'agent' which might be involved in either the initiation or promotion of cervical cancer. For example, in the *Lancet* (1988) Armstrong made the observation that:

> **"...cancer of the cervix may be due to a venereally transmitted infection is strongly suggested by its association with the number of sexual partners that a woman or her husband has had".**[138]

He went on to postulate the possible nature of this venereal contagion:

> **"...for over 20 years, herpes simplex type II was the prime candidate agent but, while a role for this virus remains possible, attention has turned recently to certain types of human papillomavirus (HPV)".**[139]

The distinction in disease states associated with these two viruses, herpes simplex II (HSV-2) and HPV, is crucial. HSV-2 is the sexually transmitted agent responsible for 95% of the cases of genital herpes, (while the remaining 5% is due to HSV-1.)[140] Symptoms of genital herpes are frequently unpleasant, even debilitating, and are sometimes associated with secondary bacteria or fungal infections. However, in commonly used medical text books such as *The Merck Manual*, cancer is not listed as a sign, symptom or complication of HSV-2 infectivity.[141]

On the other hand, HPV infectivity has potentially graver medical implications than those associated with HSV-1 & 2. There are two disease states associated with HPV infectivity. First, a woman infected with HPV may present with genital warts, known as condylomata acuminata. The subtypes of HPV which are known to cause genital warts are 1, 2, 6, 11, 16 and 18.[142] Importantly, condylomata are *benign* in nature, and therefore not of a life-threatening consequence.[143] Of greater medical significance are the HPV subtypes (16, 18, 31, 33, and 35) which can give rise to significant health sequelae. These subtypes **"have been implicated in the etiology of cervical neoplasia.".**[144] The reader will notice that there are two subtypes of HPV (16 & 18) which are common to both benign cervical warts *and* cervical cancer. This will be shown to be a most significant point when I review the research by Gitsch, Kainz *et al.*(1992).

At this stage a fundamental question arises from these considerations: is the involvement of the HPV in the etiology (causation) of cervical neoplasia one of **initiating** cancerous cellular changes independently of the presence of the pill hormones, or does the HPV act in a secondary capacity, as a **promotor** of a pill-induced cancer?

Back in 1989, it would be fair to say that the medical community was divided on the issue, with research and arguments to support both views.

For example, Chang (1989) noted that for women suffering pre-cancerous lesions of the cervix, **"those using hormone contraception had a significantly higher infection rate with HPV "** He observed further that:

> **"...if hormonal contraceptive use and simultaneous HPV infection are associated with cervical neoplasia** (cancer), **and laboratory evidence supports this thesis, then further urgent investigations are needed, for the implications are grave."**[145]
> (see glossary for H.P.V.).

The following year Chang's misgivings were confirmed. A study by Hildesheim, Reeves and co-workers in 1990 reported that women with invasive cervical cancer who had recent or long-term use of the pill, had between a 130% and 190% (2.3

& 2.9-fold respectively) increased risk of HPV infection. Furthermore they stated that:

> **"Our findings suggest either an interaction between HPV infection and oral contraceptive use in the genesis** (origin) **of cervical cancer or an increased expression of the HPV genome** (genetic material) **in neoplasms of OC users.".**[146]

Whilst not explicitly stated, this report can be interpreted as supporting the 'initiator' role of the HPV/pill complex on cervical tissue, particularly since the quote uses the word 'genesis'.

In the same year, research by Pater and co-workers (*Am. J. Obstet. Gynecol.*) concluded that:

> **"Compelling evidence supports a role of certain types of human papillomaviruses as the cause of cervical cancer. In addition to human papillomavirus, other agents, such as hormones** (i.e., the pill), **have been implicated as cofactors in this type of neoplasia.".**[147]

This research is also suggesting that HPV acts as an initiator of cervical cancer, with 'assistance' from such cofactors as the hormones, notably the progesterone component, found in the pill.

Louise Brinton (1991), writing a review paper on this topic, also supported Chang's concern about a synergistic carcinogenic interaction between the pill and HPV but tended more towards the 'promotor' theory. She stated that:

> **"A possible promotional effect of oral contraceptives is suggested by higher risks associated with recent usage… In addition, oral contraceptives may induce proliferation of HPV, the leading suspect agent in cervical cancer.".**[148]

Dr Brinton suggested a mechanism for this connection:

> **"… oral contraceptives have been associated with the production of an estral 'clear channel' mucous that could facilitate entry of**

> mutagens and with immunologic alterations that could increase
> susceptibility to viral agents. Hormones have also been found to
> enhance the transcription of the HPV genome both in vitro and
> in vivo.".[149]

In non-medical language this quote can be read as: 'the pill causes the production of a type of cervical mucus which makes it easier for cancer-causing agents to gain access to a woman's body. Hormones can also assist the copying and replication of the human papillomavirus both in the body and in the laboratory'.

As an aside, it is interesting to note the Greek and Latin origins of the term papillomavirus: *Oma* is Greek for tumour, and *virus* is Latin for poison.[150]

In 1991, Gitsch and co-workers released a milestone report which noted that:

> "... during the last few years, several studies pointed at an
> interaction between hormones and HPV infection in the
> generation of cervical dysplasia ... Our data suggest that oral
> contraceptives in interaction with HPV infection alter and
> accelerate progression of condylomatous (benign) lesions and
> mild dysplasia to moderate and severe dysplasia.".[151]

Gitsch reported that for women *not* using the pill, the highest HPV infection rates were in wart (condylomatous) lesions which were *not* cancerous, whereas for women who *had* used the pill the highest rate of HPV infection were in tissue that *were* cancerous. From this it could be concluded that the pill, in conjunction with the HPV, was responsible for altering the benign condylomatous lesions and making them cancerous.

The results from Gitsch were precisely in line with the receptor theory of causation as suggested by Louise Brinton.

> "A relationship (between pill hormones and cervical cancer) is
> biological possible, given findings of hormone receptors in
> cervical tissue and the fact that oral contraceptives have been
> found to induce cervical hyperplasia.".[152]

The following year, Gitsch published the full results of the previously cited study. I will quote extensively from this report because the evidence it presents argues strongly that the pill is responsible for the activation of HPV in cervical warts, with the result that the warts change from a benign state to a precancerous state (CIN I,II,III - see appendix 3). I shall intersperse the quotes with pertinent explanation. Whilst it is not an easy journal to source, I would heartily encourage readers to obtain a copy if it.

> **"HPV was detected in 48% of the 142 patients** (the total number in the study, selected because all had presented with condylomatous lesions with or without cervical intraepithelial neoplasia-CIN-). **Amongst the OC users a significant trend to higher HPV infection rates in high grade CIN became evident. In OC non-users the results were the other way round, the highest HPV infection rate being found in condylomas without atypia and mild dysplasia. Distribution of HPV types 6/11, 16/18 and 31/33 was similar in OC users and non-users.".**[153]

Thus, whilst both users and non-users of the pill had the same distribution of the various types of HPV, it was the pill users who had the greatest concentration of HPV in the highest grade of precancerous cervical tissue. For non-pill users, cervical tissue *most* infected with HPV existed merely as the non-malignant cervical wart. How was it that HPV could be present equally in two groups of women, but in those using the pill, the cervical tissue has become cancerous? The answer is as follows.

> **"The interaction between steroid hormones** (such as the pill), **HPV and the generation of cervical cancer has been the subject of several biological and clinical investigations. Cervical tissue has hormone receptors and administration of hormones can result in histological** (cellular) **alterations. There might be an interaction between oral contraceptives and HPV in cervical cancer since the transcriptional** (copying) **region of HPV 16 DNA contain hormone recognition elements."**[154] (HPV 16 has a site in its structure which recognises and responds to hormones in the pill).

So, it is now established that both cervical tissue *and* HPV have molecular sites within their respective structures which recognise and interact with hormones such as those in the pill. Not only are the receptors within the cervical tissue adversely influenced by hormones (as suggested by Brinton), but so also are sites within the HPV which infect the same cervical tissue. The above research suggested that the hormones stimulated an increase in the self-replication of the virus. For a pill user, this constitutes a form of double jeopardy.

But how do the researchers know this with certainty, and what hormones if any have been shown to be recognised by both cervical cells and the HPV infection within those cells?

> "In a second report (by Pater *et al*, 1990) the same group provided evidence that the oncogenic transformation (process of initiating and promoting the development of a neoplasm) of baby rat kidney cells by HPV 16 DNA ... was dependent on the presence of progesterone or its derivate, norgestrel (a common pill ingredient)... This indicates that oral contraceptive use may be a risk factor for high grade CIN and invasive cancer, possibly by enhancing the expression of the virus and increasing the likelihood that HPV will induce transformation of cervical epithelial cells.".[155]

From this it is clear that had progesterone or norgestrel not been present, the baby rat kidney cells 'infected' with HPV 16 would *not* have initiated the transformation of normal kidney cells into neoplastic tissue. Based upon this evidence alone, the pill should be contra-indicated for all women diagnosed with HPV infection.

And now to the researchers' conclusions:

> "Our data also show that HPV positivity (HPV presence) in high grade cervical dysplasia is significantly increased in OC users as compared to non-users. The high HPV detection rate in low grade CIN in non-users might suggest that HPV positive dysplasia in such patients remains stable or regress spontaneously. In the presence of HPV infection OC usage seems to make progression from low grade to high grade dysplasia

more likely with resultant increases in HPV positivity in more advanced stages of CIN. This hypothesis is supported by the fact the incidence of 'high risk' HPV types 31/33 and 16/18 was nearly equal in OC users and non-users. Our results suggest that oral contraceptives enhance the possibility of neoplastic change due to HPV infection.".[156]

As in breast cancer, the pivotal role of the pill is called into question. In this study, both users and non-users had HPV infections, but it was the pill-user group which presented with the excessively high incidence of stage 3 cervical pre-cancerous lesions. Non-users did not suffer this consequence of HPV infection. The genital warts this latter group had, whilst showing the presence of HPV, were documented to have either remained stable, that is, not become pre-cancerous, or actually regressed.

As a personal speculation, it would seem that non-pill users have the immunological capacity to control the HPV virus, as indicated by the stable/ regressive history of their genital warts. This beneficial immune response does not succeed in pill-users; their immune system appears to be 'overwhelmed' by the increase in HPV positivity (presence). The interaction between the pill hormones and HPV has led to an increase in HPV 16 replication, increased HPV positivity in cervical tissue and consequently, an increase in high grade CIN. The conclusions from this landmark study are unavoidable.

Women with HPV infectivity who did *not* take the pill did *not* experience the alteration of non-cancerous cervical warts to high grade, pre-cancerous CIN. This study supports the *initiator* role of the pill in cervical cancer because non-users with HPV infectivity did not develop high grade CIN. Indeed, for many, their health status improved because they had no pill hormones present in their body.

Diagrammatically, this study can be represented thus:

HPV infectivity in non users $\rightarrow$ non-malignant cervical warts $\rightarrow$ stability of health, even improvement.

HPV infectivity in OC users $\rightarrow$ increased cervical presence of HPV 16 $\rightarrow$ development of high grade pre-cancerous lesions.

Following on from Gitsch (1992), Brisson reported in the *American Journal of Epidemiology* (*AJE,* 1994) that:

> **"Presence of HPV 16 DNA was associated with a 8.7-fold elevation in estimated relative risk of high-grade CIN. Relative risk of high-grade CIN increased with the amount of HPV 16 DNA."**[157]

Brisson's work showed that there was a 770% increased risk of cervical pre-cancerous lesions if infected with the HPV. This study supports the findings from Gitsch that high-grade CIN is strongly linked to the presence of HPV.

During 1995 further compelling evidence was published which linked the presence of HPV and exogenous hormones in cervical tissue to the genesis of cervical cancer (see glossary).

Typical of these studies was the research from J.T. Cox, published in March 1995, who reported that:

> **"...the evidence implicating specific HPV types in the aetiology of cervical cancer is now strong enough to establish a causative role.".**[158]

Principle amongst the various features leading to this **"causative role"** were that: HPV exposure was extremely common, particularly amongst sexually active teenagers; the progression rate from low grade to high grade CIN (see appendix 3) occurred in around one third of case; HPV infection by itself was not sufficient to cause the 'jump' from high grade pre-invasive C.I.N. to invasive cervical cancer and cofactors were necessary to cause this 'jump' from pre-invasive C.I.N. 3 to the invasive state (those cofactors included smoking, hormonal effects from oral contraceptives and pregnancy, poor diet, impaired immune system and chronic inflammation).[159]

In a similar vein, Bosch and co-workers (*J Natl Cancer Inst,* 1995) reported that HPV was present in 93% of tumour specimens obtained from 1000 patients at 32 hospitals in 22 countries, leading the researchers to conclude that:

> "...the association of genital human papillomavirus (HPV) with cervical cancer is strong, independent of other risk factors, and consistent in several countries.".[160]

This exclusive role of HPV infectivity in the production of chronic cervical dysplasia, a percussor stage to invasive cervical cancer, was also reported by Ho and colleagues in Sept 1995. They linked the development of chronic cervical dysplasia with the concurrent existence of a **"high viral load.".**[161]

Park, Fujiwara and Wright, in Nov 1995, also added to the body of literature which implicated HPV in cervical cancer.

> **"Cervical cancer develops from well-defined precursor lesions referred to as either cervical intraepithelial neoplasia (CIN) or squamous intraepithelial lesions (SIL). It is now known that specific types of human papillomaviruses (HPV) are the principal etiologic agents for both cervical cancer and its precursors.".**
> [162](The terms CIN and SIL are synonymous).[163]

Of great social importance was the finding from Thomas and colleges (*AJE*, 1996) that:

> **"...the average latent period between the women's likely exposure to a sexually transmitted oncogenic agent and her diagnosis of invasive cervical cancer was a quarter of a century.".**[164]

Some cases of cervical cancer were detected within 6 years of initial infection, other cases were not detected for 45 years.[165] It will be recalled that the latent period is the time between the exposure to an injurious agent, in this case a sexually transmitted one, and a detectable side-effect, specifically cervical cancer. This lengthy latent period means that sexually active young women, or monogamous women with promiscuous partners, are exposed to an increased risk of cervical cancer which may not be detected until the women are in their 30's or early 40's. Aside from the obvious psychological and physical damage, such a diagnosis could have harmful domestic repercussions, notably in the area of marital harmony and trust.

2.7   THE PILL: BIOLOGICAL ACTIVATOR OF HPV.

Arguably the research paper which has the most potential to redefine how medicine views the safety of the pill is that from Chen and co-workers (1996). Their original work irrefutably supported the view that certain pill hormones increased the carcinogenic effects of HPV 16 (and to a lesser extent HPV 18) in cells exposed to the virus. This process is known as hormone-dependent transactivation of HPV 16.[166] In a loose sense, the pill hormones facilitate a more rapid 'blending' or incorporation of the genetic material from the virus into the genetic heritage of the host (cervical) cells.

> **"In summary, the selected progestins and estrogens induced differential stimulation of HPV gene expression. This information is exclusively important for evaluation of oral contraceptives containing these HPV-enhancing estrogens or progestins on the relative risk of cervical cancer.".**[167]

The **"differential stimulation of HPV gene expression"** by different **"contraceptive"** hormones is highly significant. As the authors noted, there have been conflicting reports on the influence of duration of use of the pill on cervical cancer, and also **"the presence and grade of HPV-associated CIN and cervical cancer.".**[168] The answer to this apparent "paradox" may be related to, and dependant upon the various hormones which are in different brands of the pill.[169] In short, different studies, using different formulations of the pill, will show results which are not always uniform. Hence in the future there is a clear need for researchers to be mindful that their results may depend on the hormonal composition of the pill that women enrolled in a study may take.

This research from Chen has in effect moved the scientific debate on from the previous position of *"does* the pill have a role in cervical cancer?" to "this is *how* it does". This shift in emphasis is notable. It clearly indicates a move from testing a scientific hypothesis to demonstrating, at a cellular level, that the hypothesis is now tenable fact. Chen's work (1996) represents a shift away from statistical epidemiology to the newer field of molecular epidemiology; an important progression. The vast bulk of the research cited in this book falls into the category of statistical or associative epidemiology.[170] That is, the majority of the research I refer to has followed the traditional method which **"looked at the correlation between risk factors and disease.".**[171] In contrast to this classical approach, the work by Chen (1996) is known as **"molecular epidemiology"**,[172] [173] a term which indicates that the study of human disease is no longer based on a nexus between risk factors and disease, but rather, on the observable behaviour, at a molecular level, of carcinogens in contact with cells. In a slightly glib sense, the test-tube has replaced the calculator. The implications of Chen's study are wide ranging.[174]

I have listed the hormones, along with related technical information, in an extensive entry in the endnotes for the obvious reason of relevance, but also because this paper was difficult to procure. By supplying such a lengthy quote I hope that others will avoid the same problems I experienced.[175] This material is more readily accessible to those with some scientific training.

Work by Kenney (Oct,1996) presented a neat overview of the current thinking on these issues.

> **"The genital human papillomavirus (HPV) is directly associated with cervical cancer, the second most common form of cancer among women... Women at highest risk for acquiring an HPV infection had (a) initiated sex before age 15, (b) more than four lifetime sex partners, (c) more than one "once only" sexual partner, and (d) chosen male sex partners who had previously had > (greater than) 16 other female sex partners. Cofactors that increased risk by possibly contributing to progression of genital HPV infection were initiating oral contraceptive use before age 15 and having more than three sexually transmitted diseases.".[176]**

In summary: there is strong evidence which implicates the hormones in the pill as the crucial link in the pill-cervical cancer nexus. The combination of HPV and the pill represents a greater increased risk of cervical cancer than does the pill alone or HPV alone.

2.8   FINAL STATEMENT.

Based upon the international medical research projects on this topic, it is puzzling that Government- approved patient information leaflets (1996) for the pill can state the following:

"At present, there is no confirmed evidence from human studies which would indicate that an increased risk of cancer is associated with oral contraceptives.".[177]

The reality is quite the opposite. The evidence does exist. One wonders why those in positions of authority in the drug regulatory agencies have not been made aware of the errors contained within the current approved medical literature.

2.9   KEY POINTS.

1. The link between the pill and cervical cancer has been established by medical researchers and is proven beyond doubt.

2. Increased cancer risk rates vary from study to study, but all are unacceptable when viewed in the context of how NOT to treat otherwise healthy women.

3. There is a substantial link between pill use, HPV and the increased risk of cervical cancer, with pill use a decisive risk factor over and above that of HPV.

4. Even relatively short use of the pill, i.e., 5-6 years, carries a high risk factor.

5. Young women are the group most at risk.

To conclude, it was certainly highly appropriate for Prof. Guillebaud (1995) to say that **"When we say the pill is safe, we don't mean it is risk free."**.[178] It may also be appropriate to question whether or not the word 'safe' should henceforth be used in the same sentence as the word 'pill'.

CHAPTER THREE.

3.   THE PILL AND BREAST CANCER.

"At present, there is no confirmed evidence from human studies which would indicate that an increased risk of cancer is associated with oral contraceptives."[179] (Government approved drug information - Trifeme®, Ayerst Laboratories - 1996).

It is impractical to review the medical research on the pill and breast cancer by employing the same time-line approach adopted for a review of cervical cancer. This is because there are a variety of separate issues related to breast cancer which emerge at different points.

I have chosen to separate each of the fundamental issues and follow them individually from the early 80's through to the present. It should be carefully noted that whilst these contributory factors are analysed individually, this must not be interpreted to mean that each or any of these factors acts in isolation. From the medical literature it is clear that there is an interactive relationship in existence which I shall highlight at different points in this chapter.

3.1   RESEARCH IN THE EARLY 1970's.

Two conspicuous features emerge from a review of the medical literature of the early 70's: (a) there is a paucity of papers on links between breast cancer and the pill and (b) what exists presents a picture sharply in contrast to our present knowledge, viz., the data either finds no link or suggests that not only was the pill safe, but its use was protective against breast cancer.

Highlighting the first point: the dearth of early research was starkly reflected in a lengthy review paper on breast cancer by Schlesselman (1989),[180] which contained a summary of only two papers from the 70's but over 40 papers covering the period 1980-88.

39

As another measure of the limited range of early research on the safety of the pill, a count of the number of references in a major research paper from each of the 70's, 80's and 90's is illuminating. Vessey's paper (1979) had a mere 21 references, Pike & Henderson *et al* (*Lancet*, 1983) cited 29 references, whilst Olsson (*Cancer*,1991) named 54 references. This is a loose criterion, but a helpful one nonetheless.

The favourable view of the pill is illustrated by the positive but qualified medical reports published by Vessey (1972) in the *British Medical Journal* and in a follow-up study published in the *Lancet* (1975). In the 1972 article Vessey concluded that:

> **"The present findings are reassuring. There is no suggestion that the use of oral contraceptives is related in any way to the risk of breast cancer in women under the age of 40, while there is some evidence that their use may actually protect against benign breast cancer in this age group, as was originally suggested by Pincus and colleagues.".**[181] (*sic*)

Vessey reiterated these views in the 1975 *Lancet* article:

> **"Our latest findings, which are based on a substantial number of patients with breast cancer, are reassuring; there is no suggestion that the use of oral contraceptives is related in any way to the risk of breast cancer in women up to 45 years of age."** Furthermore: **" the use of oral contraceptives might be more likely to reduce the risk of breast cancer than to increase it.".**[182]

Between these years, the Boston Collaborative Drug Surveillance Programme reported results similar to that of Vessey (1972):

> **"When breast cancer was studied, there was no evidence of a higher risk in oral contraceptive users relative to non-users.".**[183]

The 1975 edition of *The Pharmacological Basis of Therapeutics,* a primary text for teachers and students of pharmacology, devoted only one sentence to breast cancer:

"... extensive earlier studies in Puerto Rico and Haiti (Pincus, 1965) showed a lowered incidence of cancer of the uterus and the breast amongst users of the contraceptive.".[184]

Also, another major report by Vessey (1979) failed to find any link between the pill and cancer. In fact this report found that the pill conferred protection *from* breast cancer:

"Information on clinical stage (of cancer) was available for 487 patients with breast cancer treated before the end of 1975. Those who had never used oral contraceptives had appreciably more advanced tumours at presentation than those who had been using the pill during the year before detection of the lump, while past users of the pill occupied an intermediate position. This difference in staging (of breast cancer) was reflected in the pattern of survival. *Oral contraceptives may have had a beneficial effect on tumour growth and spread,* though diagnostic bias could not be definitely excluded." (my emphasis).[185]

A further report by Vessey (1982) again concluded that pill use protected against breast cancer:

"Data are presented on 1176 women aged 16-50 years with breast cancer, interviewed in London or Oxford, together with a like number of matched control subjects. The results are entirely reassuring, being, in fact, more compatible with protective effects than the reverse.".[186]

Yet the lack of research of itself is not an adequate explanation for the early conflicting data. To suggest that less data explains errors of omission or commission is to imply professional research incompetence. A greater scientific issue was at stake than that of professional proficiency.

What factor or factors could be operative which hampered the capacity of specialist researchers to accurately address the issue of the pill and breast cancer? Essentially there where two factors at work here. One was the latent period of the disease, while the other was the deficient statistical methodology used by researchers in the early 70's. I shall now discuss both of these factors.

3.2   THE LATENT PERIOD.

The biological concept of latent period is defined as the time taken between the exposure to an injurious drug and a detectable side-effect.[187] All drugs have a number of possible side-effects. Each side-effect will have its own latent period.

Consider, for example, the latent period of penicillins, a sub-category of antibiotics. Certain side-effects such as anaphylaxis, itchy skin and swelling occur soon after ingestion in sensitive patients, hence in these instances the latent period is short. Other side-effects such as serum sickness may not present symptomatically for 7 to 10 days,[188] hence the latent period for these side-effects is relatively longer.

The same principles apply to the pill, which belongs to a class of drugs known as steroidal hormones. The pill can cause certain frequent side-effects such as nausea, occasional vomiting, dizziness and headaches. The latent period for these side-effects is short. For other side-effects, specifically breast cancer, the latent period is very long.

Industrial medicine further validates the existence of a long latency period for certain diseases. Mine workers, for example, exposed to uranium dust, are known to develop lung cancer after **"a 15- to 20-yr latent period."**.[189]

Thus, *latent period is related to time and delayed effect.* This is the prime underlying reason why the early data on the pill was variable.

A substantial number of researchers concur on the prolonged latent period of breast cancer from pill use. Vessey, Doll and Sutton (*BMJ,* 1972), for example, commented that:

> **"Hertz (1969) pointed out that if contraceptive steroids initiate malignant changes in breast tissue de novo the consequences would probably not yet be detectable because human carcinogens seldom produce an overt effect in less than 10 years.".**[190]

Other researchers, (Vessey, *Lancet,* 1975) without specifically using the term 'latent', have clearly intimated that there is a need to observe a long period of time before declaring that the pill is not a carcinogen:

> **"It is important to remember that it must be many years before the question of the possible relationship between the use of the preparations** (the pill) **and cancer of the breast is finally settled."**[191] (see note in endnote).

Valerie Beral, reporting in the *British Medical Journal* (1980), also made a similar observation: **"... the latent period before the tumour becomes clinically apparent may be 15 years or longer.".**[192]

Klim McPherson and co-workers suggested in the *Lancet* (1983) that one of the possible explanation for their results was the existence of **"a latent period in the manifestation of any OC effect on breast cancer...".**[193].

Samuel Shapiro, writing in the *New England Journal of Medicine* (1986), advised against a premature conclusion that the pill was safe because of the long latent period:

> **"A reasonable conclusion is that the oral contraceptives used in the United States do not increase the risk of breast cancer. But there are some important qualifications: First,** *latency intervals longer than 15 years* **following the discontinuation of oral contraceptives remains to be evaluated. This is particularly important because the incidence of breast cancer climbs steeply after the age of about 40."** (Emphasis added).[194]

Klim McPherson (*British Journal Cancer*, 1987) presented an extensive and illuminating discussion on the long latent period of carcinogens, supported by pertinent historical examples and their own qualified support for the hypothesis:

> **"OCs became widely and freely available in the UK to unmarried women in the early seventies. Such women will now only (1987) be in their thirties and early forties and will be unlikely to have accumulated long term early use more than 5 or 10 years ago.**

Since the formation of a palpable breast cancer may typically take the best part of twenty years, (i.e. the time for precancerous changes plus the time for a tumour to be diagnosed) it may be too soon to expect to observe a coherent epidemiological relationship (Armenian & Lilienfeld, 1979; McPherson *et al.*, 1986).

A parallel might, perhaps, be drawn with young women exposed to radiation from the atomic bombs of Hiroshima and Nagasaki who showed a dose related increase in breast cancer incidence but not until 15-20 years after exposure (Tokunaga et al., 1979) or, equally, with pregnant women exposed to diethylstilboestrol (DES) who have been shown to have twice the ultimate breast cancer risk compared with unexposed controls (with a follow-up extending to forty years), but in whom no difference was observed until 22 years after exposure (Greenberg *et al.*, 1984) ... (Our) data suggest (but not strongly) a latent period of at least ten years for E-O pills (ethinyl estrodiol) **between long term early exposure and an increased risk of breast cancer diagnosis ... latency could plausibly be related to the apparent discrepancies in published epidemiological results ... The notion of a latent effect is consistent with the known epidemiology of breast cancer and with the observed effect of radiation and diethylstilboestrol (DES) exposure.**[195] (DES is an oestrogen).

The Swedish researcher Olsson (*Procedings of the Annual Meeting American Society Clinical Oncology,* 1989) substantiated the views of Hertz, Vessey, Beral, McPherson and Shapiro:

"Studies on the risk with modern OC use have to wait another 20 yr, due to, as yet, a too short latency time.". [196]

As well, both the 1975[197] and 1990[198] edition of *Goodman & Gilman's The Pharmacological Basis of Therapeutics* cautioned that the low number of adverse (negative) findings for the pill **"may reflect the latent period *needed* for cellular transformation"** (which leads to breast cancer).

The Australian researcher, Dr Kevin Hume (1991), noted that there was a **" long** lead time involved in the development of cancer (of the breast)."[199] He suggested further that **"new formulations must be in use for 10 to 20 years before the final pronouncement on their safety can be made."**.[200] This view is also supported by Dr R.J.B. King (1991), who has written that the latent period for breast cancer is greater than 20 years.[201]

Given that there was a substantial authoritative consensus on the latent period, it is logical to expect that health problems would only become apparent in the early 80's. The pill had not been marketed in the United States until the early 1960's,[202] and was not freely available until the late 60's and early 70's.[203] A 10, 15 or 20 year latent period, dated from the time when the pill was freely available, meant that Vessey (1972,1975,1979 & 1982) and other researchers had been looking for a disease which had had insufficient time to develop to detectable levels in a sufficiently large proportion of the female population. In short, the necessary epidemiological evidence was not yet available. This point is explicitly acknowledged by Mcpherson (1987) above.

Yet even in the 80's there was not unanimous agreement amongst researchers on the relevance of the latent period to breast cancer. In Schlesselman's review paper (1989) on cancer of the breast and the pill, he cited five papers which had failed to confirm the long-term latency period (for women with 10 or more years of pill use).[204] This would seem a strong contrary argument to that of Hertz, Vessey, Olsson, McPherson, Shapiro, Hume and Goodman & Gilman.

It is surprising, though, that Schlesselman did not actually make reference to Hertz (1969), Vessey (1975), McPherson (1983), Shapiro (1986), McPherson (1987) or the opinions of *Goodman & Gilman* (1975), all of whom did support the applicability of a long latent period in breast cancer. The inclusion of these six opposing references would have created a more balanced assessment of the medical literature and the relevance of the latent period in breast cancer. The omission of Olsson's (1989) endorsement of the latent period might be explained by a clash of publication dates: both his paper and that of Schlesselman were printed in 1989.

I cannot provide an explanation for the variation in opinions amongst researchers. This is beyond the scope of my book. I merely draw attention to the discrepancy and suggest that a divergence of views on the operation of the latent period does not mean that the concept is invalidated. To suggest that the latent period is irrelevant works against too much authoritative research.

3.3   DEFICIENCIES IN STATISTICAL METHODOLOGY.

A reading of the medical literature from the early 70's until 1996 indicates that there had been (and still is) an evolving awareness of the various statistical variables (called confounders) which can influence the collection and analysis of data.

The complexity of factors which might alter the interpretation of data include the subject's capacity to recall personal medical history (recall bias), their sexual and reproductive history, number of sexual partners, number of abortions, previous contraceptive practice, previous exposure to STD's, age at first intercourse, age at first pregnancy, age at onset of menarche, age at first use of the pill, family medical history, diet, socio-economic group, smoking history and the ability of the researchers to recruit sufficient subjects and/or controls for a study.

All of these confounders have a meaningful impact on the accurate analysis of data, but it is evident from the 'discussion of results' portion of the research literature that not all of these factors were taken into account by all researchers in all studies, a point they acknowledge.

The gradual realisation of the multi-factorial nature of data collection and analysis represents a progressive maturation in the mathematical discipline of epidemiology, that area of medicine which uses statistical analysis to examine the occurrence, distribution and causes of disease in humankind.[205] The capacity to identify and accommodate statistical confounders is a skill which has evolved. Data collection has become more all-encompassing, recall bias has slowly been eliminated and computer modelling programs have became more powerful.

The need for greater sophistication in data examination was acknowledged by Pike and Henderson (1983), who reported that their study was at variance with four earlier reports by other researchers on the pill and breast cancer. And what reason did they postulate to explain this variation?

"Much more subtle analysis is going to be required to understand

the nature of any risk associated with combined-type OC use
after age 25.".[206]

Shapiro (1986) also noted that careful attention to certain statistical confounders
was of paramount importance:

"... it may be that we still lack adequate information about certain
subgroups, such as women who begin to use oral contraceptives
soon after menarche, when the breasts are still growing
rapidly.".[207]

In summary, two valid reasons exist which explain certain discrepancies in the
early research on the pill and breast cancer: the demonstrated need to observe a
latent period of 10 to 15 years and the relative immaturity of epidemiological
techniques employed in data collection and statistical analysis during the 70's
and through to at least 1986 (also see Shapiro, *New Eng Journ Med,* 1986).

3.4   DURATION OF USE OF THE PILL.

If, as hypothesised, the pill acts as a carcinogen, then the longer a woman is
exposed to the drug, the greater will be the risk of breast cancer. Risk will increase
with time. Thus, the concept of *duration of use is related to risk measurement.*

By analogy, it is well known that continuous exposure to low levels of X-rays
have the potential for long-term genetic effects. Also, exposure on a regular
basis compounds the risk of cancer because the effects are cumulative.[208]

Yet notwithstanding the acceptance of the principle of duration-of-use within
medicine, there is some dispute amongst researchers as to the applicability of
the concept as a significant factor in the genesis of breast cancer. One who
supported the duration-of-use concept was Vessey and co-workers (1979), who
acknowledged that one of the shortcomings in their study was the *absence* of
long-term users of the pill:

"...relatively few of the women who were interviewed had had
prolonged exposure to contraceptive steroids.".[209]

Another team whose research supported the duration-of-use hypothesis was Pike & Henderson *et al* (1983), who reported on a study of 314 women under age 37 at the time of diagnosis of breast cancer. For women aged under 25 years, the short-term use of the pill with a "high" component of progestagen pill i.e., 1-24 months, had a 40% increased risk (RR 1.4), use for 25-48 months had a 140% (RR 2.4) greater risk and *long term use* (5 years) had a 310% increased risk of breast cancer (RR 4.1) when compared to never-users of the pill.[210] The merits of the 'progestagen potency' classification system used in this study have been questioned by other researchers.[211]

Klim McPherson (1983) also reported that duration of use (notably before the first full-term pregnancy) was important. The risk of breast cancer when compared to non-users of the pill was 21% greater (O.R. 1.21) for pill use of 1-12 months, 72% greater (O.R. 1.72) for pill use of 13-48 months, and 211% greater (O.R. 3.11) for pill use of 49 or more months.[212]

Three years later, Meirik and co-workers (1986) from Sweden also suggested that risk increased with duration of use *after* seven years of use of the pill, but not before this time, with the greatest risk associated with 12 or more years of pill use.

"We found no statistically significant association between the use of OCs for 7 completed years or less and premenopausal breast cancer. However, our data for long-term use of OCs beyond 7 years and particularly for 12 years or more are suggestive of an association with an increased risk of premenopausal breast cancer. The most striking finding was the statistically significant association between the duration of OC use, defined as a linear continuous variable, and breast cancer[213] ... The relative risk of breast cancer after 12 or more years of OC use was 2.2 (120% risk increase). **OC use for more than 7 years before first full-term pregnancy entailed an increased breast cancer risk (RR = 2.0) which was of borderline significance."[214]** (100 % risk increase).

Another point of interest from Meirik's research was that those using the pill for 7 years or less experienced no added risks, a finding which was at odds with the earlier work of Pike and Henderson. If, at the time, Meirik's data was accurate, his conclusion would have been welcome news, because it would have implied that short term pill users were in a type of 'safety time zone', free from the worry that long term users may experience.

Some have criticised the validity of Meirik's results on statistical grounds[215] but the fact that Meirik's results are in conformity with a substantial number of other researchers argues against this criticism.

Later research, notably that of Clair Chilvers, did not support Meririk's findings on the non-existence of risk with less than 7 years of pill use. Dr Chilvers, who released a major study on May 6, 1989 in the *Lancet,* reported on 755 cases of women diagnosed with breast cancer before age 36 and found that **"there was a *highly significant trend* in risk of breast cancer with total duration of OC".** (my emphasis).[216] Women using the pill between 49-96 months had a 43% greater risk (RR 1.43) of breast cancer, and users for more than 97 months (8 years) had a 74% greater risk (RR 1.74).

Chilvers also reported that the age at first use of the pill was an important risk factor for breast cancer, which is one of the inter-linked factors mentioned earlier. This is reviewed more thoroughly in point three (Early pill usage and breast cancer).

Further support for duration-of-use came in a paper by Miller and Rosenberg in the *American Journal of Epidemiology* (1989). This paper reported that there was a 100% increased risk (RR 2.0 95% CI, 1.4-2.9) of breast cancer which extended from 10 years of pill use down to just *3 months use of the pill:*[217] a startling result. Further, breast cancer risk was 310% increased for pill use of *more* than 10 years (RR 4.1 95% CI, 1.8-9.3), a result in line with risk increasing with duration of use. These dramatic results can be seen to vindicate Pike's earlier prophetic suggestion calling for a "much more subtle analysis".

Another source of support came from the Harvard School of Public Health (Romieu, 1990) in a review paper published in *Cancer*:

> **"...data combined from case-control studies revealed a statistically significant positive trend (P=0.001) in the risk of premenopausal breast cancer for women exposed to oral**

contraceptives for longer duration. This risk was predominate among women who used oral contraceptives for at least 4 years before their first term pregnancy (RR 1.72; 95% CI 1.36-2.19).".
[218]

This relative risk represents a 72% greater risk of breast cancer when compared to never-users.

A paper published in America by Weinstein (1991)[219] also lent support to the view that duration of use created a higher risk for pill users than for never-users.

Importantly, Olsson and co-workers (*Cancer Detection and Prevention,* 1991) reported that the duration of pill use and the risk of breast cancer **"was dependent on the age at first use. An increasing** (carcinogenic) **effect for a fixed duration was seen with lower starting age ".**[220] For example, women starting the pill at age less than 20 and taking it for less than or just on two years had a risk factor of 2.7, whereas women from within the same age bracket who took the pill for *more* than two years had a risk factor of 4.7;[221] a clear increase and an even clearer medical message. Young women should not take the pill unless the medical condition being treated has a risk of breast cancer greater than that which the treatment, the pill, may cause. That is, the disease must be more lethal than the treatment.

And finally, Rookus and co-workers (1994) from the Netherlands Oral Contraceptives and Breast Cancer Study Group reported the following:

"Our findings strongly suggest that long-term OC use is related to the risk of breast cancer and the association varies by age at cancer diagnosis. Among young women(<36 at diagnosis), the use of OCs for 4 or more years was associated with double the risk found with shorter use. No duration-response relation was found in women 36-45 years of age, but long-term OC use (>/ 12 years) was also associated with double the risk of breast cancer (related to never use) at age 46-54[222] **... We took into account all known and several susp-ected risk factors of breast cancer as potential confounders of the relation between OCs and breast cancer. Adjustment for th-ese confounders generally resulted in slight increases of the estimated RRs** (relative risk). **Thus, the**

positive association we found cannot be explained by measurement errors of these confounders.".[223]

These reports cannot be easily set aside. Too many researchers since the early 80's have observed and reported on the same findings: duration of use of the pill is a significant contributory factor in breast cancer etiology.

3.5   EARLY PILL USAGE AND BREAST CANCER.

The third of the intertwined issues pertaining to breast cancer is the disproportionate risk to women initiated onto the pill at an early age. This aspect, like most of the evidence cited above, has rarely been reported in the mainstream media outlets. This is both puzzling and worrying.

One of the significant studies to draw attention to the elevated risk associated with the early use of the pill was by Pike & Henderson *et al* (1983), who noted that:

> **"Long-term use before age 25 of combination-type OCs with a 'high' content of the progestagen component was associated with increased risk of breast cancer: the relative risk was 4 after 5 years of such use…"**[224] (a 300% risk increase).

A paper by Olsson *et al* (*Lancet,* 1985) reported that:

> **"women who had started OC use at 20-24 years of age had 3 times the risk of developing breast cancer before 46 years of age when compared to never users …Our results, taken together with earlier reports linking early OC use with breast cancer, are a matter of great concern in respect of OC use by young women."** (RR 3.3, p<0.001, CI 1.3-9.4)[225] (A 3 fold increase in risk for this age range is a risk increase of 200%).

It is important to note the language used by Olsson. A "matter of great concern" is a passionate and animated style of expression which is not normally associated with the dry, emotionally detached manner of medical journals.

Yet in the mid 80's not every researcher reported on the connection between early pill use and breast cancer. One of those who did not agree with 'age' as a co-factor in breast cancer genesis was Samuel Shapiro, who wrote in the *New England Journal of Medicine* (1986) thus:

> **"It has recently been suggested that prolonged use of oral contraceptives before the age of 25 years or by nulliparous women** (no children) **may confer an increased risk** (of breast cancer) **... Fortunately, there was sufficient data in the Cancer and Steroid Hormone Study to permit statistically stable estimates of breast cancer risk within these subgroups. Again the evidence was against an increased risk.".**[226]

From a review of the medical literature, Shapiro's findings are in sharp contrast to the preponderance of research which *does* support the view that early age pill use carries with it a high risk of cancer. Typifying this contrary view is the work of Meirik (1986), who reported that: **"long term use of OCs may increase the risk of breast cancer in young women.".**[227] This research was consistent with that of Pile & Henderson, and Olsson. Adding further support to the early age pill use-breast cancer nexus was work by Chilvers *et al* (1989), who noted that **"These results support the hypothesis that OC use and the risk of breast cancer at an early age are related.".**[228]

As well, a review paper published by Olsson (1989) stated that:

> **"... with the emphasis on early OC-use, consistent results seem to emerge showing an increased risk of premenopausal breast cancer, when the possible bias of different latency times is taken into account. Also results on breast cancer incidence in early exposed age groups, tumour biology and prognosis in early OC-users support a genuine risk relationship.".**[229]

The use of such words as 'consistent', 'genuine' and 'great concern' (Olsson 1985) are significant. They reflect a certainty of mind on the part of the author regarding the link between the pill and cancer.

A second report by Olsson (1989) further underscored the lamentable situation young women were placed in when initiated onto the pill at an early age: "**...the odds ratio for women starting OC use before 20 years of age was 5.8.**"[230] Thus, for the pre-20 year old women taking the pill, there is a 480% higher risk of breast cancer compared to never-users of the pill.

Also during 1989, Johnson published a review paper in *Family Planning Perspectives* which in part provided a "new analysis" of the Cancer and Steroid Hormone Study (CASH) . Earlier reports on the CASH study, such as that by Shapiro referred to earlier, had suggested that pill use by nulliparous women or women aged younger than 25 years was not problematic.[231] Johnson, re-analysing the same CASH data as that reviewed by Shapiro, concluded that teenage women who had used the pill had a 460% greater risk of breast cancer than never-users:

> "**... nulliparous women who had experienced menarche prior to age 13 and had used the pill for eight or more years did have a significant relative risk. Most of the increased risk was confined to women who had begun the pill as teenagers; they had a relative risk of 5.6 compared with never-users.**"[232]

The weight of evidence on early-age pill use and cancer continued to accumulate, this time from British research in 1989. A letter in the *Lancet* pointed out that: "**there was a significant trend in risk of breast cancer with total duration of OC use with relative risk 1.43 for 49-96 months use**"[233] for women aged under 36 years - a 43% risk increase.

More research by Olsson (*Cancer,* 1991) re-affirmed these findings:

> "**In 175 premenopausal breast cancer patients, a history of oral contraceptive use before 20 years of age was significantly associated with higher tumour cell proliferative activity.**"[234]

Previously the response to this mounting evidence against the pill was to discount the adverse findings by suggesting that the increased incidence of breast cancer was merely a reflection of improved diagnostic tests which detected the cancers sooner rather than later. From two sources this conclusion was shown to be inaccurate.

First, additional research published by Olsson in 1991(*Cancer Detection and Prevention,*) rejected the view that the increased incidence of breast cancer seen in young women in Sweden was due to changes in diagnostic activities or non-pill risk factors. Rather, Olsson proposed that the increase in incidence **"could be due to OC exposure"**.[235] Second, a similar observation was made by the Cancer Council of New South Wales (Aust) in its report *Cancer in NSW - Incidence and Mortality 1994*. This report **"reinforce(d) concerns that there has been a 'real' increase in breast cancer incidence in recent decades, rather than being due to earlier detection alone."**.[236]

The following year another study from Scandinavia by Ranstam (1992) reported that:

"Oral contraceptive usage before 20 years of age seemed to be related to higher risks than usage between 20 and 25.".[237]

To all those who decry the validity of this age-linked problem and the human suffering it represents, Ranstam (1992) stated the case succinctly:

"... the incidence of breast cancer has been found to be increasing in Sweden during the late 1970's and 1980's. Presently, usage of OC's is widespread and, to a high degree, initiated during adolescence".[238]

In 1993 Wingo & Lee reported that for younger users of the pill the breast cancer risk was evident, although in this study it was found to be only slight,[239] - in the order of a 40% increase risk. (OR 1.4, CI 1.0-2.1). Whilst not as dramatic as some other studies, I would contend that 40% is still unacceptable.

And now we come to 1994 and a report from the Netherlands Cancer Institute. The researchers conclude that for young women the risk was double that of never-users:

"4 or more years of OC use, especially if partly before age 20, is associated with an increased risk of breast cancer at an early age.".[240]

Whilst the aforementioned studies constitute a convincing argument for the susceptibility of early-age users of the pill to breast cancer, there is the ever-present question of 'why?' to be addressed. Arguably the most plausible reason comes from Olsson (*Cancer*,1991), already referred to on a number of occasions:

> **"Why are there higher rates of tumour cell proliferation and more patients with aneuploid tumours in young OC users? One possibility is that tumours induced in these early ages reflect the normal cell proliferation and conserve a higher proliferation rate than in tumors induced at later ages when the rate of proliferation in normal breast epithelium is low. Thus, it has been found that the cell proliferation in the normal breast is highest in teenage women.".**[241]

This hypothesis suggested that tumours, induced by the pill in young women continue to 'grow' at a rate faster than that of tumour growth induced by the pill in older women. This reflects the naturally higher cellular growth of breast tissue in young women compared to older women. It is as though the more rapid rate of breast tissue growth in young women is usurped and adopted as the 'normal' rate of cell growth by the tumour. Thus with much justification did Olsson advise that: **"The findings in this article should prompt additional investigations in patients who at an early age used OC or had a miscarriage or abortion.".**[242] This is an interesting hypothesis which may be difficult to conceptualise so I have included the following stylised diagram to assist in its understanding.

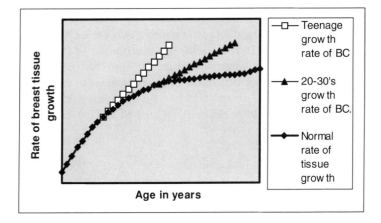

Further support for the views of Olsson, Ranstam and others was presented by Palmer and co-workers (1995), who studied the pill's effect on the risk of breast cancer in African-American women aged 25 to 59 years. Five hundred and twenty four cases of invasive breast cancer from this population were compared to 1021 controls. The researchers found that for women aged less than 45, the increased risk of breast cancer due to three or more years of pill use was 180% greater than non-users. For women aged 45-59, pill use carried little or no increased risk. As the authors noted:

> **"These findings add to the evidence from studies of White women and a recent study of Black women which have suggested an increased risk of breast cancer at young ages for moderate or long duration use of OCs.".**[243]

Also in 1995, a study from the Netherlands, which was **"initially designed to examine the relationship between diet and the incidence of cancer"**, reported a 30% increased risk for women who were under 35 when they first used the pill.[244] This result is important on its own merits, but it is also noteworthy because it was detected by the researchers almost by accident.

As they observed:

> **"...** (there were) **two important shortcomings of this study regarding exogenous** (from outside the body) **hormone use and the subsequent risk of breast cancer. First, because of the age range** (subjects in the age range 55 to 69 years had been chosen), **a relatively small percentage of the women ever used OCs. OCs were introduced on the Dutch market in the beginning of the 1960s. Even the youngest women of our cohort were then over the age of 30. Second, because of the primary interest in the relation between diet and cancer incidence, the questions on the use of exogenous hormones either as OCs or as HRT, were brief.".**[245]

The emergence of a 30% increased risk of breast cancer for young women on the pill, in what the researchers accepted was an inadequately designed study, confirms the first law of epidemiology:

"... if a causal effect is large enough, it will show up despite all the problems of performing, analysing, and interpreting observational studies on real people.".[246]

In 1996, Rosenberg and colleagues, writing in the *American Journal of Epidemiology*, reported on a study of 3,540 white women, aged 25-59 years. They used data obtained from hospitals in Boston, New York and Philadelphia between 1977-1992.[247] For women 25-34 years, there was a 70% increased risk of breast cancer for pill use of more than one year when compared to pill use of less than one year. As the authors reported, **"the results add to the evidence of an association between oral contraceptive use and an increased risk of breast cancer at young ages.".**[248]

Also during 1996 Olsson and co-workers published 'leading edge' research which verified the susceptibility of young women's bodies to the carcinogenic potential of the pill. The researchers examined breast tissue which had been removed from 58 women who had undergone a breast reduction operation. The purpose of this examination was to determine if there were different rates of cellular proliferation from amongst the samples, an important issues because:

"Knowledge about factors influencing the proliferation of normal breast epithelium is essential for understanding critical time periods for breast carcinogenesis, as there is a relationship between the proliferative rate in an organ and propensity for tumourigenesis.".[249]

Each woman was interviewed for age at menarche, menstrual cycle characteristics, family history, parity, abortions, use of drugs and use of hormones. A number of revealing results were obtained.

- **"Women who used OCs before the FFTP** (first full-term pregnancy) **had a significantly higher proliferation rate compared with never users or late users.".**[250]

- **"An especially high proliferation rate was seen in young women with both a positive family history** (for breast cancer) **and present hormonal use. Overall younger women had a higher proliferation rate than older women.".**[251]

- **"OC use before age 20 and before FFTP were associated with a higher proliferation rate.".**[252]

Whilst these results are in harmony with previous work by Olsson and others, the authors nonetheless advised that due to small number of women enrolled in the study the results should be regarded as **"preliminary"**.

From a best-practice medical perspective, the promotion of the pill to young women via teenager magazines, peer pressure and parental misguidance is a dangerous health option without objective justification. If the rationale for this approach is that the pill will act as a means of disease prevention or teenage pregnancy avoidance, then the evidence unambiguously indicates that the social experiment is an abject failure.

A feature article in the *Lancet* (1995) presented an illuminating reflection on the demographic and sociological impact of current 'pregnancy-avoidance' policies. It is a model of logic which is difficult to refute. This article is recommended to the reader.

"Although oral contraceptives are a very effective method of preventing pregnancy, numerous programmes aimed at reducing unintended adolescent pregnancy, increased access to oral contraceptives, and a widespread public perception that 'the pill' is a reliable form of birth control have had little effect in this age group.".[253]

further: **"... with regard to North America, over the past decade there has been an unprecedented epidemic of sexually transmitted diseases (STDs), especially among adolescent and young adult women"**[254] and therefore **"... physicians and policy makers must begin to consider whether the risk reduction through technological means (the pill) has been emphasised at the expense of investigating and addressing primary problematic behaviour.".**[255]

The authors then outline how some American communities have adopted a program which seeks to reduce teenage pregnancy rates by placing strong emphasis on tactics other than that of promoting the pill:

> **"Some communities have implemented educational strategies which, in addition to the goal of increasing student knowledge about sexuality and related issues, directly address behaviour by means of their explicit aim of encouraging adolescents to postpone sexual activity... By the end of the following year, there were fewer pregnancies among the programme group because there were fewer girls who were sexually involved. As a result of the success of this particular initiative, the US government is devoting $300 million to the 1000 American schools with the highest out-of-wedlock birthrates in order for them to devise their own versions of this programme."**.[256]

Based upon the preceding evidence, the administration of the pill to adolescent and young adult women is deserving of the strongest ethical reproach.

3.6   AGE AND PROGNOSIS FOR BREAST CANCER.

Superimposed upon the problem of greater susceptibility of young women to breast cancer is the research which indicates that once afflicted, these same young women have a worse prognosis. Swedish researchers have focused on this unique problem in some detail. Olsson (1989) reported that:

> "... women with breast cancer, who at an early age have used OC, have larger breast tumours... and a worse prognosis compared with later (pill users) and never users".[257]

This study finding was later corroborated by Ranstam (1991), who reported that:

> "... five-year survival was 62% among women who started to use OCs before the age of 20, 78% among those who started to use OC's between the ages of 20 and 25, and 86% among non-users (of the pill) and those who started to use OCs after the age of 25.".[258]

Put simply: the younger the pill-taking group of women were at the time of diagnosis, the greater the possibility that they would be dead within 5 years, when compared to tumour patients who had *not* taken the pill.

Supporting the work of Ransram was another study by Olsson (*Cancer*,1991) which reported that:

> "... the higher tumour proliferative activity and frequency of aneuploidy (any variation in chromosome number) in early OC users are in line with previously reported findings of worse prognostic indicators and *a worse survival in early users of OC* compared with other young women *with* breast cancer "(emphasis added).[259]

Olsson is stating that the pill caused chromosomal aberrations in the breast tissue of young female users of the pill. This result is consistent with previous findings of 'worst survival scenarios' for these women.

One of the factors which contributed to the "worse survival in early users of OC" was the **"greater incidence of axillary metastasis"** (Olsson, *J Natl Cancer Inst,* 1991).[260] That is, early age pill users presented with tumours which had spread more extensively into the lymphatic area of the armpit than that seen in nonusers.

In a separate study designed in part to reveal what the "worse survival", or dying rate was for young pill users, Olsson and co-workers (*Cancer Detection and Prevention,* 1991) reported that for those who started the pill before 20 years of age, the relative risk of dying was 820% higher than for **"healthy"** nonusers of the same age. For women who started the pill between 20-25 years of age, the risk of dying was 180% higher when compared to **"healthy"** nonusers of the same age.[261]

Olsson speculated as to the possible causes for the finding that **"early OC use increases the risk of premenopausal breast cancer..."**.[262] Only two were offered:

a) Synthetic hormones (such as those in the pill) may have a direct influence over how cells within normal breast tissue divide and grow. This synthetic hormonal effect may **"increase the potential for carcinogenesis."**.[263]

b)**"Another possible mechanism may involve permanent changes of hormonal systems or growth factors after early OC use."**.[264]

Given these results, it is not beyond the bounds of reasoned argument to suggest that this situation could be categorised as drug-induced vandalism of the female physiology. In my view, the promotion of the pill to young women, notably in the early adolescent years, constitutes a form of child abuse. Yet little or nothing is heard of this lamentable betrayal of young women's health, despite the admonishment from Olsson (*Cancer,* 1991) that:

> **"... the findings in this article should prompt additional investigations in patients who at an early age used OC or had a miscarriage or abortion... and confirm that indeed cell proliferation is higher and tumours are more aneuploid in the early exposed patient group."**.[265]

3.7   PARITY AND BREAST CANCER.

In epidemiology, parity is the classification of a woman by the number of live-born children delivered.[266] This definition varies slightly from that used in obstetrics, which counts the number of live births *and* stillbirths delivered at more than 28 weeks of gestation.[267] Women who have not given birth are referred to as *nulliparous* while those who have given birth are *parous* (Latin, *parus, bring forth*). A number of studies have indicated that child-birth protects against pill-induced breast cancer.

One such study was published by Meirik, Farley and co-workers (1989) in *Contraception*.[268] These researchers first compared women who *had used* the pill for 8 years and not given birth (nulliparous) with women who *had not used* the pill and not given birth. Those who *had* used the pill and not given birth had a 330% greater relative risk (RR 4.3) of breast cancer compared to never-users who had not given birth.

Next the researchers compared women who *had* used the pill for 8 years *prior* to giving birth (parous) with women who *had not* used the pill and given birth . Those who had used the pill had a 70% greater relative risk (RR 1.7) of breast cancer compared to never-users.

Finally, the researchers reported on the effects that pill use had *after* childbirth:

> **"... parous women who had used OCs for 12 or more years after their first full-term pregnancy had a relative risk of 3.0 (CI 1.3-7.4)."** (a 200% risk increase).[269]

The protective benefit imparted by child-birth is clearly demonstrated: 12 years of pill use after a woman had given birth is less dangerous than 8 years of pill use for a woman who had not given birth. As the researchers concluded:

> **"Nulliparous women have a higher relative risk estimate after 8 years of OC use than did parous women after 12 years of use, thus our findings indicate that a full-term pregnancy may modify any increased risk possibly induced by OCs."**[270]

It would seem that the hormones of pregnancy tend to 'correct' or 'block' any injurious cellular damage that the pill hormones might have inflicted on the developing breast tissue, particularly in young women.

Support for Meirik's findings came also from Rushton (1992), who reported:

>"... (the) **risk of breast cancer may be raised around 20% in younger, nulliparous and long use duration subgroups oral contraceptive users".**[271]

Thus the recommendation would seem to be that if a woman either cannot have or does not intend to have children, pill use should at least be strenuously discouraged. Even for parous women, a strong precautionary warning would seem advisable.

Another aspect to the interplay between parity, age and breast cancer has been discussed by Dr Graham Colditz (1996) of Harvard Medical School, Boston, Massachusetts. Dr Colditz has reported that:

>"... (the mother's) **age at first birth and the spacing of subsequent births predict the risk of breast cancer. The closer births are spaced after the first birth, the lower the risk of breast cancer.".**[272]

When Dr Colditz compared women who had multiple births - with the first birth occurring at an early age- to women with a single birth at a late age, he found that the cumulative risk of developing breast cancer for these two groups of women when they had reached age 70 was 50% less for the early age and multiple births group.

Interestingly, Dr Colditz also noted that it is now the accepted view that a woman's first pregnancy causes a brief but passing increase in the risk of breast cancer. Countering this transient increase in risk is the influence of the second and subsequent pregnancies, which are *not* associated with this temporary increased risk. In fact, the second and subsequent pregnancies confer additional *protection* from breast cancer.[273]

3.8   GENETICS AND BREAST CANCER.

During 1992, work published by Giske Ursin of the University of Southern California sought to address one of the most relevant questions in cancer research: what role does a genetic pre-disposition play in the development of cancers and how, if at all, could it be statistically accounted for?

The medical justification for this concern is strong: **"... new techniques of molecular genetics have confirmed the existence of oncogenes literally, tumour genes...** (which) **are present in everyone"**.[274]

The central question to be posed is: to what extent can the pill be classified as an environmental carcinogen which 'switches on' the oncogenes? As the *Merck Manual* (1992) had noted **"most malignancies seem to occur in genetically predisposed individuals who are at some time exposed to environmental carcinogens"**.[275]

Dr Ursin's study involved 149 women who had used the pill and had been diagnosed with premenopausal bilateral breast cancer. As matched controls, the researchers enrolled the unaffected *sisters* of the subjects. This unique inclusion conferred two important benefits.

First, since sisters have the same genetic parentage, a truer indication of the impact of certain environmental carcinogens can be more accurately assessed. Second, since unaffected sisters have been used as the controls, adverse findings about the pill cannot be easily dismissed, as any genetic pre-disposition to breast cancer can be presumed to be reasonably equal for both the affected pill user and her never-using but genetically similar sister.

The researchers acknowledged that there were certain shortcomings in their study, such as too few women taking the pill prior to their first full-term pregnancy (FFTP) and too few using one of the oestrogens (ethinyl estradiol). Nevertheless the researchers could still statistically conclude that:

> **"... restricting the analyses to women who had ever given birth yielded an odds ratio for ever-use of OC's of 2.1** (a 110% risk increase). **These results indicate an increased risk of pre-**

menopausal bilateral breast cancer associated with OC use."[276]

Since a similar genetic pre-disposition could be presumed for both the subject and her control/sister, it could reasonably be concluded that the substantial breast cancer rate was attributable in large part to the carcinogenic nature of the pill. The pill had activated the oncogenes.

As a summary of this topic, it seems the following statement, made in 1992, by Lund and co-workers accurately reflects the medical literature :

> **"Over the last few years a shift in opinion has taken place. Most reviewers now consider that long-term use of oral contra-ceptives is associated with an increased risk of premenopausal breast cancer".**[277]

This view is in contrast to that of Dr Edith Weisberg, who specialises in the area of female sexual and reproductive health and is the Medical Director, NSW Family Planning Association (Aust). In 1994 she wrote that:

> **"Despite information to the contrary, many women are still convinced that the pill causes cancer... Much misinformation exists about the pill.".**[278]

Women could be forgiven for feeling rather confused about what has been said by these two experts in this field of human sexuality. The statements are unmistakably contradictory and therefore irreconcilable. Who is to be believed? Surely the preponderance of scientific evidence weighs most heavily in favour of the majority view as expressed by Lund (1992).

3.9   BREAST FEEDING AND BREAST CANCER.

Whilst it is true that "bad" news such as the above can be turned to good use if properly acted upon, it is equally true that "good" news can be rendered mean-ingless if ignored.

Thus there is much to promote in the positive findings from Chilvers and Pike

(*Br J Cancer*, 1992) about the protective effects of breast-feeding:

> **"There was a strong trend in protection effect associated with total duration of breast feeding, and the number of children breast fed. Breast cancer risk increased with number of children not breast fed."**[279]

furthermore:

> **"Breast feeding is promoted in terms of benefit to the infant and in strengthening the bond between mother and child. Perhaps the time has come to suggest that there may be a benefit to the mother also in terms of a reduction in risk of premenopausal breast cancer".**[280]

3.10   INCIDENCE AND MORTALITY OF BREAST CANCER.

The ultimate support for the credibility of any claimed link between the pill and breast cancer can only come from longitudinal population-based cancer rates. This point is well recognised by experts in the field of female reproductive health such as Dr Edith Weisberg, who has been reported as saying that if there was any significant cancer risk **"surely we would have had some inkling of it"**.[281]

The 'inkling' does exist. The NSW Cancer Council has reported that " **between 1973-77 and 1988-91, the age-standardised rates** (of breast cancer) **rose by 25%** ... (and) **mortality rates rose by 6%"**.[282] Graph 3a presents the age-standardized rates of breast cancer with the addition of new figures for 1992-94.

Of equal concern is the data presented in graph 3b, which shows that the age-specific incidence of breast cancer increased from 1972 to 1993. As can be seen, for each age bracket except the 30-34 year age group, the age-specific incidence of breast cancer has increased in the 21 year period 1972-93.

GRAPH 3a: Age-standardised incidence of Breast Cancer (1993.NSW)[283]

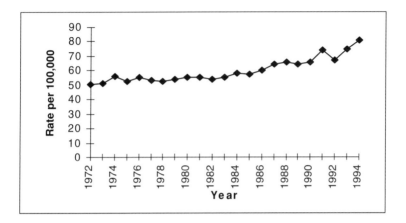

Graph 3b: Age-specific incidence of breast cancer per 100,000 women (NSW, Australia). 1972 (left column) v 1993 (right column) .

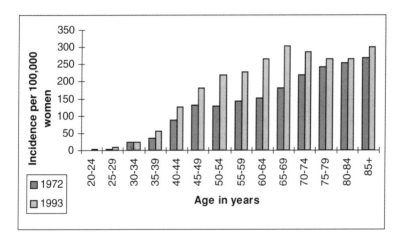

What is *not* evident from graph 3b, due to scaling of the Y 'Incidence axis', is the increase in the incidence of breast cancer in the 20-24 and 24-29 years age brackets for the years 1972 versus 1993. For the 20-24 age bracket, the incidence of breast cancer has increased 600% in 21 years, from 0.5 cases per 100,000 women in 1972 to 3 cases per 100,000 women in 1993. For the 25-29 age bracket there has also been a jump in the incidence, from 3.3 cases per 100,000 women in 1972 to 7.9 cases per 100,00 women in 1993; an increase which is in excess of 100% . These figures have been extracted and are presented in more detail in graph 3c, as well as the respective age data for 1982. The inclusion of the 1982 data gives the 1972 versus 1993 data a contextual perspective. I have placed all the data used to formulate these graphs in Appendix seven.

Graph 3c: Age-specific incidence of breast cancer per 100,000 women (NSW, Australia). 1972, 1982, 1993.

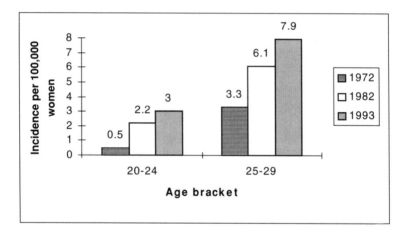

Some caution must be exercised in reading too much into these figures because the number of cases of diagnosed breast cancer for each age-bracket and year was small. Nonetheless, it is unarguable that overall there has been a significant increase, as shown by graph 3a .

What can be suggested as possible explanations for these events? Is the increased incidence only as a result of better public awareness of the need for regular breast cancer screening? Certainly this is part of the answer, but is it the full answer? As previously pointed out, the *Cancer in NSW Incidence and Mortality 1994* report had noted there was a "real" increase in the incidence of breast cancer, not an increase due to earlier detection programs alone.[284] Could the increased incidence be due to women starting the pill during mid to late adolescence when the developing breast tissue has been shown to be most susceptible to the effects of synthetic hormones? The work of Olsson (1991), Ranstam (1992) and Rookus (1994), previously discussed, supports the latter view.

More recently, the Sydney Breast Cancer Institute has also reported that **"the incidence of the disease is increasing..."**.[285] The situation in America is little different from Australia, with the annual age-specific incidence rate (1981-1985) of breast cancer showing a precipitous increase for women once they have passed age 20. Graph 4 shows this data. Media-medicos also substantiated this data. The Media Tracking Service recently reported that there had been an **"an annual rise of 3% p.a. since the mid 1980's"** in breast cancer.[286]

The probability of a woman developing breast cancer over her lifetime in the U.S.A. is one in eight; in Australia one in 16 whilst in Japan it is only one in 50. [287] Whilst some have sought to explain these international variations in breast cancer rates by attributing it to the high-fat diet in America,[288] it is equally plausible to attribute it to the fact that Japan had not, at least until the end of 1996, legalised the use of the pill.

Graph 4: Annual Age-specific Incidence Rates per 100,000 U.S. Women. 1981-85[289]

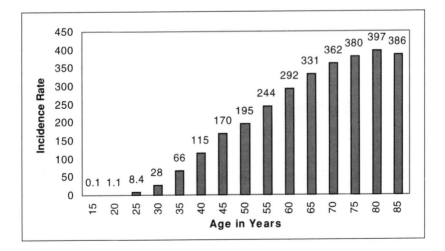

These graphs, and the study by Ursin (1992) in particular, are in line with reports by the *International Agency for Research on Cancer*, which has listed combined oral contraceptives as carcinogens, along with such well-known products as asbestos, mustard gas, tobacco smoke, arsenic and solar radiation.[290]

Moreover, according to the Associate Professor of Public Health at the University of Western Australia, Dr Konrad Jamrozik, the incidence of breast cancer is expected to rise 25-33 per cent by 2005. Amongst the various factors contributing to this problem is **"the wide-spread use of oral contraceptives".**[291]

To recap: I again quote from the beginning of this chapter so that all can decide how accurately the government-approved information reflects the reality of the medical research on this vital topic:

> **"At present, there is no confirmed evidence from human studies which would indicate that an increased risk of cancer is associated with oral contraceptives."** (Government approved drug information - Trifeme - 1996) .[292]

Is it now time for some hard questions to be asked of those in positions of authority?

3.11   KEY POINTS.

1. Early-age use of the pill carries a greater risk of breast cancer, of developing larger tumours and of having a worse prognosis..

2. Parity confers some protection from breast cancer, but the initial effects of parity are greatly reduced by long-term pill use.

3. Breast feeding confers a protective action.

4. The incidence of breast cancer is increasing in New South Wales, the largest state in Australia. This reflects similar trends in America.

5. The pill acts as a carcinogenic substance independent of any genetic predisposition a woman may have.

CHAPTER FOUR

4.   THE PILL: BLOOD CLOTS, BIRTH DEFECTS AND INFERTILITY.

"Although not risk-free, the pill's benefits far outweigh its risks. Another way of saying this is that the pill is safe - but some women are dangerous."[293] Prof. John Guillebaud, Family Planning and Health, London.

Aside from the pill's role in causing cervical and breast cancer, there are numerous other side-effects of the pill which have the capacity to seriously undermine the health status of women. The order of their presentation in this chapter are: alterations to a healthy cardio-vascular status, notably via thrombo-embolisms; birth defects attributable to pill use immediately prior to pregnancy; and the influence of the pill on cervical mucous production and the resultant deterioration in post-pill fertility, leading to a diminished capacity for conception.

4.1   THE PILL AND BLOOD CLOTS.

Concern that the pill was implicated in thrombo-embolic disorders was reflected in the medical literature as far back as 1968. In 1973, a report from the Boston Collaborative Drug Surveillance Programme noted that:

"Compared with non-users, the estimate of relative risk for thromboembolism in oral-contraceptive users was 11 and the estimated attack-rate attributable to oral contraceptives was 60 per 100,000 users per year."[294] A relative risk of 11 represents an 10 fold increase in risk, or 1,000 %.

The researchers attributed this increased risk in part to an increased blood viscosity and increased platelet stickiness. These two haematological changes were: "due to the oestrogen component of the contraceptive preparations and do not occur in patients receiving progestins alone."[295]

In 1980, Meade and co-workers reported on their analysis of data from 2,044 women who had presented with suspected cardiovascular and related reactions to a selection of formulations of the pill. Whilst they noted that **"the increased risk of cardiovascular disease in women on combined oral contraceptives is usually attributed to the oestrogenic component, "** they also suggested that **"Progestogens probably have metabolic effects that may contribute to the increased risk of cardiovascular reactions associated with combined oestrogen-progestogen oral contraceptives."**[296]

To justify this 'shifting of the blame' to the progestin component of the pill, Meade *et al* reported:

> **"There was a significant positive association between the dose of norethisterone acetate** (the progestin) **and deaths from stroke and ischaemic heart disease (IHD)."**[297]

This assigning of responsibility for thrombo-embolisms to either oestrogens or progestins is an interesting development which was to emerge repeatedly through the subsequent medical literature. The source of this conflict about culpability did not, however, lie with data collection as such, but it rather ironically reflected the fact that both drugs were culpable: that is, both hormones were eventually seen to be implicated. More will be stated on this point later.

In 1981, Layde and Beral reported on data collected from 23,000 women in the United Kingdom who had taken the pill during 1968-69. These researchers found that mortality from *all* circulatory disease was 320% higher (RR 4.2) in women taking the pill than in non-users. When the data was reviewed according to various sub-categories of disease, the risk of specifically developing cerebral thrombosis, haemorrhage and embolism was 110% higher (RR 2.1) for pill users than for never-users. The relative risk of ischaemic heart disease was 3.9 i.e., a 290 % increased risk compared to never-users.[298]

These statistics can seem rather cold and meaningless when viewed just as numbers with % signs after them. They take on a different dimension when it is pointed out that in this study, the total number of deaths for the control (non-pill-using) group was 4 but for pill users was 10. Statistics lack humanity; real people don't. Statistics don't die, but real people do.

Another important research paper during the 80's was by Susan Helmrich *et al* (1987), who reported on a study done with women admitted to hospital as a result of deep venous thrombosis (DVT, or leg clots) or pulmonary embolism (lung clots). These women had used the combined pill in the previous month. It was calculated that this study group had acquired an 710% increased risk of developing venous thromboembolism from the pill (RR 8.1).[299]

Also of major significance in this paper was the finding that lower doses of the oestrogen component may have failed to produce the expected reduction in the risk of DVT (see footnote).[300]

> **"The data suggest that the risk of venous thromboembolism is increased for recent oral contraceptive users relative to nonusers, even if women use oral contraceptives containing low doses of oestrogen... It has not yet been determined whether the reduction in the estrogen dose has indeed reduced or eliminated the risk of thromboembolic diseases in oral contraceptive users.".[301]**

This point is of much interest as it implies that it is not just the oestrogenic component of the pill which can precipitate blood clots. If, as previously reported, the progestin component also has thromboembolic potential, then it would seem that women are not safe from the pill *per se.*

Aside from a reduction in dose of the oestrogenic component of the pill, researchers sought also to reduce the cardio-vascular problems linked to 'second generation' progestins commonly in use in the 70's and 80's i.e., levonorgestrel and norethisterone, by developing new 'third-generation' progestins such as desogestrel and gestodene.

Desogestrel and gestodene had been promoted as representing a marked improvement over previous progestins. In particular, researchers had reported that these drugs had greater progestin-receptor binding capacity (causing less pill-induced acne), less impact on carbohydrate metabolism, no interference with lipoprotein metabolism and no significant alteration to blood pressure.[302] Importantly, they said, desogestrel **" has been widely shown to produce minimal changes of the coagulation and fibrinolytic systems, and it has not been associated with an increased risk of thromboembolic disorders.".**[303] The coagulation/fibrinolytic systems are the counter-balancing clotting/anti-clotting systems. They work to keep our blood in a stable, free-flowing state.

But reports during the mid-80's in West Germany suggested that this optimism was to be short-lived:

> "... cases of thrombo-embolism were reported with one of the newest micropills, Femovan (containing gestodene). Between 1987 and 1989 there were 13 cases from Germany and 8 from England, with one fatality in each country. Suspicion fell on the new progestogen, gestodene.".[304]

Another of the new generation of progestins, Marvelon® (desogestrel), was also linked to serious health questions:

> "Thrombo-embolic episodes were also recorded in England between 1982 and 1988 with another micropill, Marvelon. There were 25 cases in England, including six fatalities. In Germany between 1981 and 1988 there were 15 cases, with 2 fatalities, and in Switzerland, five with no fatalities.".[305]

In response to these new reports the Federal German Health Ministry issued a medical alert bulletin in 1989 which sought to explain the mechanism by which the third-generation progestins had caused the thrombo-embolisms:

> "The suspicion is that gestoden (the 'progesterone') in Femovan reaches high levels, that it accumulates in the duration of one dosage cycle, and therefore, breakdown of ethinyloestradiol (the 'oestrogen') by the liver is prolonged.".[306]

What this means is that the new third-generation progestogens cause a "metabolic blockage" in the liver's ability to break down ethinyloestradiol (the oestrogen). This leads to a build-up of ethinyloestradiol in a woman's body which adversely impacts upon the blood clotting mechanisms, possibly leading to the reported thromboembolic problems.

This explanation ties the earlier research together. There is an interplay between the two drugs in the pill which comes into effect when the drug passes through the liver (as all oral drugs do). I offer this as one of three hypothesis to explain the increased incidence of thrombo-embolisms in users of the combined pill. (The third hypothesis, related to clotting factor 5 and activated protein C, is the most biologically certain. It will be discussed a little further on).

The German Health Ministry report also made mention of another feature which has previously been discussed in the context of breast cancer. Many of the victims of the new third-generation progestogens were young and healthy and not taking alcohol or smoking.

There is an interesting co-incidence between these medical reports and a class action launched in England (April, 1995) by a group of women who claimed that manufacturers of the pill failed to disclose the full health implications of the drug. This legal initiative prompted TV researchers to check **"the death certificates of eight young women who died from blood clots in the last two years. The pill was the cause of each death.".**[307]

In the same newspaper piece, a world authority on the pill, Prof. John Guillebaud of London's Margaret Pyke Centre, said:

"When we say the Pill is safe, we don't mean it is risk free".[308]

Cardio-vascular problems related to the pill continued to be reported in Europe and the U.K. during the 90's. The *Lancet* (1991) published a case study on the hospital admission of a 19 year old suffering from shortness of breath. Investigation found that she was suffering from blockage in the right common iliac vein, a major blood vessel which returns blood from the legs to the heart for re-oxygenation.[309] Clot-dissolving treatments were required for 5 days, followed by 4 weeks of anti-coagulant therapy, which ultimately led to a successful recovery for this patient. In the minds of the authors of this report, no other risk factors existed which might have led to the deep venous thrombosis (DVT), other than the use of the pill.

What was most revealing from the pathology tests conducted on this woman whilst she was in hospital was that she had developed *antibodies* to cyproterone (Diane®), one of the components of her pill. The authors of this report stated that: **" Although we cannot be certain that cyproterone acetate antibodies caused the DVT, this case is very suggestive.".**[310]

Other researchers have also reported the presence of antibodies to components of the pill. Violette and Jean-Louis Beaumont (*Lancet*, 1991) stated that:

> **"in women on oestrogen-progestogen pills the antibodies det-
> ected by radioimmunoassay were usually against ethinyl-
> oestradiol ... (and) were observed in 25% of otherwise healthy
> users of OC and in 80% of users with thrombosis".**[311]

Ethinyloestradiol is one of the most common oestrogen components in contemporary pill formulations (see appendix 2).

But what does this reference to antibodies and the pill mean? An antibody is a **"specific substance produced by specialised blood cells as a reaction to an antigen** (foreign substance) **for the purpose of host defence.".**[312] In this definition I see the second of the workable hypotheses for the increased incidence of thrombo-embolism associated with the pill. The woman's body perceives the artificial hormones as a foreign substance and endeavours to eliminate them via the immune system. The interaction between the immune system and the 'foreign' drugs leads to an interference with the normal clotting mechanisms, with inconvenient and sometimes tragic consequences. I consider that this theory has more scientific validity than the previous.

To further highlight the dramatic impact of the pill on the haematological system it is relevant to review a paper published by Prof. Vandenbroucke of the Netherlands in the *Lancet* (1994):

> **"We compared 155 consecutive premenopausal women, aged 15
> to 49, who had developed deep venous thrombosis (DVT) in the
> absence of other underlying diseases, with 169 population
> controls. The risk of thrombosis among users of oral
> contraceptives was increased 4-fold."** (a 300% increase risk
> increased).[313]

More importantly, though, Vandenbroucke reported that for women who had a defective clotting factor in their blood, the risk of developing a thrombosis was more than *30-fold increased* if they took the pill when compared to the risk for women who did not have the clotting disorder and did not take the pill.

This particular blood clotting problem is known as a factor 5 Leiden mutation, and occurs in 3.5% of women in the Netherlands and 5% in Sweden. This mutation is **"a hereditary abnormality in the protein C/Protein S anticoagulant pathway which leads to increased susceptibility to venous thrombosis."**.[314]

Women suffering this deficiency do not respond to the anticoagulant effect of activated protein C (and hence are called APC resistant). As a consequence, their blood becomes 'sticky', clots more frequently and predisposes them to thrombosis[315] (see end-note for a more detailed description).[316] This problem is made much worse if the woman is also taking the pill. As the authors noted:

> **"The incidence of thrombosis increases from 0.8 per 10,000 per women per year for non users of oral contraceptives *without* the mutation to 28.5 per 10,000 for those with the mutation who also use oral contraceptives... it is clear that a young woman who starts using oral contraceptives is at a higher risk of venous thrombosis if she carries the factor 5 Leiden mutation."** (my emphasis).[317]

It would be interesting to know what percentage of women have this blood disorder in countries other than Sweden and the Netherlands, and how frequently doctors screen for this potentially fatal disorder prior to prescribing the pill.

More recent events have again brought into sharp public focus the capacity of the pill to undermine the health status of women.

On October 19th, 1995, the UK Committee on Safety of Medicines (CSM) recommended that women should change from pill formulations containing the third-generation progestins (gestodene and desogestrel) because these progestins had been shown to double a women's risk of non-fatal blood clots (thrombo-embolisms).[318][319]

The media response to this announcement was rapid. The *Times* (21.10.95) carried the headline:

> **"Three Pill studies showed increased risk of blood clots."**[320]

and the Sydney (Australia) *Sun-Herald* (22.10.95) led with:

"Pill Panic - Health warning on seven brands.".[321]

This Australian headline was followed by the lead paragraph:

"Warnings that low-dose contraceptive pills double the risk of women developing potentially fatal blood clots has caused panic around the world.".[322]

The specific focus of these public warnings pertained to the newest versions of the pill: Femoden®, Trioden®, Minulet®, Tri-Minulet® and Marvelon®, which contained either gestodene or desogestrel.

Clearly this report was a legitimate surprise for many distraught women, given the amount of radio air-time allocated to reassuring worried callers both in Sydney and in England.[323]

What may have gone unnoticed amidst the media coverage was the important point that the doubling of risk which was reported was a doubling of the pre-existing risk associated with currently used 'second-generation' progestin formulations of the pill. It was *not* a doubling of the risk when compared to that encountered by women who do not take the pill.

This point needs added emphasis: the control group against which the risk was calculated was composed of women taking the currently available, older versions of the pill [324]. It is this fact which makes the news report all the more dramatic. A doubling of risk is significant, but when that doubling of risk means a doubling of the already existing risks of the "old' but still frequently prescribed versions of the pill it becomes apparent that any delay in making the facts public is unacceptable.[325] [326]

A week after the CSM announcement an editorial in the *British Journal of Medicine* (*BMJ*) quantified the elevated risk associated with the third generation progestagens. The *BMJ* reported that the cardiovascular risks associated with the newest forms of the pill have been estimated at 30 cases of venous thromboembolism (VTE) for every 100,000 users per year, compared to only

15 cases for every 100,000 users per year of other brands.[327] These figures add an important human dimension to the 'doubling' of risk, and, in my view, validate the concerns with third generation progestagens.

Layde and Beral (*Lancet*, 1981) had previously shown that 'old' second-generation progestagens increased a woman's risk of thrombo-embolism 3- to 4-fold.[328] Therefore, the significance of the *Times* and *Sun-Herald* report lay in the fact that the public was being told that the new 'safer' pill formulae actually double the pre-existing risk factor of 3 to 4. Thus, gestodene and desogestrel could elevate a woman's risk of blood clots 6 to 8 fold when compared to the risks affecting a woman who didn't take the pill. Some research places this figure even higher: pill users can be up to 11 times more likely than non-users to have thromboembolisms.[329]

Interestingly, comment on the CSM decision in the Letters page of the *Lancet* during November 1995 was critical. One correspondent decried the CSM action as an act of **"great haste"** done in **"secret"** which **"does not provide reassurance about protection of the public health"**.[330] Another expressed the concern that whilst the controversy over third-generation progestins was substantial **"... even more important implications may arise from the effect of the media coverage of this issue on the standing of doctors"**.[331]

Furthermore, the Australian researcher, Dr Edith Weisberg even questioned the reliability of the data upon which the British government had based its decision:

> **"Thromboembolic disease is an oestrogen side-effect, and as the dose of oestrogen in the contraceptive pill has been reduced, so has the incidence of thromboembolic disease. I am not aware of any evidence in the published literature that the progestogens have any such effect ... I'm cynical enough to think that perhaps the British government is using this to get women back on to the cheaper pills.".[332]**

The so-called 'cheaper pills' to which Dr Weisberg referred to are in fact the second-generation progestagen formulae, which had been shown to be the safer type of progestagen.

Prof. Klim Mcpherson, of the London School of Hygiene and Tropical Medicine took a different view to that of Dr Weisberg. After re-analysis of the data
upon which the CSM had based its public announcements, Prof Mcpherson
stated: **"Now that the data are published, it seems clear that the Committee on
Safety of Medicines did what it had to do.".**[333] Prof. Mcpherson's justification
was based on the fact that had the CSM not made the announcements when it
did and had it delayed making the results public as some had insisted,[334] 80 new
cases of venous thromboembolism in British women on the third generation
pills pill would have occurred **"and possibly one death.".**[335]

The suggestion that 'third-generation' progestagen pill formulations may have
been incorrectly promoted as safer than 'second-generation' versions was
evident in a report published on December 16, 1995 in *The Lancet* by Bloemenkamp and co-workers. The authors of this study noted:

> **"Recent concern about the safety of combined oral contracept-
> ives (OCs) with third-generation progestagens prompted an
> examination of data from a population-based case-control study
> (Leiden Thrombophilia Study). We compared the risk of deep-
> vein thrombosis (DVT) during use of the newest OCs, contain-
> ing a third-generation progestagen, with the risk of "older"
> products... We selected 126 women with DVT and 159 controls
> aged 15-49 (mean age 34.9) and premenopausal and found, as
> compared with non-users, the highest age-adjusted relative risks
> to be that for an OC containing desogestrel and 30 micrograms
> of ethinyloestradiol (RR 8.7, 95% CI 3.9-19.3).".**[336]

This means that for third-generation progestagen gestodene users, the overall
increased risk of DVT, measured across all ages was 770% greater than that for
women who had never used the pill (non-users).

By comparison, women taking a second-generation progestagen had varyingly
between a 120% and 280% greater risk of DVT when compared to non-users.[337]
Clearly this is a diminished risk compared to gestodene-containing products.

When the data was reviewed from an age-specific perspective, younger women
exposed to a third- generation product were found to be at greater risk:

"When we restricted the analysis to the youngest women, where most new users will be found, we found the highest risks for the desogestrel-containing OC was 7-fold higher than that of the levonorgestrel-containing products; among women aged 20-24 the risk was 4-fold higher.".[338]

Note that in this instance the estimation of risk of DVT was obtained from a comparison of third and second-generation progestagen use (recall that levonorgestrel is a second- generation progestagen). This comparison leaves unanswered the important question of what might be the risk of DVT for a *young* woman taking a third-generation progestagen compared to a young women not taking *any* artificial birth regulation hormones? It is self-evident that it must be greater than the 7-fold increased risk for third versus second- generation products, but how much greater?

As a guesstimate of this latter comparative risk, it would seem reasonable to increase the 7-fold risk for third versus second-generation products by 120-280%, since these percentages represent the increased risk of DVT from second-generation products compared to pill non-users. From this computation it can be seen that women aged 15-19, taking a third-generation progestagen, may have a 15 -26 fold greater risk of DVT than women not taking any artificial birth regulation hormones.[339]

More dramatic still was the finding that there was a 50-fold increased risk of DVT for women who took 3rd-generation progestagens and were carriers of the Factor 5 Leiden mutation.[340] Summarizing their concerns the authors concluded their research with this final paragraph:

"When we come to look back on the history of oral contraception it is certain that the decrease in the dose of ethinyloestradiol (the oestrogen component of the pill) **will be seen to have contributed to a reduced thrombotic risk, especially for arterial disease. However, the use of a third-generation progestagen does seem to have led to an unexpected and yet unexplained return of a higher risk of venous thrombosis.".**[341]

During 1996 a number of further reports were published which reinforced the view that significant cardio-vascular damaged was occasioned due to the use of the pill in general, and third-generation progestagens in particular.

On January 13th, Spitzer and co-workers (*BMJ*) published an internationally conducted study into the risks of venous thromboembolic disorders from third-generation progestagens. Amongst the principal findings were: *any* oral contraceptive use versus no use carried a 300% increased risk of deep venous thrombosis (DVT) for users, second- generation products (low dose ethinyloestradiol [EE], no gestodene or desogestrel) versus *no use* carried a 220% increased risk of DVT, third-generation products (low dose EE, plus gestodene or desogestrel) versus second-generation products carried a 50% increased risk of DVT.[342]

From these figures it can be seen that:

(a) no pill use is the best way to avoid DVT
(b) third generation versions of the pill carry greater risk of DVT than do second generation products.

In summary, Spitzer and co-workers noted that:

> **" (the) probability of death due to venous thromboembolism for women using third-generation products is about 20 per million users per year, for women using second generation products it is about 14 per million users per year, and for non-users it is five per million per year.".**[343]

Spritzer referred to this increased risk as "**modest**" but nonetheless recommended that it be taken "**seriously**".

Endeavouring to place these statistics in a more meaningful context, the researchers equated the increased risk of venous thromboembolism if using a third versus second-generation progestagen with "**... the increased risk of death from cancer and heart disease if a woman smoked 10 cigarettes a year.**".[344]

At first glance the nexus between the 'equivalent' risk of smoking 10 cigarettes per year and using third-generation products as opposed to second- generation products would appear to suggest that the real-life risks associated with third versus second-generation progestagens is, as Spitzer had said, "**modest**". In response I would suggest that it is only a modest risk if you are a man and not related to a victim. For women, and victims' relatives, the **'modest'** rate death of up to 20 women per million per annum is not a trifling matter.

In the same edition of the *British Medical Journal* (1996) Lewis and co-workers reported on a study done in 16 centres in Austria, France, Germany, Switzerland and the U.K. The study specifically investigated whether there was a link between third-generation progestagens and the cardiovascular problem known as myocardial infarction (MI- see glossary). Their results indicated that second - generation products increased a woman's risk of MI by 211% compared to non-users and, third-generation products marginally *decreased* a woman's risk of MI compared to second-generation pill users.[345]

Lewis acknowledged the surprising nature of his findings by stating: **"This finding from an interim analysis should be interpreted with caution.".**[346]

In August 1996, Vandenbroucke (*Lancet*) reported results contrary to those of Lewis regarding the protection from MI afforded by third-generation progest-agens. Vandenbroucke analysed the mortality data related to MI for men and women aged 15-49 in the Netherlands and found that:

> **"Among men aged 15-49, we see a continuing reduction in mortality, that had already started in the early 1980s... Among women, there was an initial decrease, followed by an upturn in mortality... Although it is likely that changes in smoking patterns may have affected the trends for MI (not for venous thromboembolism, for which smoking is not a risk factor) the mortality data *do not* suggest a protective effect of third-generation contraceptives against MI at the population level."**[347] (my emphasis).

The only information missing from the above quote was the data related to the mortality rates, which I now present in graph 5.

GRAPH 5.

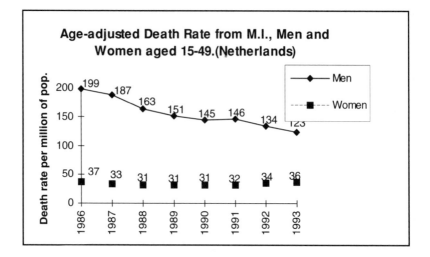

An explanation for this decrease, followed by an increase in mortality for women from MI is given by the authors of this report:

> **"Although a desogestrel-containing contraceptive was already available in the Netherlands from the early 1980s, the market share of third-generation contraceptives has been increasing since the late 1980's when competing gestoden-containing products were introduced.".**[348]

This observation by Vandenbroucke was in agreement with the reports, previously mentioned, which had noted problems with third-generation progestagens in West Germany, England, Wales and Switzerland. The emergence of a similar problem in yet another country which had introduced these products strongly suggests a causal link between the drug and the cardio-vascular problems.

Vandenbroucke's study (*Lancet*, 1996) also reported that there was an increased mortality rate from venous thromboembolism (VTE). In 1980, the female mortality rate was 5.2 deaths per million person-years. Whilst this figure dropped to its lowest point of 3.3 deaths per million person-years in 1984 there was, subsequent to this date, a steady increase in the death rate, reaching 7.5 women per million person-years in 1995.[349]

Further substantial research published in August 1996, this time by Thomas (*Lancet*), highlighted a theme encountered elsewhere in this book: the deleterious impact artificial hormones had on young women. Thomas reported that during the period 1984-86, the mortality rate from venous thromboembolism (VTE) for women aged 15-29 was 1.8 per million. For the years 1990-92 it had increased to 4.2 per million.[350] These results are consistent with those from Vandenbroucke, previously discussed.

In this same report by Thomas (*Lancet,* 1996), the changing death rate for women aged 30-44 from venous thromboembolism was also disconcerting. Between the years 1984-92 there was a downward, then upward trend; again, a cause for serious re-evaluation of the motives fuelling the enthusiastic promotion of these potent drugs. The data pertaining to these two age brackets of women is presented in graph 6.

GRAPH 6. [351]

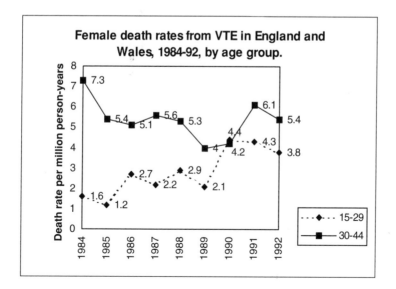

Thomas also reported on the influence of third-generation progestagens and MI, but concluded that the data and findings were insufficient to make any firm observations:

> **"If preparations containing desogestrel and gestodene were confirmed to carry a reduced risk of MI, their use might reduce overall mortality in this group. Currently, however, there is** *inadequate* **evidence to substantiate this."**[352] (emphasis added).

Thomas, whilst noting that deaths from MI and VTE are rare events in women of childbearing age, and that **"the data have limited value for studying the effects of new drugs on mortality"**[353] due to, amongst other factors, human error in accurately diagnosis the cause of death, nonetheless proffered a rationale as to why young women seem disproportionately represented as 'death' statistics:

> **"The increase in mortality from venous thromboembolism in younger women is of concern. Although these data do not prove cause and effect, the observed increase in fatal thromboembolism is consistent with the increased odds-ratio** (measure of increased risk) **of non-fatal thromboembolism associated with desogestrel-containing or gestodene-containing preparations found in epidemiological studies. The larger increase in mortality in younger women would be anticipated because they are** *most* **exposed to oral contraceptives and likely to have received the highest proportion of the newer preparations."**.[354] (emphasis added).

Shortly after the report by Thomas (*Lancet*, 1996), proof for, and an explanation of the cause-effect relationship between pill use and venous thrombosis was announced by Rosing and colleagues in the *British Journal of Haematology* (April, 1997). I take the view that this report is of such gravity that it justifies the removal of third-generation products from distribution. The evidence presented in this study makes it the most convincing of the three hypotheses linking the pill to blood clots.

To conduct the study, the researchers collected blood samples from a variety of patients, both male and female, comprised of the following; 40 healthy females not taking the pill and 50 males, 24 women who had taken a triphasic pill, 32 women who used a monophasic second- generation pill, 40 women who used a third- generation pill (gestodene, desogestrel or norgestimate), and 17 women with the factor V (5) Leiden mutation. Tests were performed to determine the clot-forming capacity of the various blood samples.

To understand the merits of this research it is beneficial to recall the interactive roles of factor 5, activated protein C (APC) and thrombin. Briefly, **"factor V is a blood-clotting factor that occurs in normal plasma... It is needed to change prothrombin rapidly to thrombin.".**[355] Thrombin causes fibrinogen to change to fibrin, which is essential in the formation of a clot.[356] As can be seen, there is a interactive 'domino' like effect operative between the various components of the blood-clotting system. Naturally a substance is needed to counteract the blood-clotting process, least an unrelenting process of clot formation take places, which could be serious if not fatal.

One such component of the blood system is known as activated protein C, or APC. It is the role of APC to inactivate factor 5, which in turn will stop the formation of thrombin and, ultimately, clot formation. Via a genetic mutation, some people are born with a defective factor 5. This is known as factor 5 Leiden mutation. This mutation means that the blood coagulating factor 5 is not as readily neutralized by APC.[357] Such people are known as APC-resistant. This genetic impairment to factor 5 **"probably explains the increased risk of venous thromboembolism in APC-resistant individuals"**[358] who do not take the pill.

The work by Rosing (*Br J Haem*) was startling because it showed that women with no pre-existing genetic defect in their factor V nonetheless had developed APC resistance. That is, whilst they had been born with a properly functioning clotting/anti-clotting system, exposure to the pill had made this system defective, with a significant shift in tendency towards clotting. The defect was an *acquired* one due to pill ingestion. It was not an *inherited* defect:

> **"In this paper we report a substantial change of a haemostatic variable** (a variable which alters the flow of blood) **in women using OC which appears to be much more sensitive and that may be indicative for the existence of a prothrombotic** (increased clotting) **state in OC user... Screening a population of women who use or do not use OC shows that OC therapy induces** *acquired* **APC resistance. Significant differences in sensitivities to APC**

were observed between women not using OC and women on OC therapy independent of the type of OC users... We propose that decreased sensitivity to APC (acquired APC resistance) in OC users may, at least in part, explain the higher risk of thrombo-embolic disease of women taking OC... Until now, the increased risk for venous thrombosis during OC therapy has always been linked to effects of oestrogen on the coagulation system. Our study provides the *first* example of a biological effect of the progestogen component on haemostasis and shows that, with respect to the risk of venous thrombosis, the role of progesterone *cannot* be ignored."[359] (emphasis added).

Rosing and co-workers, subsequent to demonstrating that women on the pill can acquire APC resistance, also proffered a powerful reason why these facts must be swiftly conveyed to prospective users of the pill: the effect of OC therapy on the blood clotting response **"takes place within a few days after starting OC therapy…"**.[360] The tragic consequences of this rapid interference with the blood-clotting mechanisms is set out in the case studies at the end of this discussion. As well, there are significant implications in this finding for the promotion of the pill as a 'morning-after' pill.

It is interesting that Rosing made the point that **"the role of progesterone** (in blood clot formation) **cannot be ignored"** because according to a letter from J.P.Vandenbroucke (*Lancet*,1997) this is precisely what appeared to have happened in the interval between the CSM decision of 18 October 1995 and April 1997. Vandenbroucke's views are expressed in a manner atypical of those seen in journals such as the *Lancet*. The normative form for '*Letters*' is one of respectfully correction or gentle disagreement tempered by an apologetic tone. Vandenbroucke's divergence from this style indicated, at least in my view, an anger barely concealed. Is his sharp, thinly concealed criticism justified? The answer is evident in the following quote.

"For over a year the epidemiological findings pointing at an increased risk with some third-generation oral contraceptives have either been ignored or downplayed ("small effects"), or have been denied ("bias, confounding"). The objection that the third-generation effect was merely a matter of "starters" and "healthy users" had been completely countered by several data analyses

restricted to first-time or recent users. Prescription bias had been countered by the fact that all risk factors that can predict a first venous thrombosis in healthy young women had been accounted for. Nevertheless, "experts" continued to sow confusion, at their best with data and analyses less adequate, than those showing the hazard, but most often by mere repetition of arguments. It is rare in the history of epidemiology that a biological explanation emerges in the middle of controversy, thereby permitting immediate separation of epidemiological chaff from wheat.".[361]

Aside from this criticism levelled at those who sought to subvert the CSM decision of October, 1995, Vandenbroucke made a strong case for a re-examination of the current system of peer-only review of medical data:

"The main beneficiaries of this new finding (from Rosing) **will be women: with the prospect of a causal explanation that fits the epidemiology, drug-regulatory agencies can no longer postpone decisions: clear prescription guidelines should be discussed** [362] **... Women who have lost out are those who have, in the meantime, developed severe venous thrombosis on the highly thrombogenic pills - especially since the warning about third-generation contraceptives containing gestodene or desogestrel by the British Committee on Safety of Medicines of October 18, 1995, did not lead to sufficiently similar regulatory action in all European countries. In particular, the European Agency for the Evaluation of Medicinal Products (CPMP) has been too willing to postpone action by demanding "more evidence" in the face of a rather complete epidemiological file. For the future, greater involvement of independent consumer boards or patient platforms in drug-safety regulation might be an option to consider. Such boards might be able to resist pressures better, and help to make safety decisions that are free from other considerations.".**[363]

This view has much merit. The unfortunate consistency seen in these studies by Bloemenkamp, Vandenbroucke, Thomas and Rosing suggests that if there has been a deliberate strategy to market the third-generation progestagens to young women, then that strategy was a success, gauging by the increasing incidence of various cardiovascular problems.

This, though, is not the limit of the adverse impact of third- generation progestagens, either on the cardiovascular system or on specific age groups of women. Two reports by Poulter (*Lancet*, 1996) indicated that pill use by women over 35 years exposed that age-bracket of users to a 100% increased risk of haemorrhagic stroke [364] and that women in a 20-44 year age bracket, who were current users of the pill, had a 199% higher risk of ischaemic stroke[365] (see glossary).

4.1.1 CASE STUDIES.

Earlier in this chapter I suggested that 'the **'modest'** death rate of up to 20 women per million per annum is not a trifling matter'. The three following case studies illustrate the human suffering caused by pill-induced cardio-vascular problems.

The CSM decision of October 1995 was, regretfully, made too late for British teenager, Caroline Bacon, who died from a stroke in May 1994, aged 16.[366][367] Caroline was 14 when a family planning clinic doctor prescribed Femoden® for her. It is reported that within six months of starting Femoden®, Caroline was **"suffering from headaches, numbness to her right side and hands, and seeing flashing lights".**[368] After spending some days in a coma, Caroline regained consciousness, but could only move her eyes. She was in this state for 11 months, until her death. According to her mother, **"my daughter had circulatory problems which the pill aggravated".**[369]

News reports from Britain indicated that this has not been the only fatality arising from the use of a version of the pill. *UK News* (5/2/97, Issue 621) reported that Christina Roberts, a 17 year old was prescribed Dianette™ for mild acne on her face, arms and back. She died after a series of heart attacks.[370] It will be recalled that Dianette contains ethinyloestradiol and cyproterone, drugs previously mentioned in *Lancet* articles because they were implicated in cardio-vascular complications.

In Canada, stroke victim Judy Mozersky, aged 19, must send a code to her nurse via a blinking eye movement. The nurse deciphers the code and relays Judy's message to the judge. Judy is involved in a legal action against the doctor who prescribed the pill to her.[371] The outcome of this case will have far-reaching ramifications.

4.1.2 CONCLUSION.

Against the background of the above medical literature, and prompted by the recent alarm raised by Trioden®, Femoden®, Marvelon®, Minulet® and Tri-Minulet®, it is appropriate to quote from the *Times*:

> " ... the government decided that public safety took precedence over scientific protocol. Most women - and their families - would probably agree with it".[372]

It is for women such as Caroline, Christina and Judy that I write this book.

4.2   THE PILL AND BIRTH DEFECTS.

Another area of major concern is the pill's capacity to inflict birth defects upon the developing baby. A report from America highlights the damage that taking the pill *during* pregnancy can cause. This report has significant implications for any moves to make the pill a non-prescription, over-the-counter (OTC) purchase.

Dr Kim reported on a *male* infant born with full *female* genitalia as well as camptomelic syndrome, which is characterised by severe bowing and shortening of limbs, rib cage curvage, a shortened neck, and a softening of the larynx and trachea. This last complication was the ultimate cause of death for the infant at 3 & 1/2 months.

A review of the mother's history indicated that she was healthy, aged 21, with no history of exposure to drugs, infectious agents or radiation. The only significant feature was that she was taking the 'pill' known as Ortho-Novum® (0.5mg-1mg of norethindone, and 0.035mg of ethinyl estradiol) for 18 months prior to conception, and for 6 months *into* the pregnancy.[373]

The authors of this study noted that this was the *second* such report of sex reversal and camptomelic syndrome in an infant exposed to the pill in the early part of pregnancy. This report highlights the powerful nature of the pill hormones. It also indicates that the current classification of the pill by the Australian authorities may need to be re-evaluated. Currently the pill is ranked as a 'B3' drug (see appendix 4). Based upon the preceding study, it may be more appropriate to classify the pill in category D, which is the equivalent of the American classification of 'X' for the pill (see appendix 5).

It is of interest to note that the Food and Drug Administration have previously issued a **"... warning of teratogenicity in fetuses of women who conceived immediately after stopping oral contraceptives"**.[374]

Prof. Rahwan also has written on this point:

> **"Patients should be instructed that it is important to discontinue the oral contraceptive about 3 months prior to conceiving, since there is emerging evidence that chromosomal abnormalities are higher in pregnancies that begin the month following discontinuation of the pill.".[375]**

As well, he has warned of problems related to transplacental teratogenesis (birth defects due to hormones crossing to the baby via the placenta). He sees the progestins as clearly implicated in birth defects:

> **"... recent studies indicate that if used during the early months of pregnancy progestins quintuple the usual risk of harm to the fetus of deformities of the arms and legs ... a higher incidence (>10%) of cardiovascular malformations has also been reported in offspring's prenatally exposed to sex steroids (particularly progestins)... The overall incidence of major malformations is 26%, and that of minor malformations is 33% higher, in offspring's prenatally exposed to female sex steroids as compared to the general population.".[376]**

The list of birth defects recorded in the medical literature extends to many other problems. The following list is taken from *Martindale-The Extra Pharmacopoea,* a principle texts for pharmacists in both England and Australia.

"**Pregnancy and the Neonate- Effects on the Foetus.**
In Hungary where 30% of all pregnant women were given
hormonal support therapy with progestogens during the early
1980s, a case-control study suggested that there was a causal
relationship between such treatment and hypospadias in their
offspring. (1) Reports of abnormalities in infants following
exposure in utero to progestogens have included hypospadias (2)
with norethisterone and hydroxyprogesterone, other genito-
urinary anomalies with dydrogesterone (3) and hydroxy-
progesterone, (4) tetralogy of Fallot (5) and adreocortical
carcinoma (6) with hydroxyprogesterone, foetal masculinisat-
ion (7) with norethisterone, norethynodrel, and ethisterone,
meningomyelocele or hydrocephalus (8) with norethisterone and
ethisterone, and neonatal choreoathetosis (9) with
norethisterone."[377] (see glossary).

The litigious implications of inappropriately labelling a drug's capacity for causing birth defects (teratogenicity) is an issue which manufacturers would be well advised to re-consider. The aforementioned problems with *in utero* exposure to sex hormones also have significant legal implications in view of the current world-wide push to make "post-coital contraceptives" a non prescription over-the-counter purchase.

4.3   THE PILL AND INFERTILITY.

Impairment to fertility diminishes with time, but "**may be evident up to 30 months after cessation of the pill in women who have not previously had children**".[378] For certain subgroups of women the return to fertility will be longer:

"**In nulliparous women aged 25 to 29 years impairment of**
fertility was more severe but the effect had almost entirely
disappeared after 48 months. In the older, aged 30 to 34 years,
nulliparous women there was even more impairment of fertility
but this was not permanent as by 72 months [6 years] after
stopping oral contraceptive use the numbers of women who had
not conceived were comparable to a group who had previously
used non-hormonal methods of contraception.".[379]

The obvious question is: Why is there this substantial delay?

Some of the answers to this question have been uncovered by Prof. Erik Odeblad, Department of Medical Biophysics, University of Umea, Sweden, who has spent more than 30 years researching the impact of the pill on women's fertility. He has placed particular emphasis on hormonal interference with the various types of mucus secreted by the cervix. It would be accurate to say that Prof. Odeblad is at the forefront of research into this area of female fertility. He has identified three different types of cervical mucus.[380]

First, there is the highly viscous (thick) G mucus, which causes the cervix to be closed during most of the cycle, except of course, during menstruation and around the time of ovulation. Sperm cannot swim though G mucus, hence this type of mucus acts as a naturally occurring barrier contraceptive.

The second type is called L mucus, and is partly responsible for trapping low-quality spermatozoa.

Finally there is S mucus, which is watery, and greatly facilitates the movement of sperm through the vagina into the cervix, whence fertilization may take place. Most of the damage to a woman's fertility occurs in relation to the S mucus.

> **"Following the use of contraceptive pills, there is an inactivation of the S mucus producing crypts** (skin folds in the womb) **which undergo atrophy** (shrinking or wastage). **Coming off the pill, some women have difficulty in restoring the S mucus production and restoration of an *optimum quality* of the S mucus. Such women may have their ovulations but still have less probability to conceive because their S mucus does not show the optimum fertility conditions."** (emphasis added).[381]

Thus, a return to ovulation when the pill is stopped does not mean that a woman has had a return to fertility. The woman's body must restart production of the S mucus, both in terms of quantity and quality. The lingering damage to the S mucus-producing glands is the weak link in the chain of events necessary for fertilization, the true measure of fertility.

There is a secondary factor which complicates the return to normal fertility. The pill also causes an over-stimulation of G mucus, which may persist for some time *past* the time when ingestion of the pill has stopped.[382] To recall, G mucus impedes sperm mobility, and hence fertilization.

These two interlinked actions of the pill on mucus production, rather than any long-term effects upon ovulation, are the cause of a delay in the return to pre-pill fertility.

Following on from these findings, it *is* quite reasonable to describe the pill's impact on the health status of women as bad medicine. The ancient medical rule was, and still is, "First do no harm". It would appear scandalous to advise healthy women to risk becoming unhealthy, and sometimes fatally so.

4.4   KEY POINTS.

1.   The use of third-generation progestogens such as gestodene or deso-gestrel have been proven beyond rational refutation to be linked to the increased risk of DVT and MI.

2.   Young women are most at risk, though not exclusively so.

3.   Because of the capacity of progestogens to cause acquired APC resistance and hence blood clots, their promotion as a 'morning-after' therapy has significant medical consequences and legal implications.

4.   The capacity of the pill to cause a variety of birth defects also suggests that there are potential legal   problems associated with the promotion of easy access to the 'morning-after' pill.

5.   The pill has a proven capacity to cause long-term impairment to woman's fertility.

CHAPTER FIVE.

5.   DEPO-PROVERA.

"If our results are confirmed the indications for using medroxyprogesterone will need to be reassessed."Dr. Charlotte Paul. *British Medical Journal.* 1989 [383]

5.1   INTRODUCTION.

This chapter will review some of the medical literature related to Depo-Provera® (Depo-P, DMPA, medroxyprogesterone) and also highlight the health implications for women from this drug delivery system. Special emphasis will be placed on the relevance of animal studies as a means of acquiring data relevant to human health and the parallel problems between Depo-Provera and the pill. I have allocated a chapter to Depo-Provera® because (a) it is a unique drug delivery system and (b) it uses an artificial hormone which is different from those used in various formulas of the pill and Norplant. To include Depo-Provera® in another chapter would create too many occasions of confusion and disharmony in analysing the pertinent medical research. It is relevant to note that DMPA achieves its 'contraceptive' effect by inhibition of ovulation, thickening of cervical mucus, premature luteolysis and the creation of a thinning endometrium. [384] The latter effect upon the lining of the womb would make implantation physiologically difficult.[385]

5.2   THE MARKETING OF DEPO-PROVERA.

Depo-Provera® is an injectable form of synthetic progesterone called medroxyprogesterone acetate, or DMPA. The marketing history of Depo-Provera® is a chequered one, but illustrative of the manifold health problems for women from medically unjustified pharmaceutical ingestion. The drug's release/withdrawal/re-release is interesting, since it acts as a gauge for the level of apprehension on the part of the American regulatory body, the Food and Drug Authority (FDA).

The following historical perspective is presented so that readers can have a sense of the unease which the FDA harboured about Depo-Provera. It is a *verbatim* copy from Micromedex®, a clinical drug data base collated in and distributed from America.

"**Q. What is the main controversy that has delayed the approval of medroxyprogesterone (Depo Provera, DMPA) as a long-term contraceptive in the US?**

R. Upjohn initially applied for FDA approval of Depo-Provera(R) as a CONTRACEPTIVE in 1967 and subsequently started 2 long-term animal studies to determine the safety of the drug (Richard & Lasagna, 1987). In 1974, the FDA proposed the approval of Depo-Provera(R) for contraceptive use only in patients unable to tolerate other methods of contraception and those that were institutionalized. In less than 2 months, this recommendation was revoked because of concerns that the drug may be carcinogenic (Anon, 1982). Powell & Seymour (1971) reported adverse reactions in 1123 patients receiving MEDROXY-PROGESTERONE for periods of 3 to 54 months as a contraceptive. Abnormal CERVICAL CYTOLOGY (as indicated by a rate higher than the general population) was reported in 11 patients. Dabancens et al (1974) observed the incidence of cervical NEOPLASTIC LESIONS in women treated with Medroxyprogesterone and IUDs. Neoplastic lesions were reported to be prevalent in 36 of 2239 female patients, with the occurrence of the lesions significantly higher than in users of IUDs. Addison et al (1979) presented a case report of a patient who exhibited a recurrence of endometriosis in the rectovaginal septum following a dramatic response to hormonal pseudo-pregnancy. During progestational therapy with medroxy-progesterone, malignant transformation in the area of endo-metriosis occurred; however, a definite causal relationship between the neoplastic lesions and the drug could not be stated. Upjohn also intensified the issue in 1978 with animal data from their 10-year study with rhesus monkeys that showed an increase in the incidence of endometrial CANCER in rhesus monkeys administered 50 times the normal human dose of

medroxyprogesterone as compared to controls (Anon, 1982).

In another animal study sponsored by the manufacturer, malignant neoplasms in the mammary glands of 2 of 16 beagle dogs exposed long-term to medroxyprogesterone were detected.

On March 7, 1978, the FDA notified Upjohn that approval for medroxyprogesterone for contraception had been denied on the basis that benefits for this purpose do not justify the risks.

The FDA's disapproval was based on the following issues:

a) safety questions raised by studies in dogs that showed an increase in the incidence of mammary tumours have not been resolved;

b) a number of safer alternative methods of contraception are available;

c) irregular bleeding disturbances caused by the drug may require the administration of estrogens which imposes an added risk factor and decreases the benefits of a progesterone-only contraceptive;

d) exposure of the fetus to medroxyprogesterone, if the drug fails and pregnancy occurs, poses a potential risk of congenital malformation (this risk is enhanced by prolonged use of the drug);

e) postmarketing studies to monitor the risk of breast and cervical carcinoma were considered a practical impossibility (FDA Drug Bull, 1978) .

Upjohn issued a letter to the FDA denouncing that the drug is carcinogenic in response to the FDA's disapproval for contraceptive use and questioned the significance of applying the animal data to humans (Richard & Lasagna, 1987)." [386]

Given this questionable background, it is instructive to look at what subsequent research data has found.

5.3   DEPO-PROVERA AND BREAST CANCER.

Dr Charlotte Paul (1989) reported in the *British Medical Journal* that young women were most at risk of breast cancer from DMPA. When the data was analysed according to age at which the women first used DMPA it was found that:

> **"In women who had first used it before age 25 the relative risk** (of breast cancer) **was 1.5** (a 50% increase). **Again the highest risk was in women in this group who had used it for six years or longer: their risk was raised significantly (relative risk 4.2; 1.1 to 16.2)."** (a relative risk of 4.2 is a 320% risk increase).[387]

Dr Paul also reported on the broader impact that DMPA has on young women. The result was consistent with the work on early age-use of the pill and breast cancer:

> **"Use for two years or longer before age 25 was associated with a significantly increased risk of breast cancer (RR 4.6, CI 1.4-15.1)."**.[388]

This relative risk equates to a 360% increase in the risk of breast cancer for early age, long-term users of Depo-Provera when compared to non-users of the same age. Dr Paul observed that since the number of patients in this particular sub-category was small, the result could only be viewed as suggestive, not conclusive. Nevertheless, the results are worrying for three reasons.

First, the magnitude of the risk which Dr Paul's research revealed is considerable. Another researcher has suggested that Dr Paul's work highlighted a **"significantly increased relative risk of breast cancer"** for recent or current use of Depo-Provera.[389] A risk of almost 5-fold would seem to be a gamble of substantive proportions, particularly when this risk is being taken by healthy women.

Second, the results of Dr Paul's study confirm the forewarning from animal studies which Upjohn Pharmaceuticals rejected. Their rejection begs the question of the relevance of doing animal studies if the results are then deemed to be inconsequential. Cross-species susceptibility to drug side-effects may not allow for an absolute extrapolation, but this case (and others) highlights the fact that there is a reasonable measure of certainty which can be presumed when applying the lessons learnt from animal studies.[390][391]

Third, the susceptibility of a *young* woman's body to the potent effects of artificially elevated and altered hormone levels is by now a familiar theme. It pervades the whole area of female reproductive health. As a medical event it cannot be a surprise. As King has observed:

> **"... breast epithelium** (tissue) **from young women is more sensitive to female sex steroids** (hormones) **than that from older women..."**.[392] furthermore: **"... existing data suggests that both combined and progestin-only oral contraceptives increases epithelial proliferation in-vivo** (in the body) **over that seen in the natural cycle."**.[393]

The National Association of Breast Cancer Organisations concurs: **"progestins stimulate the growth of breast tissue"**.[394] Therefore, when scientific studies report adverse findings from drugs such as Depo-Provera (a synthetic progesterone), disbelief is a scientifically illogical reaction, given that: **"medroxyprogesterone is a potent progestogen, which is delivered to the body in relatively high concentrations"**[395] (N.B. see glossary re. progestins and progestogens).

The only difference between the synthetic progesterone-only pill and DMPA is the method of drug delivery into the woman's body, which results in no difference at all at a cellular level. The cells of a woman's body cannot biologically discern the mode of delivery of an artificial hormone. These breast cells react in the same deleterious manner irrespective of who manufactured the drug and in what format it is administered.

Dr Paul's work is not the only study which has pointed to problems associated with DMPA use. A multi-centre, multinational WHO study (1991) re-stated the risks which young women are preferentially susceptible to. The WHO report noted that: **"there is an apparent trend of increased risk with duration of use before age 25"**[396] (the relative risk was 2.41, a 141% risk increase).

The authors of this report made some interesting observations and comments on the mechanisms by which breast cancer might 'occur' in young women and importantly, the different biological effects on breast tissue from naturally produced (endogenous) progesterone versus artificial (exogenous) progestogens such as DMPA: Briefly, artificial progestogens stimulate a greater growth response in breast tissue than that seen from the natural progesterone produced by the woman's body.[397]

Natural progesterone, secreted by the *corpus luteum* after ovulation stimulates cellular activity in breast tissue as do artificial progestogens, but artificial progestogens produce *more* cellular activity than do the natural hormones, leading to a higher level of cellular activity. Greater cellular activity, if uncontrolled, may shift into cancerous cellular activity.

Other reports have also testied to the problems which younger women encounter from Depo-Provera. The *Australian Prescription Products Guide* (1995) states that:

> **"... an increased relative risk of 2.19 has been associated with use of Depo-P in women whose first exposure to the drug was within the previous 4 years and were under 35 years of age..."** [398]
> (a 119% increase).

What are the implications of this?

> **"The Australian Institute of Health & Welfare report , between 1983 to 1985, an average incidence rate of breast cancer in Australian women, age 30 to 34 years, of 20.97/100,000. A relative risk of 2.19 thus increases the possible risk of 20.97 to 45.92 cases per 100,000 women. The attribute risk, therefore, is 24.95 per 100,000 women per year."** [399]

Based upon these reports as many as 25 women per 100,000 using Depo-Provera may contract breast cancer (45.92-20.97). If Depo-Provera was not a 'sexual' drug with its attendant mortality rate, it would encounter resistance to its registration from the Therapeutic Goods Administration (TGA) division of the Australian Department of Health.

The existence of this double standard of acceptable safety of a drug is a medical and ethical scandal which is difficult to fathom. To say the least, a greater measure of objectivity is needed when standards are set for drug safety. It is irrelevant that a drug is a 'sexual' or a 'non-sexual' drug. The same degree of vigilance and scrutiny of the medical literature should be operative for both classes of drugs.

5.4 DEPO-PROVERA AND BONE-DENSITY.

Another important health issue caused by Depo-Provera® use was discussed at the 27th Annual Meeting of the *Society of Adolescent Medicine* (1995). This conference reported that contraceptive injections, specifically medroxy-progesterone acetate (DMPA), **"may suppress skeletal bone mineralization in growing adolescent females"**.[400] A report in the *Lancet* (1995) further supported the concern over the effects of Depo-Provera® on bone mineralization.[401] These skeletal effects may make young women more susceptible to osteoporosis in the menopause.

Consider this irony: A pre-menopausal woman is first assaulted by the carcino-genic risks of Depo-Provera® *and* its capacity to "suppress skeletal bone mineral-ization" and then during menopause medicine strongly advocates the restorative use of HRT to improve her bone-density status.[402] As a consequence of this necessary corrective drug therapy, she is further assaulted by the carcinogenic effects of the hormones in HRT (see Colditz, Chapter 10). The exposure to powerful, artificial hormones during adolescence, and their remedial use again during menopause, amounts to the unwarranted pollution of a healthy bio-mechanical environmental system known as a woman. Rainforests would not be treated thus.

What can be said for those women currently using Depo-Provera who are concerned about its effects upon their on-going health ? It is reassuring to know that if DMPA use is stopped, the increased risk of breast cancer is non-existent after 5 years,[403] a result echoed in the work of Colditz (See Chapter 10). It would seem likely that the removal of the excessively stimulatory effect of the progestagen on breast tissue will allow cellular growth to return to a normal, non-carcinogenic rate.

Yet the full range of results of DMPA use is not yet known. The 'biological plausibility' of breast cancer promotion from exogenous progestogens suggests that there are still unknown dangers connected with DMPA. Since one of the largest markets in the world, America, only licensed the drug's use in 1992, and since the epidemiological evidence on DMPA and breast cancer is sparse, conflicting[404] and inconsistent[405] medical vigilance is a prudent form of protection. The unfolding epidemiological 'story line' of the pill, taken together with the need to observe the latent period discussed extensively in chapters 2 and 3, suggest that the safety of DMPA is not a finally resolved issue.

5.5   CASE STUDY: DEPO-PROVERA INDUCED COMA.

On March 28, 1997, the *Binghamton Press & Sun* reported that an 18 year old woman, who had recently given birth, suffered a severe allergic reaction to DMPA and lapsed into a coma. It was reported that she bled internally to such an extent that blood flowed from her eyes, nose and mouth. Fortunately she regained consciousness and suffered no apparent long term damage.[406]

5.6   KEY POINTS.

1. The official approval, then disapproval, then re-approval of Depo-Provera gives cause for considerable public concern with the process of drug safety appraisal.

2. As was the case with the pill, young women are the most 'at risk' group, notably in the areas of their increased susceptibilty to breast cancer and bone-thinning.

3. As highlighted in the above case study, unpredictable side-effects, including coma, are medical emergencies that both current and propective users of this drug delivery system must be mindful.

CHAPTER SIX.

6.   NORPLANT .

"I would not tell my worst enemy to get the Norplant."[407]
Jessica Ann Shipe - Norplant user for 2 years.

6.1   INTRODUCTION.

The search for new, innovative, reliable and safe forms of fertility regulation is an unrelenting process. Drug companies strive to gain market share by releasing products which offer a perceived user advantage but which also possess a reduced list of side-effects when compared to the products of rival manufactures. This chapter will review one such product, known as Norplant®.

6.2   DESCRIPTION.

Norplant® is a new form of birth-control developed by the American-based Population Council and manufactured by Wyeth-Ayerst Pharmaceuticals. Norplant® **"has been estimated to cost around $8.50 to manufacture"**[408] but is sold for $US365. Wyeth pays $14.60 per sale in royalties to the Population Council.[409] The Population Council's International Committee for Contraceptive Research, a co-operative research group, **"has done virtually all the bio-chemical and clinical investigation required for the development of Norplant."**.[410] The Population Council (PC) is a non-profit organisation whose *raison d'etre* is the promotion of drugs and surgical procedures to women who do not wish to become 'pregnant'[411] or stay pregnant. The Population Council is ideologically aligned with the pro-abortion movement[412] and a multitude of family planning organisations.

Norplant® comprises six rods, each of which is impregnated with 36mg of an artificial progesterone called levonorgestrel. The rods are inserted under the skin on the inside of a woman's upper arm. As a method of birth control Norplant® must be classified as an abortifacient because ovulation occurs in up to 41% of women,[413] yet the drug has an annual observed pregnancy rate over 5 years of only 0.3 per 100 women[414] to 3.5 per 100 women[415].

The product is currently unavailable in Australia. A review of its brief but troubled history will clearly set out why Norplant's limited international availability represents a positive health outcome and why it is reasonable to hope that Australia's regulatory authorities will never give permission for its introduction.

6.3   THE MARKETING OF NORPLANT.

On December 6, 1990, *USA Today* proclaimed that the soon-to-be licensed Norplant was **"as perfect a method as you can have".**[416] When approval was granted on December 10, Norplant was regarded as a **"dream method"**[417] of birth control. Similar positive sentiments were expressed in England when Norplant was released in October 1993; it was claimed that it would give women **"complete peace of mind".**[418]

The justification for this unrestrained enthusiasm was the many perceived advantages which Norplant allegedly possessed. These included: ease of insertion, five years of contraceptive efficacy, apparent ease of removal of the rods if a woman was dissatisfied (**"removing the capsules takes 15-20 minutes"**)[419] and a high level of patient compliance because **"the method is not coitally dependant".**[420]

Patient safety was considered to be a forgone conclusion, since Norplant had been through a most rigorous testing procedure. It was, its proponents claimed, **"the most extensively tested contraceptive implant, with nearly 60,000 women participating in clinical** (pre-marketing) **trials..."**.[421]

By any measure, this positive *curriculum vitae* would be expected to generate nothing but long-term profits, patient confidence and market approval. Yet a mere three years later a *Chicago Tribune* headline read: **"No Panacea: Norplant (law) suit charges failure to educate patients".**[422]

The substance of the joint action by the four American plaintiffs in the suit were listed as heavy and continual menstruation, weight gain of 20 pounds, severe headaches, excessive hair growth, numbness and pain in the left arm (the site of insertion), migraines, mood changes, decreased libido and multiple failed attempts to remove the rods leading to severe scarring on the arm.[423]

Reports from England mirrored those in America, with headlines reading **"Spare the rod"**[424] and **"Agony of women who used Pill implants."**.[425] British women reported mood swings, exhaustion and an inability to care for their children, excessive bleeding, hair loss, violence towards their partner, weight gain, severe PMT and depression.[426][427]

Other media outlets had also reported similar patient problems and an associated increase in the number of litigious actions. *America Online* informed its audience that:

> **"thousands of women from around the country have filed suit against the makers of the implant contraceptive. The women's suit against the Norplant makers seeks compensation for the harmful effects of the drug...** (which) **is said to have dangerous side-effects... The most common complaint about the implants is the painful procedure required to remove the contraceptive."**.[428]

On August 22nd, 1995, *USA Today* reported that law suits against Norplant totaled 200, and involved 26,000 women.[429] By March 12, 1996, the number of American women who had hired lawyers had increased to 50,000, in 5,227 separate federal cases.[430]

In Britain, litigious action also began. The British lawyers acting for aggrieved U.K. women - The Norplant Action Group - had planned to bring legal action against Hoechst Marion Roussel under consumer protection legislation, citing deficient product information.[431]

6.4   ROD REMOVAL OF NORPLANT.

6.4.1 CASE STUDIES.

The experience of British women who request rod removal is disturbing. Caroline Foster, 28, was referred to two separate specialists in an attempt to remove her Norplant rods after her own doctor failed to locate them.[432] The specialists could only remove four of the rods and as a consequence: **"... almost a year later** (she) **had to undergo a general anaesthetic to get the final implants removed".**[433]

As Caroline Foster said: **"No one seemed to know what they were doing and even after the operation I have still got one of the rods left in my arm because it is so deeply embedded it's impossible to remove.".**[434]

Another woman, Helen Irwin, 19, from Stanford-le-Hope, Essex, threatened to sue her GP, who had refused to remove the rods on the grounds that he was **"not trained to take it out and referred me to a family planning clinic. They also refused and told me that the person who fitted it had to remove it.".**[435]

A review of the medical literature authenticates the experiences of these American and British women. Doctors Thomas and LeMelle reported that:

> **"Removal can be difficult even if a well-trained clinician has exercised meticulous care to ensure appropriate capsule placement... Difficult removals have been reported in 13.2% of patients participating in clinical trials.".**[436]

In human terms this 13.2% means that one in every eight women experienced more than the originally claimed 'easy' removal. Other researchers have also noted the same problem:

> **"Norplant removal has been much more difficult for many physicians than might have been anticipated.".**[437]

As Caroline Foater's case illustrates, one of the most troublesome aspects of Norplant removal is actually locating the rods' precise position in the woman's arm, due either to inappropriately deep insertion or migration of one or more rods. The British marketing agents of Norplant, Hoechst Marion Roussel, offer training courses for doctors, but some GPs are reluctant to attend it, **"either because they lack experience or because they will not be reimbursed in the same way as they are for other forms of contraception such as IUDs"**.[438]

Poor physician training has also been highlighted by researchers who surveyed family practice physicians in Ohio. Their study results showed:

> **"... only 35% of those inserting Norplant had been trained in a formal instructional setting, and 32% described themselves as 'self-taught,' ie, having received neither formal or informal instruction.".**[439]

One solution to this problem, an option not readily available in Third World countries, is the use of an ultrasound transducer to first locate and then visualise the Norplant rods,[440] although this approach is not always successful. Steadman and co-workers have reported that **"the levonorgestrel-releasing silastic implants may not show on radiographs and, if improperly inserted, may be difficult to palpate prior to removal.".**[441] If successfully located using these imaging techniques, surgical removal can then follow.

6.5   IRREGULAR MENSTRUATION AND NORPLANT.

Another area of major concern for women using Norplant® was: **"the high incidence of irregular bleeding"**[442] with **"the overall incidence of menstrual irregularities in the first year** (of) **between 60 and 70 percent"**,[443] leading one in ten women to request removal for this reason alone.[444] The British reports indicate that women have suffered greatly due to menstrual disruptions. Becky Stewart, 22, from Oxford says: **"I bled permanently... you bleed all the time, you feel miserable and look bad"**.[445]

To cope with this medical problem, one of the proffered solutions was **"careful patient screening and counselling"** because, amongst other considerations, **"women differ in their sensitivity to nuisance side effects and in their ability to tolerate even simple types of outpatient surgery"**[446] such as Norplant removal. The classification of irregular menstrual bleeding as a 'nuisance side effect' is misogynous and insulting. It bears a strikingly similarity to an editorial comment in the *New England Journal of Medicine* in 1986 which stated, in the context of the pill and breast cancer, that **"we tend selectively to notice and remember the victims and not the beneficiaries".**[447] It is a matter of some concern that there appears to be such a paternalistic mentality towards women when it comes to the impact of new reproductive drug strategies.

Unfortunately the menstrual side-effects generated by Norplant® have in their turn generated a fresh set of problems. The treatment regimes for the side-effects suggested by advocates of Norplant® may exacerbate, not ameliorate, the situation. Instead of Norplant removal, which is the cause of the side-effects, Norplant supporters such as Dr. Thomas (1995) suggested the administration of *extra drugs* as a curative approach to Norplant's® side-effects:

> **"If prolonged bleeding is a problem for a patient, clinicians also should be aware that treatments are available to help control irregular bleeding during the first year of use of the method, after which time menstrual patterns will become more regular. These treatments include use of ethinyl estradiol, nonsteroidal anti-inflammatory drugs** (such as ibuprofen), **and the progestin levonorgestrel.".**[448]

The approach of Dr. Thomas' is known as poly-pharmacy, a term which means the administration of a variety of drugs for the same medical problem. As a solution to the distressing side-effects of Norplant® the advocating of poly-pharmacy would seem a backward step. It raises the possibility of further side-effects from the new drugs to correct the problems caused by Norplant®. Ibuprofen, for example, has the capacity to affect platelet function.[449] It also increases the possibility of drug/drug interactions. The proper course of action would be the removal of the original offending drug, a more logical and humane approach, rather than the over-medicalisaton of women's bodies.

6.6   INTRACRANIAL HYPERTENSION AND NORPLANT.

Thus far the problems attributable to Norplant® have not been surprising either in origin or outcome. A brief reading of any standard medical or pharmacy text book would show that side-effects from synthetic progesterones are well-documented. Menstrual disorders, mood changes, weight gain, unusual tiredness, acne, increased body and facial hair and trouble in sleeping are foreseen problems caused by progesterone ingestion.[450][451][452] Some of these problems were mentioned in the quoted extract from the law suits.

What has surprised some are certain other problems attributable to Norplant®: side-effects which are not predictable in view of the known pharmacology of progesterone.[453] One such unpredictable side-effect is intracranial hypertension (increased pressure inside the skull), reported in the *New England Journal of Medicine* (*NEJM*, 1995) by Doctor's Alder and Fraunfelder.[454] They reported on two young women aged 16 and 19 years:

> **"... in whom disk edema occurred four to five months after the implantation of levonorgestrel. Neither was obese, had prior medical problems, or used other medications that have been associated with intracranial hypertension.".**[455]

Both young women originally presented with symptoms of visual impairment, severe headaches, or emesis (vomiting). Removal of Norplant permitted the 19-year old to recover but the 16-year-old had 3 recurrences over a period of 18 months which were controlled with acetazolamide,[456] a diuretic drug used to treat glaucoma, congestive heart failure, edema and seizures.[457]

Some might rush in and claim that these are isolated cases and that in the context of the large number of women using Norplant® they constitute a non-issue. The adverse-drug notification records from the WHO, FDA and the National Registry of Drug-Induced Ocular Side-effects say otherwise. There have actually been **"56 cases of intracranial pressure or disk edema"**[458] related to Norplant use.

Whilst the Norplant manufacturer (Wyeth-Ayerst) has tried to qualify these numbers in a letter printed in the *NEJM*, it must be obvious that 56 cases is 56 cases too many for a drug that is being given to healthy young women.

A proportional risk of developing intracranial hypertension might be acceptable in the context of treating a women with a serious, debilitating medical problem but normal fertility hardly qualifies as a disease state. As well, a woman's health is not an incidental commodity which should be dismantled by a drug delivery system of questionable benefit or merit.

6.7   SILICONE DISEASE AND NORPLANT.

Aside from the foreseen and unforeseen problems due to the synthetic progesterone in Norplant®, worrying issues have also arisen because of the material composition of the rods *per se*. The specific focus of concern is the silicone content of the implants.

Unlike breast implants, which contained between 250 to 500gm of silicon, Norplant contains only 0.75gm.[459] Presumably the manufacturers concluded that because there was such a large discrepancy between the amount of silicon used in the two artificial implant systems, a wide margin of safety for Norplant users would automatically be generated. But if recent patient complaints are dependable, there may only need to be a small quantity of this foreign substance present inside a woman's body for it to cause problems.

This would appear to be the view of the Triad Silicone Network, a group which represents women who believe they are victims of silicone disease. The Network claims that **"... women with Norplant suffered from 'joint pains, muscle pain, infections, lots of scar tissue', the same thing that happened... with breast implants"**.[460]

In an attempt to reduce the silicone problem caused by the original version of Norplant, a new version of the implant has been trialed. This new version, Norplant 2, has also encountered problems due to the manufacturer's inability to devise a composition which is free from materials of a teratogenic potential:

> **"Production of Norplant-2 has recently been curtailed due to the withdrawal of polydimethylsiloxone** (silicone) **used in the core of the implant. This measure was necessary as it was expensive to produce and due to the potential side effects of ... stannous octo-** ate (part of the plastic rod). **Tests have indicated that stannous octoate may produce teratological defects in rat fetuses."**.[461]

Since silicon would seem to be an essential material component of the rod structure, it appears that Wyeth-Ayerst, Norplant's manufacturer, was unrealistic in expecting that there would be no problems with this particular substance. Certainly this is the view of *Martindale®, the 'bible' of pharmaceutical reference texts:

"**Foreign-body reactions have been reported following their (silicone) use as joint implants. Other implants, usually for cosmetic purposes, carry the risk of migration of silicone, with cyst formation and other complications; accidental transvascular injection has been fatal ... many of the reports of adverse effects to silicones are concerned with their use by injection or implantation for cosmetic purposes. Reactions range from cysts and granulomatous reactions to pneumonitis and pulmonary oedema. Fatalities have occurred. (A) silicone wound dressing was withdrawn from the German market because of possible animal carcinogenicity.".**[462]

Articles in both the *Journal of the American Medical Association* (*JAMA.*, 1988)[463] and the *New England Journal of Medicine* (*NEJM*, 1983)[464] have also indicated that cautious use of silicone is a prudent medical policy.

This insurmountable technical problem will probably finish Norplant as a product even if Wyeth-Ayerst can finance the escalating costs of litigation.

6.8   CLINICAL TRIALS OF NORPLANT.

Having reviewed the pharmaceutical and medical problems associated with Norplant®, the question arises as to why this plethora of difficulties was not uncovered during the pre-marketing clinical trials of the implant. Clinical trials exist precisely to fulfil this investigative function.

The usual procedure with any new drug is that trials are conducted in a number of countries, data from the research centres are collated, and the results are presented to the relevant regularity authorities who determine if the drug is suitable for approval. Upon approval a new drug is permitted to be prescribed by medical practitioners.

To assist in this procedure with Norplant, a large number of countries participated in the clinical trials: sufficient, one would have thought, to reveal the previously mentioned and documented side-effects of synthetic progesterone. These countries included Brazil, China, Bangladesh, Egypt, Colombia, Ghana, Haiti, Kenya, Indonesia, Dominican Republic, Mexico, Nepal, Nigeria, Senegal, Thailand, America and Zambia.[465] [466] They were enlisted by the International Committee for Contraceptive Research, **"a network of collaborating centres funded by the PC"**,[467] the promoters of Norplant.

Careful note should be made of the preponderance of countries which would be classified as Third World. It is significant that this socio-economic category was preferentially selected. 'Third World' countries have a number of common features, including illiteracy and a dearth of consumer-rights agencies. These detrimental social characteristics are germane to understanding how it was possible for Norplant® promoters to present 'favourable' data when the clinical trials in these impoverished countries were over. I shall shortly explain this point more fully.

For now, it is worth noting that the suspicious and questionable dominance of third world countries in the Norplant® trials led feminist groups such as the WEMOS/HAI International Group on Women and Pharmaceuticals to voice strong concern about the Norplant marketing approach. In its review of the Norplant experience, the board stated that it was:

> **"... concerned about the widespread distribution of Norplant in Family Planning programs in developing countries, while iss-ues concerning the ethical administration, safety of the method, and service delivery have not yet been resolved ... women in developing countries living in remote areas, moreover, are more likely to suffer from anaemia and to have or have had liver diseases. These conditions, which require extra medical attention, make rational use of implants especially difficult.".**[468]

This quote hints at certain irregularities in the 'acquisition' of clinical data. The following is a detailed analysis of these irregularities.

6.9   EXPLOITATION IN BRAZIL.

In the opinion of medical writer Ana Regina Gomes Dos Reis of Salvador (Brazil), there was a cover-up of the disturbing results experienced by participants in the trial. For this reason the nature and extent of many problems with Norplant® were 'hidden' until *after* the product's release in America.

The following extensive summary of an article by Reis, published by *Pergamon Press* in 1990, catalogues *eight* major procedural irregularities in the Norplant trials in Brazil.

The *first* issue raised by Reis is the parlous level of civilian participation in an evaluation of the proposed drug trials, and hence an inappropriate level of accountability. It is usual practise for hospital and university ethics' committees to include non-medical personnel. This did not occur in Brazil.

> **"The Brazilian Ministry of Health gave permission for the testing of the long-acting implantation contraceptive Norplant on Brazilian women in 1984, at a time when the country was living under a military dictatorship and the public had no opportunity to participate in, or even be informed of, many government decisions. The following year, political changes allowing more democratic participation enabled feminist groups to exert an influence on government actions regarding fertility control. A Committee for Studies of Human Reproductive Rights was formed in the Brazilian Ministry of Health, composed of representatives of the Ministries of Education, Foreign Affairs, and Social Welfare, and the National Council of Women's Rights, the Federal Medical Council, as well as feminists and congresswomen. Once this committee evaluated the Norplant trials, *finding many irregularities, contradictions, and methodological errors*, the Medicaments Division of the Brazilian Ministry of Health cancelled its authorisation of the Norplant trials in January 1986."** [469] (emphasis added).

The *second* problem area in the Brazilian Norplant® trials identified by Reis was the potential for a conflict of interest on the part of some personnel involved in running the trials. She considered it to be inappropriate to have an overlapping of personnel associated with both the development and the later testing of Norplant:

> "... a close relationship exits between universities and international population control agencies. For example, the president of the University of Campinas (Brazil) at the time Norplant tests began, Jose Pinotti, was a former member of the board of trustees of the Population Council.".[470]

The *third* criticism made by Reis was the inadequate attention paid to the criteria associated with the selection of candidates for implantation, most notably the age of the recipients:

> "...of the 3589 women using the implants, there were seven girls under the age of 14 and 301 between the ages of 15 and 19".[471]

These figures pose many serious ethical questions about informed consent and the capacity of very young women to understand the implications of medical information given to them. Also, ethical questions arise concerning the morality of inserted long-acting hormones into the developing bodies of teenagers. The health consequences of such actions are as relevant for Norplant users as they are for young women initiated onto the pill, an issue previously covered in chapters 2 & 3. Whether a woman is exposed to levonorgestrel via Norplant or via the pill is biologically irrelevant. It is the same drug; hence the consequences are the same (see footnote for American example of misuse of Norplant).[472]

The *fourth* issue discussed by Reis is the flagrant breach of protocol on the part of some of those who conducted the trials in Brazil. One of the fundamental aspects of any clinical trial is that the patient *must* be permitted to make a free and informed decision about participation. My own involvement as an investigator in clinical trials with nicotine-impregnated patches for smoking cessation studies affirms this point. Yet as Reis documented:

> "Statements taken by feminists groups have revealed that several women did not know that they were taking part in research and that the method was given as an alternative form of contraception; the clinics did not fulfil the criteria for test participation and very often the method was imposed on the women (Brazilian Health Ministry Workgroup, 1987).".[473]

The *fifth* difficulty outlined by Reis is that of illiteracy and poor consumer-rights awareness in third world countries. It would seem that scant regard was paid to these issues by some investigators involved in the trials. The normal procedure, not followed in Brazil, is for women to sign **"a document legally declaring knowledge of risk, internationally known as informed consent"**.[474]

Maria Almeida was a Norplant® recipient. Her case is representative in showing that some women were duped into signing a document called a **"term of responsibility"** which was **"an attempt to pass to them** (the women) **the onus of possible harm caused by Norplant®"**.[475]

The obvious intention behind the substitution of an 'informed consent' form with a 'term of responsibility' form was to negate any legal rights which the women in the trials might have sought to exercise if serious, unanticipated problems arose during the trials.

The *sixth* procedural error discussed by Reis also involved the 'term of responsibility' form. The form stated that the patient had received **"detailed explanations about all contraceptive measures in the clinic"**.[476] Upon closer investigation, it was discovered that in fact the 'contraceptive' options were limited to the much-discredited IUD or Norplant®. In effect, this was no choice, since it involved selecting from the undesirable and the unknown. Diaphragms, condoms or the Billings method were not options available for the women to select from,[477] despite the fact that the WHO have found the Billings method to be 97% effective.[478] This lack of choice violated the approved protocol which the promoters of Norplant had been granted prior to commencing the trials.

Clearly the health of the women was a secondary issue in these trials. The first consideration was the accumulation of research data for Norplant® approval purposes. As Maria Almeida said: **"What they** (the researchers) **mostly said was not to have children"**.[479] Any pregnancies would spoil the statistical results for the Norplant® researchers.

And how was this flagrant breach of fundamental human rights promoted unfettered and concealed? Simply by exploiting the ignorance of women involved in the trials - the *seventh* of the issues canvassed by Reis. As Maria Almeida said in an interview with Reis: **"I think they chose poor people because** they imagined that we are badly informed and don't try and find out more about it (Norplant)".[480]

The *eighth* major area which Reis criticised was the corrupt ethical standards which permitted the manipulation of data and the minimization of side-effects with the intention of fabricating a report which would give Norplant® a favourable reputation with no basis in fact.

The following are examples of how the researchers from the Population Council (PC) attempted to gloss over serious problems with Norplant® when preparing the final report on the Brazilian trials of the drug. Of specific interest are the vague side-effect classifications of 'increased bleeding' and 'weight gain' listed in the PC report. When the civilian government investigated these results, a different and rather callous picture emerged. As the government investigators observed:

> "Behind the term increased bleeding are hidden blood losses that would be considered pathological if the classic gynaecological terms and concepts, such as menorrhoea and hypermenorrhoea, were used. Interviews with Norplant® users taped by feminist groups reveal that many women had continuous bleeding lasting 20 or even 30 days. The impact of these "irregularities" on these women's day-to-day life and health was ignored.".[481]

And what of the problems of weight gain so coyly listed in the Population Council report? Again, the civilian government investigation team discovered that this reference in the final PC report was an understatement of substantial proportions. As the civilian investigators discovered:

> "... women in Rio de Janeiro showed 'dramatic' changes in weight. One woman gained 38kg in 9 months and then started to drink too much, the study noted. Another had an immediate weight gain of 2 kg in the first week, 3kg in the second, and also developed depression and respiratory problems. A third woman gained 26 kg after Norplant was removed. In a fourth, the extra 27 kg was gained over a four-month period (Brazilian Health Ministry

Working Group, 1987).".[482]

To this Reis responded: **"These dramatic alterations in women's bodies are minimized by the way they are shown in the researchers' final report...".** For the women involved, these and many other serious side-effects placed a great burden and strain on inter-personal relationships. For the Population Council researchers, however, **"those symptoms** (were) **only 'causes for removal,' factors reducing the method's continuation rates".**[483]

6.10   EXPLOITATION IN BANGLADESH.

Given the problems outlined in Brazil, it would seem reasonable to at least ask: 'Did data falsification and patient exploitation occur in other countries participating in the Norplant trials'? Based upon reports from Bangladesh, the answer is YES.

The problems experienced by Bangladeshi recipients of Norplant make a strong supportive case *against* Norplant use in third world countries and again highlight the uncharitable pharmaceutical exploitation of ill-informed and poorly educated people for the sake of concocting data to support a first-world promotion of a new drug. The following quote indicates that there was an unfortunate multi-national similarity to the policies effected by those responsible for the trials of Norplant®. Anwara and Rabia, women from the Bangladeshi village of Gazaria tell a story strikingly identical to that of Maria Almeida from Brazil:

"Presently in Bangladesh, it is being used in more than 20,000 women all over the country...The women in Gazaria do not know that the method is on trial. They are not told anything beyond a few sentences... when Anwara could not bear this bleeding any more, she went to the hospital and requested medicine to stop the bleeding, as well as removal of the method. She told them, ' I am dying please remove it.' The doctor said 'There is no medicine for stopping bleeding (caused by Norplant), so we cannot give any medicine. And removal of the method? Let us know when you die, we will take it out'"... Rabia, another client in the same village has taken Norplant for 2 years. She knows the family planning

worker who comes to her village. The family planning worker assured her that if it is too difficult for her then she will help her remove the method. For the past year Rabia has repeatedly requested removal, but in vain. Her husband also wants her to remove it... but the doctors told him ... he must pay Tk. 2000.00 in order to remove it. Rabia's husband is very poor; he will not be able to manage 2000.00Tk...The doctors become furious: 'How dare they can talk about removal when such an expensive medicine is given free of cost to these women.' The women wonder, 'we have taken this medicine for our own good. We were told that if we stop childbirth we will be happy. Our health will be good if we do not become pregnant. But we are experiencing a very difficult life... we did not ask for this expensive and coercive medicine.".[484]

6.11 CONCLUSION.

Given these documented attempts at suppressing the significant problems and deficiencies of Norplant, it is not surprising that the initial delight with this new style of 'contraceptive' evaporated when the truth became evident in a more open society such as America.

The structures to lodge notice of dissatisfaction with new drug delivery systems clearly do not adequately exist in Third World countries, leading to a violation of essential human rights. In a countries like the U.S. or England, well known for their zealous commitment to litigious actions as a defence against pharmaceutical exploitation, the situation is obviously very different.

The ultimate question in this pathetic saga of deceit is 'Why?'. According to the *New York Times*, a major reason for the alleged cover-up was financial:

"... the Population Council, which designed the device... has yet to recoup the $25 million it spent to develop the drug, and it stands to lose millions of dollars in future royalties... because of the falloff in Norplant's popularity.".[485]

And yet, if recent reports about Norplant are to believed, a change in medical policy may be redundant for two reasons. First, sales of the drug have fallen from **"a robust 800 a day to about 60"**.[486] By current estimates, this makes Norplant as unpopular as the heavily litigated IUD and barrier contraceptives such as spermicidal foams.

Second, combined with this fall in sales, and hence revenue, there has been an increase in expensive litigation:

> **"...the number of lawsuits against American Home Products and its Wyeth-Ayerst Home Products division skyrocketed from 20 in the first three years that Norplant was on the market to 180 in the last year, including 46 class-action suits."**.[487]

Taken together, a strategic withdrawal from the market-place may be the best option available to the Population Council.

6.12 KEY POINTS.

1.The developmental testing of Norplant is reported to have been done by exploiting women in third world countries.

2. The promises made at the time of the Norplant launch have subsequently been shown to be without foundation. The rods *are* very difficult to remove, weight gain and mood disturbances *are* significant, and menstrual irregularities *are* so extensive as to cause unacceptable levels of emotional, physical and marital distress.

3. Other health problems for women, such as visual impairment, severe headaches, and vomiting, have been documented in the *New England Journal of Medicine*.

4. Bodily reactions to the silicone component of the Norplant rods are reported to be similar to those seen in women who have had reactions to silicone breast implants.

5. There are many thousands of law suits against Norplant.

CHAPTER SEVEN

7. BARRIER METHODS OF CONTRACEPTION.

"I find absurd the notion that condoms allow one to safely engage in sexual relations with HIV carriers."[488] C.M.Rowland Ph.D., editor of the journal *Rubber Chemistry and Technology.*

7.1 INTRODUCTION.

This chapter will review two major barrier contraceptives: spermicides and condoms. As this chapter title suggests these products act as a physical barrier to conception. i.e., they impede the unification of sperm and ovum in the female reproductive tract. I have chosen not to discuss the diaphragm, although it is properly called a contraceptive, as it rates lower than the withdrawal method in order of popularity,[489] and is of only minor historical curiosity.

In Chapter One it was shown that the linguistic and embryological facts, as well as widespread medical consensus, pointed to an acceptance of the view that only drugs or devices which act before fertilization, not after, are entitled to the title of contraceptive.

What then is the need for a chapter on such products? Are not condoms and spermicides innocuous, even safe products?

From my clinical experience I would suggest that barrier-contraceptive 'safety' is a commonly held community attitude which also extends to a belief in the success of these methods in preventing pregnancy and disease. Both of these societal beliefs are flawed: hence the need for a review of pertinent medical literature on barrier methods, the substantial failure rates of these methods and the manner in which they are unambiguously implicated in both the spreading of disease and in the generation of many illnesses.

7.2   SPERMICIDES.

Nonoxynol-9 is the principal active ingredient in a diverse range of spermicidal products which are commercially available i.e., Delfen Foam® and Delfen Vaginal Cream® (Aust. & Canada), Conceptrol® gel and suppositories (U.S.A.), Semicid® vaginal tablets (U.S.A.), Today® sponge (Canada), Gynol II® vaginal jelly (U.S.A) and Ortho-Creme® (U.S.A.).

Nonoxynol-9 acts as a contraceptive by killing sperm deposited into the vaginal canal during intercourse, thus reducing the possibility of fertilization. As well as its spermicidal action, nonoxynol-9 has been shown to inhibit the growth of a variety of STD pathogens including *Chlamydia trachomatis, Gardnerella vaginalis, Mycoplasma hominis, Neisseria gonorrhoea, Trichomonas vaginalis, Ureaplasma urealyticumis*, decrease the infectivity of *Treponemea pallidum* (syphilis) and inactivate HIV.[490]

Spermicides can be used as a sole method of contraception, although the high failure rate of 30%[491] means that they are more commonly used in combination with other methods such as condoms or with the Billings' method of natural family planning (NFP). The Billings method, even without recourse to spermicides, has been rated by the WHO as more effective than the mini-pill and on a par with the combined pill for reliability.[492]

One of the reasons for the high failure rate of spermicides is that most of them must be inserted not more than one hour in advance of intercourse. If intercourse is delayed longer than one hour, a fresh application must be made.[493] This rigorous protocol is not compatible with human nature, which is both passionate and forgetful.

Spermicides cause a variety of side-effects for both sexual partners. Some are of a temporary, annoying nature, whilst others can be life-threatening. Significantly, it is women who are most at risk from the serious side-effects.

7.2.1 COMMON MINOR SIDE-EFFECTS OF SPERMICIDES.

The most frequently reported side-effects from spermicides for both partners are vaginal and penile discomfort, irritation, soreness, or itching. The frequency of these minor and discomforting side-effects is in the range of 6-11%.[494]

For women only, genito-urinary complications including vaginal discharge, dryness, burning and dysuria (painful urination) occur. Part of the explanation for these female-specific problems is nonoxynol-9's selective toxic effect against *L. acidophilus*, an organism which normally lives within the vagina. A reduction in the cell count of *L. acidophilus* leads to an overgrowth of *E.coli,*[495] which is a causative factor in vulvovaginitis, an infectious disease affecting the vaginal mucosa. One of the symptoms of vulvovaginitis is vaginal discharge.[496] The manufacturers of spermicides recommend discontinuation of the product if this side-effect occurs.[497]

7.2.2 TOXIC SHOCK SYNDROME (TSS) AND SPERMICIDES.

More serious side-effects have been linked with the spermicidal product known as Today® vaginal sponge. These sponges are promoted on the basis of their longer duration of spermicidal activity compared to the foams and creams. They can be inserted and left in place for 24 hours without removal, irrespective of the number of acts of intercourse.

The relative long-term effectiveness of the sponge, compared with the 1 hour protection from the foams, would seem a clear patient benefit, yet this is not the case. The medical literature indicates that this marketing advantage is actually disadvantageous: toxic shock syndrome (TSS) has been reported in at least 13 women who used the sponge.[498] TSS is defined as " **a syndrome characterized by high fever, vomiting, diarrhoea, confusion, and skin rash that may rapidly progress to severe and intractable shock".**[499]

The cause of TSS for these 13 women was attributed to a number of factors including prolonged wearing of the spermicidal sponge, menstruation whilst the sponge was in place, and traumatic manipulation whilst inserting or removing the sponge, causing damage to the lining of the vaginal canal. This last point is significant, since it has a bearing not only on a woman's susceptibility to TSS from spermicidal sponges but will also be shown to be a pivotal factor in her vulnerability to AIDS.

7.2.3 BIRTH DEFECTS AND SPERMICIDES.

"A doubling of major congenital anomalies (limb deformities, neoplasms, hypospadias - displaced urethral opening - chromosomal aberration syndromes) and a doubling of spontaneous abortions as compared to controls occurs in pregnancies associated with the use of spermicidal gels, foams, or creams containing nonoxynol-9 or octoxynol (another spermicide), but not when the spermicide is discontinued one month before conception."[500]

7.2.4 A.I.D.S. AND SPERMICIDES.

Whilst the above list of side-effects are distressing, they are also medically treatable. The same remedial approach does not exist for women infected with AIDS as a consequence of spermicidal use.

This fatal consequence was highlighted at the 5th International Conference on AIDS in Montreal (1989), where it was reported that prostitutes in Nairobi using nonoxynol-9- based products had a *higher* incidence of HIV seroconversion (presence of HIV in the blood) and an *increased* incidence of genital ulceration compared to prostitutes *not* using nonoxynol-9 products.[501]

This report would appear, at first glance, to be contradictory to the previously mentioned wide biological spectrum of activity of nonoxynol-9. How is it possible for this spermicidal product to *increase* HIV transmission, given that the AIDS virus lives within the seminal fluid which nonoxynol-9 is active against?

There are two reasons for the higher rate of HIV seroconversion with nonoxynol-9 users compared to non-users. *First*, nonoxynol-9 has the " **potential to induce impairment of local immunity via toxic effects on lymphocytes**".[502] This means that nonoxynol-9 interferes with the immune response system located within the cells of the vaginal canal. The role of these vaginal immune defence cells is to destroy any invading bacteria, fungi or virus.

The Montreal report suggested that nonoxynol-9 reduced the number of immune (T4) lymphocytes by up to 35%, thereby impairing the immune response of the woman's body. Consequently, the spreading of HIV into the woman's body is made easier. [503] The role of T4 lymphocytes is crucial to host defence:

" ... the complete spectrum of immunological dysfunction in AIDS can be explained by the loss of the critically important T4 helper lymphocytes.".[504]

This report from Montreal is not an isolated example. Other investigators have also questioned the suitability and safety of spermicides. In a letter to the *British Medical Journal*, Jeffries(1988)[505] expressed concern at the capacity of nonoxynol-9 to increase the risk of HIV infection by inactivating T4 lymphocytes. So significant is the deleterious impact of nonoxynol-9 on the T4 lymphocytes of the vaginal immune system that the suggested use of this product for rape victims has been criticized by researchers in letters to both the *Journal of the American Medical Association* (Murphy and Munday 1989) and the *British Medical Journal* (Murphy and Munday 1990).[506] The administration of non-oxynol-9 in these circumstances would further *increase* the rape victims' risk of contracting AIDS via its chemical interference with the T4 lymphocytes.

Second, the irritant action of nonoxynol-9 causes micro-tears to occur in the woman's first line of defence: the skin. In this particular case, the skin damaged is that which lines the vagina. Normally the unbroken surface of the skin acts as a physical barrier to entry by infectious agents. Under the caustic effects of the spermicide this skin protection barrier is compromised. When this effect is coupled with an impaired T-cell immune response also caused by nonoxynol-9 it is easy to see how this spermicide facilitates the spread of the virus at the site of the break in the skin lining the vagina.

The implications from this Montreal report are wide-ranging. Nonoxynol-9 has clearly demonstrated its capacity to damage the defence mechanisms of the vaginal immune system . Therefore, as a method of disease prevention and control, spermicidal products of this type represent a poor health option.

Further proof that the promotion of spermicides is an invalid health option was presented in a report in *The Lancet* (1997) entitled *"Nonoxynol-9 fails to protect against HIV-1"*. [507] The following quote is the full text as downloaded from the *Lancet's* web site:

"A study of prostitutes indicates that the incidence of sexually transmitted diseases (STD's), in particular HIV-1, is not reduced by nonoxynol-9 (N-9), announced the US National Institute of Allergy and Infectious Diseases on April 3.

In a randomised placebo-controlled double-blind study (see glossary) done by Family Health International and the Cameroon Ministry of Health, female prostitutes in Yaounde and Douala received monthly medical examinations, treatment for STDs, counselling about STD risks, supplies of male condoms, and supplies of a contraceptive film containing either N-9 or placebo.

For women given N-9 film and condoms, the infection rates were 6-7 cases of HIV-1 per 100 women-years, 33.3 of gonorrhoea, and 20.6 of Chlamydia. For those receiving placebo film and condoms, the numbers were 6.6, 31, and 22.2 cases per 100 women-years of HIV-1, gonorrhoea, and Chlamydia, respectively. The overall HIV-1 transmission rate was reduced by about half by the programme but the lack of effect of N-9 on HIV-1 transmission rates was disappointing given that, in vitro, N-9 film can completely inactivate HIV-1.".[508]

7.2.5 SPERMICIDES AND URINARY TRACT INFECTIONS (UTI).

Further reinforcing the view that the use of spermicides is harmful to a woman's health was a study in the *American Journal of Epidemiology* (1996) which reported that the incidence of UTI's increased with a woman's exposure to spermicide-coated condoms. The authors of this study reported that **"exposure to spermicide-coated condoms conferred a higher risk of UTI..."** and the risk of a UTI increased with exposure.[509] For women exposed to spermicide-coated condoms more than once per week, the risk of developing a UTI was 234% greater then for women not exposed to the spermicide-coated condom. For exposure greater then twice weekly, the risk of a UTI was 465% higher for women who used spermicidal style condoms when compared to women not using such condoms. The authors concluded that **"spermicide-coated condoms were responsible for 42% of the UTI's among women who were exposed to these products.".**[510]

7.3   CONDOMS AND SAFE SEX.

The singular focus of the anti-AIDS campaign over the last 10 years has been on the protective qualities of condoms as a means of insulating people from a variety of sexually transmitted diseases (STD). Over this decade, condoms and 'safe-sex' became synonymous. The clear and unambiguous message was that 'condom sex = safe sex'.

The *"Grim Reaper"* and *"If it's not on, it's not on"* promotions sought to reinforce this same message. And yet, if 'safe' is to be understood in the traditional sense of the word - that is, free from hurt, injury, exposure to danger, or risk- [511] [512] then the pertinent question to ask is, "How accurate is this description"?

In part, an answer can be gleaned from the hesitant tone of a notification letter sent to all American condom manufacturers on April 7, 1987, by that country's drug regulatory authority, the Food & Drug Administration (FDA). The FDA instructed that:

> **"It would be acceptable to state on the labelling for latex condoms that when used properly, they may prevent the transmission of many sexually transmitted diseases such as syphilis, gonorrhoea, chlamydial infections, genital herpes and AIDS, although condoms cannot eliminate the risk.".**[513]

The three key phrases to note are 'used properly', 'may prevent' and 'cannot eliminate the risk'. These are all terms of qualification, uncertainty, reservation and caution. They are not terms of unbridled confidence in the safety and efficacy of the product being considered.

Two further caveats *should* be added to the above list.

The first is that condoms must be 'stored and transported properly'. It has been reported by experts in the area of HIV/AIDS epidemiology that latex is heat, cold, light and pressure sensitive as well as being adversely affected by humidity, ozone , air pollution and deterioration due to the passage of time.[514] Keeping a condom in a wallet, purse or car glove-box 'just in case' would appear to violate the stringent storage conditions required.

The second is that condoms are frequently *not* made to a sufficiently high standard. Condoms numbering in the millions have been found to be faulty. The FDA has seized 45,000 defective condoms in 1988, Philadelphia health officials confiscated 600,000 in 1990-91, and New York health officials recalled 750,000 in 1990.[515] Recall notices have also occurred in Australia on at least three occasions, with newspaper advertisements retrospectively informing condom users of risks they have unknowingly experienced.

These product recalls are ongoing events and occur with a frequency which is unsettling. Despite this frequency there is, from my experience, a sense of surprise bordering on disbelief whenever the 'safety' announcements are made. It is as though condom perfection is viewed as a *fait accompli*. Any news to the contrary is a source of astonishment. Yet to those familiar with the medical literature, such recalls are entirely to be expected.

The following outlines an experiment on condom leakage which is typical of the disturbing but rarely aired research in this area of human health.

7.3.1 CONDOM LEAKAGE.

In the following experiment, the researchers filled condoms with liquid which contained plastic molecules analogous to the AIDS virus: i.e., they were similar in shape and size. These plastic particles were placed inside a condom with a glass plunger inside the condom. This arrangement was designed to imitate many of the 'environmental' factors operative during intercourse:

> **"Condoms were tested in an active in-vitro** (test tube) **system simulating key physical conditions that can influence viral particle leakage through condoms during actual coitus. The system quantitatively addresses pressure, pH, temperature, surfactant properties** (surface tension) **and anatomical geometry. A suspension of fluorescence-labelled, 110-nm polystyrene microspheres models** (resembling in size and shape) **free human immunodeficiency virus (HIV) in semen, and condom leakage is detected spectroflurometrically. Leakage of HIV-sized particles**

through latex condoms was detectable for as many as 29 out of the 89 condoms tested.".[516]

This result represents a failure rate of 30%. If health protocols which determine safety standards accept a 30% failure rate, then it is an imprecise and dangerous standard.

Highly qualified researchers in the field of latex technology have called into question the merit of promoting condoms as a method of *stopping* the transmission of HIV-AIDS. C.M.Rowland, Ph.D., editor of the journal *Rubber Chemistry and Technology,* wrote to the *Washington Post* (1992) thus:

"... Electron micrographs reveal voids (holes) 5 microns in size (50 times larger than the virus), while fracture mechanics analyses, sensitive to the largest flaws present, suggest inherent flaws as large as 50 microns (500 times the size of the virus).".[517]

This means that even a properly made condom can have naturally occurring channels which are at least 50 times larger than the AIDS virus.

Aside from this problem of manufacture, there have been deficiencies in the technical capacity to actually identify problems with poorly made condoms. Rowland points out that even the FDA testing standards (as of Dec, 1992) could *not* detect holes in condoms if the holes were smaller than 10 microns. The AIDS virus is **"only 0.1 microns in size".** [518][519] Thus, the FDA tests could only detect holes if they were 100 times larger than the size of the AIDS virus.

The same expert is also quoted as having said: **" I find absurd the notion that condoms allow one to safely engage in sexual relations with HIV carriers.".** [520]

In the interests of balance, it should be noted that some researchers, Conat (1986) for example, have suggested that condoms are impenetrable to the AIDS virus.[521] But more recent research has challenged the accuracy of this report, citing errors in the way the study was conducted as the reason its results could not be accepted.[522]

Work by Voeller and co-workers (1994), who performed permeability tests on 31 different styles of condoms using laboratory equipment designed to simulate intercourse, have dramatically highlighted the dangers associated with condom use. Their results indicated that:

"per cent leakage ranged from 0.9 to 22.8%; 100% of the specimens of one profoundly flawed brand leaked.".[523]

A letter in *Pediatrics* (1996) by Friedman and Trivelli also reported that: **"with regard to HIV, they** (condoms) **are not impermeable"**.[524] These reports place a grave measure of doubt upon the medical correctness of the "safe-sex" campaign, particularly in light of the dissimilarity between the 'demands'' placed upon a condom in a laboratory setting using glass plungers etc, and the real world of enthusiastic and sometimes hastily arranged sexual activity. Indeed, since **"the condom failure rate for pregnancy is 10-30%"**,[525 526] it is reasonable to presume a much higher rate for sexually transmitted diseases (STD's). The latter can be contracted every day of the month whereas a woman can only become pregnant during the 5-7 mid-cycle days of the month (see explanatory footnote).[527]

Irrespective of what the failure rate of condoms are, a 10,20 or 30% figure is merely a global statistical guesstimate devoid of any attentiveness to the human suffering that it may represent. People do not contract a percentage of AIDS. They either don't contract it, or they contract 100% of it.

Unlike the varying degrees of sunburn that an unprotected swimmer may 'contract', AIDS infection is an absolute result. Thus, to dishonestly imply societal safety by this barrier method is, in my view, to deprive people, particularly women, of information they need to make good health choices.

7.3.2 DIFFICULTIES WITH CONDOM USAGE.

Aside from the question of latex condom permeability, and flawed production standards, there are also 'condom failure' issues in terms of practical application. Consequently, the FDA has cautioned against an undisciplined 'user' technique:

"condoms may still fail to prevent the spread of AIDS for other reasons:

* Failure to apply the condom before pre-ejaculatory fluid appears.
* Failure to assure the condom does not fall off or tear during intercourse
* Utilization of condoms during sexual intercourse, but then engaging in oral sex
* There is no evidence that the condom's membrane can withstand anal sex
* Some lubricants (i.e., petroleum jelly, liquid petrolatum, and other oils) may alter the permeability of the condom.".[528]

7.3.3 EPIDEMIOLOGICAL ASSESSMENT OF THE CONDOM.

Further evidence has recently been published in Australia which argues against the oft-repeated medical cliché that condom sex is safe sex:

"... more than 10 years of safe sex campaigns, which have helped contain the spread of HIV, have failed to stop the spread of genital herpes, with one in five Australians now infected... (and a) ten-fold increase in people with genital herpes since 1973".[529]

There are two points to note here. First, to "contain the spread of HIV", whilst a laudable and necessary health protocol, is not equivalent to *stopping* the spread of a disease. To "contain" is a loose and ambiguous term which may mean that the spread of HIV continues within pre-defined limits of the number of persons infected. To 'contain' unwittingly implies safety. It should not be viewed in this way.

Society errs if it concludes that condom use is the medical equivalent of a preventative protocol such as a vaccination program. Vaccination programs stop the spread of a disease by presenting a 'deactivated' virus for the body to immunize itself against. Condoms do not *stop* the spread of a disease because they risk exposing the body to a live virus against which immunity is impossible. The fact that genital herpes is increasing and HIV is only 'contained' proves this point.

The second critical point is that the incidence of genital herpes, caused by the herpes simplex virus (HSV2), is escalating at an unconscionable rate of 900%: i.e., a tenfold increase.

In the light of the previously discussed research, however, it may be time to question the assumption of condom safety and, accordingly, pose a different question: How safe are condoms? This has already happened in the person of Associate Prof. Basil Donovan, of the Sydney Sexual Health Centre at Sydney Hospital, who stated in 1995 that **"we don't know how effective condoms are. No-one has ever studied them before"**.[530]

To this end W.R.Archer, Deputy Assistant Secretary for Population Affairs, U.S.Department of Health & Human Services, has indicated that unfortunately the determination of condom safety and efficacy may be impossible to verify, since:

> **"The** (American) **Centres for Disease Control have concluded that studies of the risk of HIV infection for condom users are ' too dangerous to undertake... for ethical reasons'."**.[531]

The medical community is thus presented with a conundrum. It knows that condoms leak, break, become fragile and susceptible to tears, can never be made impermeable and, as a result, can only be expected to slow the spread of various STD's. Yet the health message of 'safe-sex' is still the same.

If the normal standards of best-practice medicine applied, the advice to the public would be 'use at your own risk', particularly since the medical evidence indicates that women more readily contract A.I.D.S. from infected men than vice versa.[532] As Grimes (1995) has stated:

> **"Biologically, the efficacy of male-to-female transmission is greater than that of female-to-male transmission, presumably due to the mucosal surface area of the vagina."**.[533]

7.3.4 THE FEMALE CONDOM.

The female condom known as Reality® is commercially available in America, and in England it is known as Femidom™. Trials of the device have been conducted in Australia but it is not currently available. Reality® is described as:

> "... a lubricated polyurethane sheath with a ring on each end that is inserted into the vagina ... No clinical studies have been completed to define protection from HIV infection or other S-TDs. However, an evaluation of the female condom's effectiveness in pregnancy prevention was conducted during a 6-month period for 147 women in the United States. The estimated 12-month failure rate for pregnancy prevention among the 147 women was 26%. Of the 86 women who used this condom consistently and correctly, the estimated 12-month failure rate was 11%.".[534]

If the estimated 12-month failure rate of 11% is used as a benchmark of efficacy in pregnancy, then it is reasonable to deduce that the actual users' failure rate for STD prevention would be four times this figure: i.e., 44%. To recall from the earlier part of this chapter: a woman is only fertile for one quarter of her cycle. Thus the pregnancy rate, as a measure of the condom failure rate, can only reflect the condom failure rate for one quarter of a cycle.

The health implications of this high failure rate are dramatic. If a woman used this method for one year, she might contract an STD every second time she had intercourse, since 44% is close to 50%, or 1 in 2. As a method of life preservation, any item with a proven failure rate of 11%, and a suspected possible maximum failure rate of 44% has little to recommend it.

7.3.5 BARRIER CONTRACEPTIVES AND PRE-CLAMPSIA IN PREGNANCY.

Another serious side-effect common to both spermicides and condoms is pre-clampsia, an abnormal condition of pregnancy, beginning around the 20th week, in which a woman suffers from high blood pressure. This condition occurs in 5% to 7% of pregnancies, with treatment ranging from bed rest to sedatives and antihypertensives.[535] Until recently the cause of pre-clampsia remained unknown **"despite 100 years of research by thousands of investigators"**.[536]

An indication of why pre-clampsia occurs in certain categories of women has been suggested by two articles in the *Journal of the American Medical Association* (1989).[537][538] It was reported by researchers that women who had used barrier methods of contraception (spermicides, condoms) up to one month prior to pregnancy had a 2.4 times greater risk of developing pre-clampsia. This is a 140% greater risk. The association of immediate pre-pregnancy contraceptive practice with pre-clampsia occurrence has allowed for an unravelling of the complex but interesting reason for this medical condition. The precise biological mechanism leading to pre-clampsia is explained by Prof. Rahwan:

> **"... Barrier contraceptives... prevent uterine exposure to sperm and seminal fluid [and] do not allow the female immunological system to develop gradual tolerance to male antigens on sperm and seminal fluid that would otherwise normally develop upon repeated exposure to these foreign antigens. As a consequence, a subsequent pregnancy in a female who previously used barrier methods of contraception will lead to an immunological attack against the (foetus) which carry the sperm antigens to which the female was not previously exposed as a result of the barrier contraceptive. The resulting maternal immunological attack against the invading placental tissue (which originates from the conceptus) results in placental damage and liberation of vasoactive substances (including prostaglandins) that may be responsible for the early onset of labour in these patients.".**[539]

This disruption to the 'delicate balance' of the naturally occurring hormones which are responsible for the control of blood pressure leads to a dominance by the hormones which cause blood vessels to constrict. When blood vessels constrict, there is an elevation in blood pressure which in the pregnant woman is known as pre-clampsia. Given the complexity of the biochemical interactions, it is understandable that the explanation and the link with recent use of spermicides has taken so long to establish.

In summary: the view that barrier methods are safe or dependable has no basis in fact. Pregnancy, disease (both minor and serious) and significant medical conditions are clearly attributable to the use of spermicides and condoms. The propagation of contrary views is an erroneous activity devoid of any rational underpinning. As such, the current public health policy on reproductive and sexual health stands condemned for its promotion of spermicides and condoms as positive health options. It is time for a serious and honest reappraisal of the evidence by government health regulatory authorities.

7.4   KEY POINTS.

1. Spermicides have a high pregnancy failure rate of 30%.

2. Spermicidal sponges cause serious side-effects such as Toxic Shock Syndrome. They also impair the T4 lymphocytes and damage the lining of the vagina, thereby increasing the risk of AIDS.

3. Condoms cannot be made without naturally occurring 'holes'. The AIDS virus is smaller than these 'holes'.

4. Leading experts have criticised the suitability of condoms as a prevention against STD's.

5. Laboratory testing confirms that condoms leak. Quality assurance is not high.

6. The female condom has an estimated failure rate in preventing STD's of almost 50%.

7. Barrier methods are linked with significant medical conditions such as pre-clampsia, birth defects and higher rates of spontaneous abortion.

CHAPTER EIGHT.

8. FERTILITY DRUGS.

"... ovarian cancer is the leading cause of death from gynaecological malignancies in the United States". Feehery K & Benjamin MD (1995)[540]

8.1 INTRODUCTION.

There are four reasons for a chapter on IVF drugs. First, there is the increasing use of IVF procedures to treat various types of infertility .[541] Second, there is an increasing body of evidence which links fertility drugs to ovarian cancer. A significant portion of that medical literature cites clomiphene as part of the treatment. Third, ovarian cancer is a serious medical problem. It accounts for 18% of all gynaecological cancers, is difficult to detect in 70 to 80% of patients until it has become extensive within or beyond the pelvis[542] and has an overall 5 year survival rate without evidence of recurrence of 15-45%[543] (for common epithelial tumours). Ovarian cancer caused by fertility drugs *is* a cancer of the epithelium.[544] Finally, the magnitude of the fatal problems associated with fertility drugs is not consistently mentioned in the approved product information (PI) or other approved patient information materials.

8.2 DEFINITION AND CAUSES OF INFERTILITY.

Infertility is defined as the **"absence of conception after 1 year of regular intercourse without use of contraceptives"**.[545] It differs from sterility which is **"the inability to ovulate"**.[546] Either medical situation may or may not be reversible.

From a female perspective, a multitude of factors may cause infertility. Various disorders of the female reproductive tract (infections, polycystic ovaries, Fallopian tube obstruction or inflammation, abnormalities of the uterus and cervix), as well as hormonal imbalances, vaginitis, diabetes, and antisperm

139

antibodies are causative factors.[547] But the event singularly crucial for conception is ovulation.

A woman might not suffer from any of the aforementioned factors of infertility, but if she is unable to ovulate, then a functional reproductive system counts for nought. Therefore, this chapter will focus on the issue of infertility and the drug therapies employed to ameliorate this condition. As well, it will present key medical research which outlines the manifest problems with infertility drugs.

8.3   OVARIAN CANCER AND FERTILITY DRUGS.

The use of clomiphene (Clomid®, Serophene®) to stimulate ovulation was shown to be a successful treatment for infertility by Greenblatt and co-workers as far back as 1962.[548] A dose of 50mg daily for 5 days, starting on the fifth day of the cycle, was recommended. Problems with clomiphene included gastric irritation, hot flushes, skin rashes and visual disturbances.[549] Amongst the side-effects observed at higher doses was excessive enlargement of the ovaries (ovarian hyperstimulation syndrome - OHSS) leading to the formation of ovarian cysts.[550] This side-effect has dramatic ramifications which I will discuss later in this chapter.

Concern over the prudence of hormonal treatment for infertility was indirectly signalled by Egyptian gynaecologist Dr M.F.Fathalla in 1971. He noted that in animals there was a link between the frequency of ovulation and the incidence of ovarian cancer.[551] Human studies supported these observations:

> **"Epidemiological data in human beings may also be suggestive of a possible relationship between the process of ovulation and the development of common ovarian neoplasms. In the absence of ovulation - before puberty and in patients with gonadal** (ovarian) **dysfunction - ovarian neoplasms of surface epithelial origin are extremely rare.".**[552]

Conversely Fathalla noted that for women who experienced no **"ovarian physiological rest periods afforded by pregnancy - nuns and unmarried and infertile women -** (there was) **a higher incidence of ovarian cancer".**[553] At an individual level, the untimely death from ovarian cancer of the Jewish philosopher, Gillian Rose, **"a great scholar in her prime,"** lends poignant support to these observations by Fathalla.[554] Gillian Rose died, aged 48, childless.

In the context of fertility drugs, it is important to understand the significance of these quotes. Dr Fathalla was suggesting that the cause of ovarian cancer was that the female ovaries did not experience certain periods of 'rest' from the physiological action of ovulation. Continual ovulation with no 'rest' was linked with cancer. A 'rest' from ovulation was associated with a decrease in ovarian cancer. The clear inference one can draw from Dr Fathalla is that if normal ovulation without 'rest' periods is associated with ovarian cancer, then excess ovulation due to fertility drugs raises many serious questions concerning the possibility of even greater risks of ovarian cancer.

But what are the mechanisms associated with continuous ovulation which induced this radical cellular change? Dr. Fathalla suggested two hypotheses: the *first* proposed that, **"the process of ovulation involves repeated minor trauma of the covering epithelium** (tissue)"[555] of the ovary. This process is referred to as the 'incessant ovulation theory', or the Fathalla hypothesis. Well-documented evidence suggests that because both pregnancy and the pill confer a 'rest' from ovulation, there is an associated decrease in ovarian cancer (Casagrande,1979[556] Lowry, 199[557]). Less ovulation means less damage to the surface tissue of the ovaries and hence less cancer.[558]

Also adding credence to Fathalla's hypothesis were the results of a study conducted in Shanghai, China, by Shu and co-workers, and published in 1989. These researchers reported that early menarche and late menopause, which both exposed a woman to an *increased* number of ovulations, were associated with an increased risk of ovarian cancer.[559]

Part of the physiological problem with fertility drugs is that they can cause a woman to have the same number of follicles breaking through the surface of the ovarian tissue *in a single drug stimulated cycle* as a normally ovulating woman might experience in two years of natural menstrual cycles (Fishel, 1989).[560] This of course means that the ovarian surface tissue is subjected to vastly increased numbers of micro tears. Instead of the usual single monthly follicle being released by the ovary, resulting in one tissue breakage needing repair, a woman on fertility drugs may experience twenty four follicle ruptures in a single cycle, resulting in substantially greater tissue damage to the ovary.

Further support for the first of the Fathalla hypotheses on ovarian cancer came at an international conference on ovarian cancer in 1991.[561] At this conference, it was suggested that unrelenting or "incessant" ovulation due to fertility drugs caused an increased number of tears in the ovarian tissue, hence a corresponding increase in the demand for cellular repair for these tears. It was proposed that this repetitive cellular proliferation and repair allowed for the proliferation of cells which contain a *defective* tumour-suppressing gene. The increased number of these defective tumour-suppressing genes, over and above the number that would be present in a woman ovulating at a natural rate, meant that tumours could develop more readily. Were it not for the enforced excessive ovulation due to fertility drugs, the ovarian cancer might not occur. The defective tumour-suppressing gene would not have had the artificially created opportunity to replicate so rapidly.

The *second hypothesis* from Fathalla suggested that the reason for the link between fertility drugs and ovarian cancer is that ovulation **"also involves repeated exposure of the ovarian surface to the oestrogen-rich viscous follicular fluid".**[562] Fertility drug-influenced ovulation leads to the ovaries being awash with 'unnaturally' high levels of oestrogen: i.e., levels of oestrogen not experienced during a normal cycle. The reader will recall that oestrogen has a stimulatory effect upon cell growth within the reproductive and sexual organs, with excessive levels of oestrogen being implicated in ovarian carcinoma.[563] Immoderate levels of oestrogen may also have an excessive stimulatory effect on the growth in numbers of defective tumour-suppressor genes.[564]

There would appear to be only a short latent period between the administration of fertility drugs and adverse changes to the ovaries, a situation rather different from that of breast or cervical cancer. Writing in the *Lancet* (1991), J Dietl noted that:

> **"there is a direct chronological relation between hormonal stimulation of previously unremarkable ovaries** (no evident ovarian problems) **and the development of ovarian carcinoma"**.[565]

Three patients involved in this report had been exposed to no more than a few months of clomiphene in addition to other stimulatory hormones. A fourth patient developed '**a tumour mass affecting both ovaries...**'[566] after fertility drug use of 2 years.[567] The reader may recall that for breast and cervical cancer, researchers needed to wait 15-20 years for 'contraceptive' drugs to cause a detectable disease. The reason for such a short latent period with fertility drugs is unclear. The fact that it is short is not.

8.4   'INCESSANT OVULATION' AND OVARIAN CANCER.

The reports by Casagrande (1979), Fishel(1989), Dietl(1991), and Lowry (1991) are not isolated examples. Dr Alice S. Whittlemore has published a review paper in the *American Journal of Epidemiology* (1992) which summarized the findings of 12 American studies conducted between the years 1956-86. A total of 2,197 women and 8,893 controls were involved in these studies.

Amongst the principal findings from Dr Whittlemore was that **"... women who had used fertility medications had almost three times the risk of women with no history of infertility".**[568]

This translates into almost a 200% increase in risk of ovarian cancer due to fertility drugs. It should be pointed out that this result is a global figure. It comprises women who had used fertility drugs and never conceived (nulligravid) *and* women who had used fertility drugs and conceived (gravid). This clarification is relevant and significant. If the data is broken down according to these two sub-groups of women, it can be seen that conception *per se* reduces the risk of ovarian cancer.

The first sub-group of women were those who had used fertility drugs but had never experienced pregnancy (conceived). They had a 2,600% increase in the risk of ovarian cancer compared to never users of fertility drugs (OR 27.0, CI 95% 2.3-315.6). This finding is consistent with the 'incessant ovulation' theory as advocated by Fathalla, although some doubt is raised about such a high relative risk, due to the wide confidence interval ie 2.3- 315.6. The closer these two numbers are, the more reliable is the data. The wider apart they are, as in this study, the less reliable is the data.

The second sub-group of women were those who had used fertility drugs and conceived. They only had a 40% increased risk (OR 1.4. CI 95% 0.52-3.6).569 From this it is clear that whilst enforced ovulation caused substantial ovarian tissue damage, the consequent conception reduced the cancer risk because it created a physiological 'rest' time. The over-stimulated ovaries are allowed time to repair, since no more fertility drugs would be given whilst there was an on-going pregnancy.

8.5   'REST' FROM OVULATION AND REDUCED CANCER RATES.

This last point is not mere speculation. It is borne out by other findings from this study which testify to the natural capacity of the female body to safeguard it-self from disease. Pregnancy, for example, conferred a demonstrable protective effect from ovarian cancer. The first term pregnancy conferred a 40 percent reduction in risk, and **"each additional pregnancy after the first confers the same per cent risk reduction, estimated to be 14 percent"**.[570]

Furthermore, breast feeding, particularly during the first six months after delivery, conferred a protective effect.[571] This is because breast feeding causes a cessation in ovulation which can extend for many months. This gives the ovaries the physiological 'rest' referred to earlier.

'Failed pregnancies' in women who had previously given birth (parous) was also associated with a decreased incidence in ovarian cancer because the woman's body had a 'rest' from ovulation during the months the pregnancy was viable.

> **"Separate analysis suggests that the protective effects of failed pregnancies are consistent among parous women regardless of the number of term pregnancies, although such protection was not evident among the nulliparous. The risk reduction per pregnancy is smaller in magnitude for failed pregnancies than for term pregnancies."**.[572]

The conclusions of Dr Whittlemore have received support from colleagues in this field of research. Dr. Robert Spirtas (1993) observed: **"the primary strength of the COCG** (Collaborative Ovarian Cancer Group) **fertility drug results is their biological plausibility"**.[573]

'Biological plausibility' means that the results are consistent with the preceding years of research, with the current knowledge of drug side-effects and with the dynamics of ovarian physiology. It means that there is nothing in the results which is unexplainable or surprising.

The research by Whittlemore has received further epidemiological support from other research centres:

> "The plausibility of these results is also bolstered by the eight malignant ovarian cases and one benign ovarian tumour report published to date (in the USA)...five other cases of ovarian epithelial carcinoma ... have also been reported to the Food and Drug Administration ... Finally, 12 ovarian tumours have been reported to have followed ovulation induction in France."[574]

Notwithstanding this professional endorsement, Dr Spirtas indicated a number of shortcomings in Dr Whittlemore's analysis, including the study's small numbers (resulting in the very wide confidence levels), failure to note the type of infertility the women suffered from, fertility drug combinations being taken, treatment dosage and duration, and the specific type of ovarian cancer induced by the drugs.[575]

Dr. Spirtas recalculated some of Dr Whittlemore's data and endeavoured to present results which more accurately accounted for these methodological 'blemishes'. The new results indicated no change in the original global figure calculated by Whittlemore: i.e., the risk for women who had used fertility drugs remained 200% higher than for non-users.

But amongst the sub-group of women who had used fertility drugs and *not* conceived, the risk of ovarian cancer reduced from 2,600% to 1,100% (RR 12.0, 95% CI 1.4- 268.0). This is a substantial drop, but the new result is still of an unacceptable magnitude. Dr Spirtas suggested that this revised figure " **does not change the overall conclusions with respect to invasive ovarian cancer**"[576] which Dr Whittlemore had made.

The editorial staff of MicroMedex®, a major international drug data base, have also concluded that even allowing for the aforementioned shortcomings in Dr Whittlemore's report, **"Overall, the results of the study sound a note of caution about possible long-term consequences of fertility drug use"**.[577]

Further supportive evidence of this causal link has come from Dr Mary Anne

Rossing (1994), writing in the *New England Journal of Medicine*. Her research involved 3837 women who had been taking clomiphene for infertility. As a general finding, Rossing reported that:

"... the risk of a borderline tumour was substantially higher than that expected on the basis of rates in the general population of women".[578] The incidence ratio was 3.3 (95% CI 1.1-7.8) - a 230 % greater risk. Furthermore:

"The women who had used clomiphene or other ovulation-induction agents were at increased risk, whereas little increase in risk was observed among women with no history of exposure to these drugs.".[579] The increased risk for clomiphene users was 210%.

Dr Rossing found that the length of use of the drugs was important:

"When we examined the risk associated with the duration of use, we noted no increase in risk associated with the use of clomi-phene for less than 12 menstrual cycles, whereas the women who used the drug for 12 or more cycles were at considerable increased risk.".[580]

The increased risk of ovarian cancer for users of clomiphene of more than 12 months was 1,000% more than non-users (RR 11.0 95% CI 1.5-82.3). Women who had used another fertility drug combination, hMG/FSH,[581] had nearly five times higher incidence of ovarian cancer than population figures would have predicted. (Age standardised incidence ratio 5.6 95% CI 0.1-31.0) -a 460% risk increase.

Commenting on these new results, Dr Alice Whittlemore was reported by the *New York Times* (22.9.94) as saying that Dr Rossing's study changed a causal link between fertility drugs and ovarian cancer "**from the possible to a probable one**" and her results were considered to be "**substantial**".[582] Elsewhere, Dr Whittlemore has observed: "**...the findings from this study buttress the exist-ing data in support of a causal link**".[583] It should be noted that the subsequent edition of the *New England Journal of Medicine*, (vol. 332, # 19), carried letters which both criticised the findings of Dr. Rossing,[584][585][586] and a reply by Dr. Rossing, who refuted all bar one of the criticisms made of her study.[587]

In 1996, Shushan and co-workers (*Fertility and Sterility*) published further clinical evidence which firmed the link between the use of fertility drug treatments and ovarian cancer. After obtaining the names of 200 women with some form of ovarian cancer from the Israel Cancer Registry, researchers conducted interviews with these women. Two controls (women who had not used fertility drugs) were matched to each of the 200 cases (women who had used fertility drugs). Shushan and co-workers reported thus:

> **"Compared with untreated women, women who had reported ever having used hMG, in any combination with other** (fertility) **drugs and for any period, had a higher risk of having epithelial ovarian cancer (crude OR 3.95, 95% CI 1.22 to 12.02). Adjusting for the variables noted above** (age, parity, body mass, region of birth, education, family history and interviewer) **resulted in an OR of 3.19 (95% CI 0.86 to 11.82).".**[588]

The 'crude OR' in the above quote refers to the odds ratio, a measure of the 'chance' of a cancer developing *after* fertility therapy. A crude OR of 3.95 means that the women in this study had a 295% increased risk of developing ovarian cancer. This risk reduced to 3.19, or 219% after certain mentioned factors (variables), which may have influenced the result, were statistically accounted for.

The fertility drug hMG is known by the full name of 'human menopausal gonadotropin'. It is the derived and purified hormonal extract from the urine of postmenopausal women. It is **"a mixture of equal activity of follicle stimulating hormone (FSH) and luteinizing hormone (LH). These hormones have specific actions necessary for the development, maturation and release of ova from the ovaries...".**[589]

The researchers noted that their project did suffer from some limitations, such as recall bias (did the women correctly recall their past treatment history accurately), an inability of the women in the treatment group to recall the precise cause of their infertility, and a difference in country of origin for the cases and the controls. Yet despite these limitations, the researchers felt sufficiently confident to state:

> **"On the other hand, the plausibility of these results is heightened by biologic theory, epidemiological findings, and other recent**

studies that have suggested that fertility drugs might have neoplastic (abnormal new tissue growth) effects. Of particular interest has been Fathalla's theory that "extravagant" and incessant ovulation in women may be an inciting factor for the development of epithelial ovarian cancer. According to this hypothesis, each ovulation causes minor trauma to the surface of the ovary, and the recurrent trauma increases the risk for cancerous changes within the epithelium. Epidemiologic studies have supported this theory.".[590]

One of the touchstones of well-conducted research is that a study arrives at the same conclusions as those that pre-date it. Such is the case with the work of Shushan and co-workers. **"Our results therefore may be in concordance with those reported by Rossing *et al*, suggesting that the *length of treatment* with ovulation induction agents, rather than the drug per se, may constitute a major risk factor."** [591] (my emphasis). The results of Shushan are also consistent with a case of ovarian cancer in a 40 year old woman following the use of hMG.[592]

In closing off their report, the authors noted an important medical/demographic trend which gave cause for considerable worry.

"The suggestion that prolonged use of ovulation induction is associated with ovarian tumours is of particular importance in light of the increasing popularity of fertility and assisted reproduction clinics. In 1988, in the United States, approximately 2 million women reported previous exposure to fertility drugs. Furthermore, whereas in the past these drugs were given only to women with anovulatory infertility (see glossary)**, today the tendency is to treat even normally-ovulating women to induce superovulation.".[593]**

Finally, the researchers made a point which is the central tenant of this book, and which is discussed at length in the last chapter: the need for informed patient consent:

"... we believe that in view of these concerns it might be advisable to provide women with this relevant information and obtain

informed consent before ovulation induction is administered.".[594]

This, one would have thought, is unnecessarily stating the obvious. Yet Shushan and co-workers have clearly marked it as a key medical pre-requisite, indicating that its prior absence in this area of medicine is a practice in need of rectification.

8.6   CASE STUDIES: UNREPORTED DEATHS FROM FERTILITY DRUGS.

To briefly summarized the situation thus far: it has been shown that there is a logical basis in ovarian physiology for concern to arise with regard to fertility drugs. Subsequently, experts in epidemiology have conducted research which concretized the earlier hypothesising into data which was unequivocal. Fertility drugs have a pernicious effect upon the health status of women. The work by Shushan (1996), Rossing (1994), Whittlemore(1992,1994) Spirtas (1993), Dietl (1991), Lowry (1991) Fishel (1989), and Casagrande (1979) all testify to this.

Yet there are grounds for believing that the incriminating data on fertility drugs might be understated. An article in the *Lancet* (1995) indicated that there has been a serious level of under-reporting of the adverse drug reactions from fertility drugs. The *Lancet* published the results of a two year study by the Australian National Health & Medical Research Council (NH & MRC) into the **"long-term effects of assisted conception".**[595] The terminology of the report, notably the use of the word 'scant', suggests that the NH & MRC doubted that the reports lodged with it fully reflected the magnitude of the problems that patients and physicians had experienced during 'assisted conception' procedures.

The voluntary notification of adverse drug reactions by I.V.F. practitioners, as reported to the NH&MRC, comprised a **"scant 37 reports of suspected reactions to drugs used during assisted conception".**[596]   Some of the serious problems associated with I.V.F. included:

"... a wide variety of complications, including two deaths because of accidental failure to deliver oxygen during general anaesthesia, visceral (organ) injuries during egg retrievals, pelvic abscesses, serious infections, five serious vascular complications -

one with residual hemiplegia, torsion(twisting) **of the ovary, and cancers discovered during or after treatment.".**[597]

The medical literature indicated that the fatalities reported to the NH & MRC might not be the sum total of deaths from fertility drugs.

According to a separate *Lancet* report (22.7.95), there was one, and possibly two, further cases of death from IVF drugs. The degree of uncertainty as to whether or not these deaths were the same as those reported by the NH&MRC is, in part, a measure of the poor level of reporting of adverse drug reactions to fertility drugs.

One of these two (new) cases was uncovered by the careful investigative work of a Canadian researcher, Laura Shanner, at the Centre for Bio-Ethics and Department of Philosophy, University of Toronto. The hitherto unreported event took place in 1988, when a woman died. Cause of death was **"due to a stroke after OHSS (Ovarian hyper stimulation syndrome) in an IVF clinic".**[598]

The second death occurred in 1993:

"... a New Zealand woman (died) **due to a cerebral infarction secondary to ovarian hyperstimulation syndrome shortly after in-vitro fertilization treatment.".**[599]

An obvious question to pose at this point is, 'Why the lack of certainty and clarity over these serious problems'? The answer lies in the specific details recorded by an attending physician on a patient's death certificate. The immediate cause of death (i.e. cerebral infarction) may be the only entry listed, with no link made back to the underlying cause, the fertility drugs. As Laura Shanner pointed out:

"Incomplete reporting of the causal linkages (of adverse drug reactions) **raises further problems. For example, there may indeed be more cases of stroke after OHSS but if the cause of death is simply given as stroke the link with OHSS may not be explicit.".**[600]

This inadequate reporting acts as a barrier to a more accurate presentation of the facts and **" patients may agree to treatments that they would reject if given more accurate outcome probabilities".**[601] As a consequence there is a climate of deformed consent for a woman, since she is not properly appraised of the facts.

The comments by Laura Shanner (*Lancet*, 22.7.95) are an appropriate finale to this chapter. They have implications for the whole area of female reproductive health:

> **"It is a physician's duty to ensure the safety and efficacy of a drug, device, or protocol before offering it to a patient, and the many problems in retrieving reports of side-effects do not relieve the clinician of that obligation. In the absence of conclusive studies confirming safety and efficacy clinicians talking to patients must be explicit about what is unknown.".**[602]

8.7   KEY POINTS

1. The frequency of ovarian cancer is linked to the frequency of ovulation.

2. A physiological 'rest' from ovulation is associated with a substantial decrease in the incidence of ovarian cancer.

3. Pregnancy, child-birth, breast-feeding and oral contraceptive use[603] provide a physiological 'rest' from ovulation.

4. The risk of ovarian cancer increases with increasing exposure to fertility drugs.

CHAPTER NINE.

9. PREGNANCY TERMINATION DRUGS: "POST COITAL CONTRACEPTION"(PCC), RU-486 AND METHOTREXATE.

"The cost of RU 486/PG abortion, for example, is not cheaper for women, but is much cheaper for the hospitals and clinics.". [604] R. Klein, J. Raymond and L Dumble. *RU-486: Misconceptions, Myths and Morals* (Spinfex Press,1991).

9.1 INTRODUCTION.

This chapter will examine the abortifacient action of the above- named drugs. As well, it will present a large body of evidence which indicates that these three methods are harmful to the integrity of a woman's health. Also within each of these topics there will be consideration given to various legal problems associated with these drugs.

9.2 PCC DRUGS AS ABORTIFACIENTS.

The everyday use of the term 'post-coital contraception' is inappropriate as it may lead to misunderstanding about the nature of these drugs. In particular, it may be concluded that PCC represents the development of a *new* drug from within the broad category of 'oral contraceptives', or that PCC's may be a totally new category of drugs which previously had not existed.

Neither of these alternatives is correct. I have chosen to employ the term PCC because it is the only one which is commonly used by the medical community and society to refer to a particular drug regimen. However, it must be stated at the outset that this is an imprecise term, since only in the rarest of circumstances are PCC drugs used as contraceptives.[605]

The drugs used after coitus are a form of the currently available formulations of the pill. To achieve a post-coital 'contraceptive' action, the pill is administered in high doses over a period of 72 hours. Three alternative drug regimes exist: the ingestion of a progestagen alone, or an oestrogen alone, or more commonly, the taking of both an oestrogen and a progestagen.

There are four possible mechanisms of action of post-coital contraception: inhibition of ovulation, effect on tubal transit time of the ovum, alteration to the normal cycle pattern and prevention of implantation due to damage to the endometrium. A scientific paper produced by the FDA, and released on 27th February, 1997 does *not* list cycle disruption as one of the methods by which PCC's 'work'.[606]

If post-coital drugs acted exclusively to inhibit ovulation, then the term 'contraceptive' would be accurate. But research published by Grou (1994) in the *American Journal of Obstetrics and Gynaecology* has concluded that post-coital drugs act principally to terminate a viable pregnancy by interfering with the endometrium:

> **"... this mode of action could explain the majority of cases where pregnancies are prevented by the morning-after pill".**[607]

Harper and co-workers, writing in *Family Planning Perspective's* (1995), made the same observation:

> **"Emergency contraceptive pills, also known as morning-after pills, are a postcoital hormonal treatment that appears to inhibit implantation of the fertilized ovum."**.[608]

Dr Diana Rabone of New Zealand also concurred with this view:

> **"In general the studies suggest the mode of action is due to variable luteal phase dysfunction, and out of phase endometrial development - a 'histologic desynchronisation of the endometrium' - such that implantation is unlikely to occur."**.[609]

Martindale - The Extra Pharmacopoeia, an internationally respected text on matters pharmaceutical, and a compulsory text for Australian pharmacists details in an unambiguously manner how PCC exerts its effect:

"Methods of contraception which prevent implantation of a fertilised ovum include progestogen-releasing intra-uterine devices and postcoital oral contraception (the Yuzpe regimen or so called 'morning after pill').".[610]

Therefore, this method of birth regulation should be re-named 'drug-induced abortion'. As Prof. Rahwan has said:

"Contraception involves the prevention of conception by interference with any step prior to fertilization of the ovum. Contraceptive mechanisms would include...interference with sperm mobility, ... inhibition of ovulation, or interference with the encounter between sperm and ovum by physical barriers. Interception involves interference with the implantation (nidation) of the already fertilized ovum, and, from a biological stand-point, must therefore be considered an early abortifacient approach.".[611]

9.2.1 SIDE-EFFECTS OF PCC.

When oestrogens alone are used as a post-coital 'contraceptive', the major problems relate to the excessively high doses given, with the attendant risks and side-effects: the prescribed regime of 5mg /day for 5 days of ethinyl estradiol or conjugated oestrogens at 30mg/day for 5 days **"represents the equivalent of 2 years' use of 50ug/day combined oral contraceptive.".**[612] Studies done using these high doses of oestrogen found that nausea occurred in 70% and vomiting in 33% of all patients.[613] Questions of concern are also raised about the damage to a woman's life supply of eggs occasioned by the ingestion of such a large dose of a female hormone.

Progestagens have also been used, especially norgestrel, although most experience with these agents involve long-term postcoital birth control and not emergency, single exposure situations. Doses ranging from 0.35 milligram to 1 milligram have been effective, producing corrected failure rates of 2.2 and 2.8 per 100 woman years, respectively.[614]

The most commonly used post-coital contraception drugs are the combination of ethinyl estradiol and levonorgestrel. The necessary two doses of these drugs are usually taken 12 hours apart, and within 72 hours of intercourse. This method is known as the Yuzpe regimen. Approximately 66% of the patients experienced nausea and 19% vomiting. Breast tenderness is also a side-effect. It has been suggested that the side-effects of the Yuzpe method are sufficiently unpleasant to **"discourage over-reliance on the method"**.[615]

Aside from these unpleasant side-effects, more serious consequences such as ectopic pregnancy have been reported:

> **"There is some evidence that there is a higher incidence of ectopic pregnancy , up to 1% in those pregnancies which did occur."**.[616]

As well, the medical literature noted that the incidence potential for blood clot formation was increased because of the higher doses administered to a woman.[617] The work by Rossing (*Br J Haemat,*1997*),* referred to in chapter four, is also pertinent in the context of the zealous promotion of the 'morning-after' pill. High-dose usage of the pill as a 'morning-after' therapy may lead to acquired APC resistance, and hence and increased incidence of DVT.

9.2.2 PCC AND OVER-THE-COUNTER (OTC) PURCHASE OF THE PILL.

At the time of writing (June 1997) the employment of the pill in high doses to act as a PCC is receiving much active promotion, and in Australia at least, is occurring without offical approval from the Therapeutic Goods Administration (the Australian equivalent of the FDA). For a doctor to prescribe the pill at PCC doses means prescribing outside of the approved guidelines (referred to as off-licence prescribing). This style of prescribing leaves the physician legally vulnerable if a patient has a significant adverse drug reaction (ADR). Prescribing within the approved guidelines of a drug's therapeutic use profile is a doctor's safeguard from litigation and a tangible demonstration of a duty-of-care.

The legal implications of pill use as a post-coital contraceptive are further expanded by the current 'push' in Australia, America and Great Britain to de-schedule the pill from the current prescription-only category to that of a non-prescription over-the-counter (OTC) line.

The enthusiasm from promoters of this change has not been matched with equal enthusiasm from those who would be legally and ethically held to account if a woman suffered an ADR from PCC: pharmacists and drug manufacturers. The reason for this diminished ebullience is not difficult to understand. The potent capacity of female hormones to affect every aspect of a woman's body demands that a detailed case history and physical examination be performed, including the ascertaining of pregnancy.[618]

These are mandatory pre-requisites. Only a doctor can meet these criteria. Any move away from this model of health-care is foolish in the extreme. De-scheduling of the pill would only trivialize its complex side-effects and, consequently, belittle the dignity of women. It implies that women are not worth worrying about.

9.2.3 PCC DRUGS AS CONTRACEPTIVES.

It is possible to take the morning-after pill as a contraceptive, but this is not a common or easy procedure as there are two conditions which must be considered together for a complete and accurate diagnosis. First, a woman must have an accurate awareness of what stage of her cycle she is at. Second, according to Dr Gerald J McShane of St. Francis Hospital, Peoria, Illinios, a urine and blood test must be done to check for the pre-ovulatory LH surge or post-ovulatory progesterone levels.[619] These tests confirm the woman's own assessment of her cycle status.

Precise awareness of cycle status can be an inaccurate guide to the possibility of pregnancy unless a woman has a particular reason for keeping a daily record of her monthly cycle length via one of the natural family planning (NFP) techniques (changes in cervical mucus during cycle, urine sample detection of mid-cycle LH surge, increase in body temperature and/or abdominal pain at ovulation). As well, a large measure of personal motivation is necessary to correctly determine cycle status. Women engaged in high level sport or couples practising the Billings method of natural family planning would be two groups typically given to this daily monitoring. If a woman meets this pre-requisite, then the blood test will confirm the accuracy of her personal monitoring.

What then might the blood tests reveal? If a woman believes that she is at an early stage in her cycle (day 1-9), the luteinizing hormone (LH) and progesterone levels would be low. If she is close to mid-cycle (10-12), then the oestrogen levels would be rapidly increasing as a precursor to the **"massive release of LH by the pituitary gland"** which causes ovulation 16-32 hours later.[620] At the time of ovulation (day 14) the progesterone levels would still be quite low.

The LH surge typically lasts 36-48 hours,[621] and then the levels drop dramatically. If a woman is some days post-ovulation, then the LH levels would be rapidly declining whilst progesterone, secreted from the corpus luteum - the name given to the ovarian follicle after it has released the ovum - would be increasing to a peak around day 21-22. Subsequently, there is a decline in progesterone as menstruation begins.

For women who fulfil the criteria of accurate cycle monitoring and supportive blood tests, the morning-after pill could be given early in a cycle and it would act as a contraceptive: i.e., the high doses might either stop or delay ovulation to such an extent that fertilization is not possible.

To maintain a truly contraceptive action, the morning-after pill cannot be given close to the usual day of ovulation. If the pill failed to prevent ovulation, fertilization might occur, with a consequent loss of the foetus some days later due to the pill's deleterious effects upon the endometrium.

For women at or a few days past ovulation, the morning-after pill could not be used as a contraceptive for the same reason: the possibility of fertilization coupled with an impaired endometrium could result in loss of the embryo. For women who are more than 4 days past ovulation, no drugs need be given as the ovum would have died and fertilization would be impossible.[622]

Clearly, the adherence to a strict symptomatic observation of the signs of fertility is not the norm. Post- coital contraception is more usually requested because of human error or misjudgment. The treatment is requested as a 'quick-fix' to a worrying problem confronting a woman. In my experience the women involved are often young, understandably agitated and frequently alone. The male is often sheepishly absent post-coitus.

9.3   RU-486.

9.3.1 HISTORY.

RU-486 is the acronym for an anti-progesterone known as mifepristone. The drug was developed by a research team comprised of George Teutsch and Daniel Philibert of the French pharmaceutical company Roussel-Uclaf (hence the letters RU) and French scientist Etienne-Emile Baulieu. The drug was synthesised in April 1980.

RU-486 was first licensed for use in France in September, 1988. Rather sensationally, the Chairman of Roussel-Uclaf, Edouard Sakiz, suspended the sales of RU-486 on 26th October of 1988:

> **"The press claimed that Sakiz' action was due to anti-abortionist threats to the company and its employees.".**[623]

The threats related to a commercial boycott of Roussels' pharmaceutical products. A mere two days later, the French Government, which has a 36% share in Roussel-Uclaf, ordered that the drug be re-released.

Since that time, RU-486 has been officially released in Britain and Sweden, with a Chinese version released in 1995.[624] In America, the Population Council gained the US patent rights from Hoechst, the German parent company of Roussel-Uclaf in 1994, and obtained interim *Food and Drug Administration* marketing approval for the RU-486/misoprostol combination on September 18th, 1996.[625] Oddly, in the FDA announcement of the 18th there was *no* mention of the cardiac problems or deaths attributed to the RU-486/prostaglandin cocktail.

In another development, Reuters (April 10th, 1997) reported that Hoechst **"will stop manufacturing the abortifacient mifepristone (RU-486), and give RU-486 patents in Europe to a new company being formed by Dr. Edouard Sakiz, a developer of the drug.".**[626] This new company was reported to be named Exelgyn. In the words of Dr. Sakiz: **"We've got to take this step, because the product is worth it... It is a magnificent French discovery which I don't want to see buried.".**[627]

According to the Reuters report the boycott of Hoechst's large range of pharmaceutical preparations was possibly behind the sell-off of the RU-486 patent rights. Peter Blair, stock analyst for Salomon Brothers (London), was quoted as saying that it (RU-486) has been **"a thorn in the company's flesh that it would rather have removed."**.[628]

9.3.2 NATURE AND OPERATION OF RU-486.

In the context of the pro/anti abortion debate, RU-486 has been variously described as "the moral property of women,"[629] a magic bullet, and a human pesticide. These titles tend to further an ideological argument rather than a scientific one.

RU-486 is classified as synthetic steroid (hormone) which has an anti-progesterone effect.[630] To understand the relevance of this classification, it is helpful to be fully aware of the role of progesterone.

When a woman ovulates, a structure known as the corpus luteum (*L.* body, yellow) remains, which secretes progesterone. If fertilization takes place, the corpus luteum continues to secrete progesterone for some months, after which the placenta takes over the role. The role of progesterone in pregnancy viability is so vital it is colloquially known as the pregnancy hormone. Without progesterone, the endometrium structure and function ends. The embryo is deprived of its source of nutrition and oxygen, and therefore dies. In women who suffer from spontaneous miscarriage, progesterone has been used to maintain the endometrium and hence the pregnancy.[631]

As an anti-progesterone, RU-486 'works' by blocking the chemical sites on the lining of the endometrium known as receptors. By blocking these receptors, progesterone cannot interact with the cells of the endometrium. Deprived of the hormonal interaction from progesterone, the endometrium degenerates.

If a woman has conceived but implantation has not yet occurred, RU-486 causes the endometrium to break down. When the embryo arrives in the womb some 5-7 days after fertilization, the endometrium is not in the necessary state for implantation to take place. The embryo dies. Alternately, if implantation has occurred prior to RU-486 ingestion, the drug will quickly begin to block progesterone from interacting with the endometrium. Again, the endometrium shrivels up, causing the expulsion of the already implanted developing embryo.

9.3.3 SUCCESS RATE OF RU-486.

Used by itself, RU-486 is not remarkably successful at causing an abortion of the embryo. Studies vary in their reporting of how successful it is - the range can be as low as 54%, up to a high of 90% [632][633][634] when given within seven weeks of pregnancy, and reduces to "only" 60% when given at nine weeks of amenorrhoea.[635] Other researchers, such as French abortionist Dr Giles Sourny of Lyon, suggested that only 15-20% of women abort when given RU-486 alone.[636] This is a view which is contrary to the majority opinion. If RU 486 fails to induce an abortion, the woman must do what she originally sought to avoid: have a surgical abortion.

Herein lies a biting irony. The intention of developing RU-486 was that it would be offered as a pharmaceutical alternative to surgical abortion. The inability of this new approach to match the 99% termination rate of surgical abortion meant that RU-486 was unacceptable. To improve the abortifacient rate of RU-486, its developers decided on the novel approach of making the RU-486 procedure a two- drug method of abortion. The second drug which was added was a prostaglandin.

9.3.4 PROSTAGLANDINS AND RU-486.

Prostaglandins are potent hormone-like chemicals, made within the body, which act in exceedingly low concentrations on specific target organs. They cause a vast range of clinically significant effects, including changes in vasomotor tone (blood pressure), capillary permeability, smooth muscle tone (e.g., the uterus and stomach), hormonal function, central nervous system activity and impact on the nerves which control muscle 'alertness'.[637]

To mimic the powerful effects of endogenous (naturally produced) prostaglandins, scientists tested a selection of synthetic prostaglandins as an adjunct to RU-486. These included Nalador® (Sulprostone[638]), Cytotec® (Misoprostol[639]) and Cervagem® pessaries (Gemeprost [640]). The pharmaceutical rationale for using a prostaglandin was that because they cause powerful uterine contractions, this characteristic could be employed to assist in the emptying of the womb of the foetus which had been killed by RU-486. The results were varied and sometimes fatal. I will discuss this point more in the section on side-effects.

The administration of RU-486 and a prostaglandin is a four- step procedure:

1. On the first visit to a clinic, the pregnancy is confirmed by a blood test, a pelvic exam and **"often an ultrasound exam via a probe inserted into the vagina".**[641]

2. The woman must then wait between two and seven days before returning to the clinic for the administration of three RU-486 tablets (600mg). Because stringent regulatory controls exist, the patient must sign for each individually numbered tablet.

3. The woman returns a third time to the clinic, 36-48 hours after taking the tablets, for the prostaglandin (either as an injection, vaginal pessary or tablet) which will induce uterine contractions. At this stage **"another pelvic examination is done, the second in 48 hours".**[642] The woman must remain in the clinic for 4 hours so that she can be monitored by doctors. Three out of four women abort whilst in the clinic. Those who don't abort at the clinic return home, where the abortion may take place.

4. Seven days later, the woman returns to the clinic for the fourth time to ascertain that the abortion is complete and to have her bleeding monitored.[643] This may necessitate a third pelvic examination.[644]

The normal cut-off time for use of the drug is 49 days after the last menstrual period,[645] although a U.K. Multicentre Trial set the cut-off point at 63 days.[646] This extended time frame has led some researchers to suggest that:

> **"...there is also the grisly possibility that a woman will deliver her tiny but unrecognisable dead fetus of 6-12 weeks' development alone and at home".**[647]

This consequence has also been noted by other writers.[648] [649] To some, an abortion at home may constitute a form of privacy, but it also condemns a woman to loneliness, isolation and total moral responsibility for her action.

This grim assessment has received support from the president of Roussel-Uclaf, Edouard Sakiz, who acknowledges that the RU-486 procedure is a traumatic one. He has described the RU-486 procedure as: **"an appalling psychological ordeal" because the woman ... has to 'live' with her abortion for at least a week using this technique".**[650]

9.3.5 CASE STUDIES: SIDE-EFFECTS OF RU-486/PG.

FATALITIES.
The description of RU-486 as a 'magic bullet' was originally intended to refer to its effect upon the foetus. Unfortunately the title backfired when Nadine Walkowiak, a French mother of eleven died as a result of the RU486/PG procedure. The prostaglandin Nalador®, which was given as an injection, caused cardiovascular shock (failure of the heart and circulation). This event was reported by *AAP* (25.3.91), the *Australian* (13-14th April 1991), *Daytona Daily News* (9th April 1991)[651] and confirmed on 8 April 1991 by the French Ministry of Health in an official *Communique.*[652] Recent private correspondence from France reported that the Administrative Court of Lille ordered Lens Hospital pay compensation of $100,000 to the spouse and family of Nadine Walkowiak.[653]

This is not the first fatality attributed to Nalador. The medical literature indicates that at least one,[654] and possible three other deaths had been caused by this prostaglandin. Four additional women have suffered non-fatal heart attacks due to it.[655 656 657 658 659] The dates of these latter events are difficult to ascertain.

Subsequent to these deaths, Roussel-Uclaff made the decision to recommend against Nalador as the prostaglandin to be used with RU-486. Gemeprost was substituted. To date, no fatalities have been reported with it.

SERIOUS BLOOD LOSS.
This is not, however, the end of the serious problems associated with RU-486/PG. Post-abortion bleeding can be significant in 10% of women,[660] lasting from 3-43 days.[661 662] Klein and co-authors, in their book *RU-486; Misconceptions, Myths and Morals* (Spinifex Press 1991), cited a graphic case which indicates that the propaganda and the reality of RU-486 are sharply contradictory :

"A nurse who was part of the US trials undertaken by David Grimes in Southern California relates - in a letter to the *Los Angeles Times* - that she was one of the non-success stories of the US abortion pill experiment. After 12 hours of severe cramping and vomiting, she went to the County university emergency room where she was given an excruciating pelvic examination, a shot of Demerol (a narcotic analgesic), and a prostaglandin inhibitor to slow down the contractions. Then after mild bleeding for six more days, she haemorrhaged. She continued to bleed for six more months... She choose chemical abortion because it was presented to her as a 'relatively benign experience' and because she thought it would advance the causes of both women and science.".[663]

Other reports have confirmed that haemorrhage is a major problem. In a study submitted by Roussel to the British Health Department, seven women out of 950 in a trial required a transfusion.[664] The *New England Journal of Medicine* (1995) also reported that:

"... haemorrhage requiring transfusion is a recognized side effect of medical as well surgical abortion. Although this complication is uncommon, the possibility of haemorrhage with medical abortion highlights the need for vigilance and ready access to medical help".[665]

This need for ready access to a high level of medical treatment would seem to negate the use of RU 486 in Third World countries.

Aside from problems of death, cardiovascular anomalies and haemorrhage, substantial pain accompanies the uterine contractions caused by the prostaglandins. In the same Roussel study done for the British Health Department, 270 out of 950 required narcotics, and 280 required less potent pain relievers. An article in the *British Journal of Obstetrics and Gynaecology* (1990) reported on a woman who suffered uterine rupture due to gemeprost, resulting in a total abdominal hysterectomy.[666]

9.3.6 PAIN FROM RU-486/PG.

A brief word should be said about the pain experienced by women using RU-486/PG. It has been said by some advocates of this new pregnancy termination technique that the uterine contractions caused by the prostaglandins are akin to what a woman might experience during a heavy period. For two reasons, the Roussel trials indicate that this assertion is an understatement.

First, if 270 out of 950 women required narcotics for the pain, then the pain was of unbearable proportions, and *ipso facto* totally dissimilar to that normally suffered as period pain.

Second, the number of women experiencing this level of pain is staggering - 270 out of 950 women is 24.5%: i.e., one in four. I would confidently assert that within the general female population, one in every four women do not require narcotics for period pain.

To sharpen our focus on the 'pain' issue, I would suggest that *if* the prostaglandin- induced pain was the equivalent of period pain, our hospital system could not cope with the level of monthly hospitalizations. Furthermore, our drug rehabilitation clinics would be overwhelmed with the number of women addicted to their monthly 'hit' of narcotics and in need of rehabilitation.

I have pushed this point somewhat absurdly I realise, but I have done this to show that the paralleling of RU- 486/PG 'pain' and menstruation pain is both trite and offensive nonsense. A more accurate reflection of the pain experienced is reported by women who liken the pain to that of the uterine contractions of child-birth.[667] One RU-496/PG patient, named Aimee, said of her experience:

> **"I felt like I was dying... it hurt so much. I had contractions coming so fast, and I was sick to my stomach and dry heaving. I couldn't stop trembling and I felt so hot.".**[668]

9.3.7 MINOR SIDE-EFFECTS OF RU-486/PG.

Prostaglandins have also been reported to cause vomiting, diarrhoea, fever, nausea,[669][670] fainting, fatigue, bronchospasm[671] and excessive thirst.[672] Dr Lyn Dumble, senior research Fellow at Royal Melbourne Hospital, attributed the problem of excessive thirst to the interaction of the prostaglandins on the hypothalamus, that portion of the brain which controls sleep, appetite, body temperature and many hormonally- activated body functions.

The ubiquitous and diverse nature of side-effects from prostaglandins indicates that these are powerful chemicals. The list of medical conditions and disease states (contraindications) which exclude many women from using the RU-486/ PG procedure lends further support to this view.

9.3.8 CONTRAINDICATIONS OF RU-486/PG.

The initial promise by the advocates of RU-486 was that it would be a safe, chemical alternative to surgical abortion of 'take-home and use' ease of administration. The ever -increasing list of women who can't use this drug combination throws serious doubt on the veracity of this assurance.

Prominent amongst the pre-existing conditions which exclude women from using RU 486 are: women who are smokers, women over thirty -five,[673] women under 18 years,[674] those who suffer from asthma, obesity, high blood pressure, fibroids, glaucoma, ulcers, colitis, arthritis, epilepsy, kidney disease, pulmonary and cardio-vascular disorders.[675][676] This list seems to *include* only the very fit between 18 and 35. From a marketing point of view this is a very narrow and limited demographic.

So what justification is there for the near hysterical fervour which some proponents of RU- 486, notably Prof. Bailleau have exhibited? The evidence would indicate that there is a heavy influence of both a pecuniary and an ideological dimension, with female health an also-ran:

> "The cost of RU 486/PG abortion, for example, is not cheaper for *women*, but is much cheaper for the hospitals and clinics...The UK Women's Health and Reproductive Rights Information Centre *Newsletter* reports that the NHS (National Health Service) in

Britain will save 15-20 million pounds per year when England begins to use RU 486/PG.".[677]

Also of some interest is the misogynist manner in which researchers down-play the significance of difficulties experienced by women. The following quote highlighted this issue.

> **"Six patients had an incomplete abortion and in one the pregnancy continued unaffected. Side effects included intense uterine pain after the prostaglandin administration (16%), vomiting associated with the antiprogestin (RU 486) intake (9%), and after the prostaglandin administration (9%). One woman needed emergency curettage due to heavy bleeding. Six percent of the treated patients had a decrease in haemoglobin exceeding 20g/l during the first week but no patient needed blood transfusion. *No serious side effects were recorded.*"** (sic).[678]

If these problems are not viewed as 'serious side-effects', then it would be instructive to ascertain what actually constitutes 'serious'. My view is that since so much money, time and personal professional reputation is on the line, RU- 486 must be a success at any cost, even if the price is women's health.

9.3.9 USE OF RU-486/PG IN THE THIRD WORLD.

Earlier in this chapter it was noted that RU- 486 alone could not be offered as an alternative to surgical abortion because it failed too frequently to cause a chemical abortion. The proffered solution was the addition of a prostaglandin, selected after a slip-shod trial and error process. From the promoters' perspective the results with this new drug cocktail have been poorer than expected.

Incomplete abortion or an ongoing pregnancy have been reported, ranging from a high of 13.4% to a mid-range of 5% to a low value of 2%. The latter figure is a result close to that of surgical abortion.[679 680] Incomplete chemical abortion necessitates a surgical abortion to remove the fetus and/or the placenta. If this is not done, there is the risk of infection, infertility and even uterine cancer, caused by remnant uterine material.[681]

The group of women for whom RU- 486/PG is a failure are placed in a position of double risk. They are first exposed to potential harm from a potent drug mixture. Then they incur the attendant risks of anaesthesia and a surgical abortion. I suspect that these health-debilitating risk factors of RU- 486/PG are not common knowledge.

Obviously these stringent contra-indications and requirements of further surgery mean that RU-486 will not be a "take home" abortion tablet or be used as a monthly "menstrual regulator", advantages hinted at by some of its advocates. To limit the international distribution of RU-486 to developed countries, the French Ministry of Health issued a memo stipulating that diagnostic equipment such as an ECG, re-animation cardio-respiratory equipment, injectable Calcium antagonists, and a defibrillator be on hand.[682]

Another impediment is that one of the 'safe' prostaglandins, gemeprost, is too expensive and requires **"specific conditions for storage and transfer, which may hinder its use in other parts of the world"**.[683] Thus it is with good reason that Joan Dunlop of the International Women's Health Coalition described the use of RU-486 in Third World countries as **"fantasy."**.[684]

9.3.10 BIRTH DEFECTS AND RU-486/PG.

Given the many difficulties, side-effects and contra-indications associated with a chemical abortion from RU- 486/PG, how do pharmaceutical manufacturers protect themselves? Their solution is to request that the patient sign a contract to the effect that she will have a surgical abortion if RU-486 fails to cause a pharmaceutical abortion[685 686 687 688] This agreement, **"although not strictly speaking a legally binding document, ... is nevertheless a safeguard for the drug's manufacturers"**.[689]

From a financial perspective, there is a logic behind this 'request'. Women who have given to birth to babies deformed by RU- 486/PG may seek redress via the courts. Animal studies support the view that RU-486 is damaging to the unborn child which survives *in utero* exposure. For example, malformations have been seen in full-term rabbit foetuses exposed to RU-486 *in utero*.[690]

The prostaglandin component of the procedure has also been the cause of foetal abnormalities. There have been many reports from Brazil of major birth defects attributable to prostaglandins, involving scalp, cranium and limb abnormalities.[691 692 693 694 695] The *Journal of Pediatrics* (1983) has reported a case of an infant born with hydrocephalus and abnormal digits after a failed first trimester abortion attempt using a prostaglandin.[696]

Beside the problems related to the individual drugs, the medical literature indicates that babies who survive the combined RU-486/PG procedure may suffer substantial birth defects. One such case, is that of a woman who underwent the RU-486 procedure which failed to cause a pharmaceutical abortion. Initially the woman refused the follow-up surgical abortion, until an ultrasound test revealed that the child had incurred substantial developmental abnormalities due to the *in-utero* exposure to RU-486. The baby was subsequently surgically aborted and found to have no kidneys, and its legs had fused together.[697 698 699] This condition is known as sirenomelia, or mermaid syndrome.

The problems of drugs or devices causing birth defects, and the ensuing large litigation payout, are not without precedent. A.H.Robbins, the manufacturers of the Dalkon Shield (I.U.D.), incurred a damages bill of $2.5 BILLION because of the injury caused by the IUD.[700 701] Roussel-Uclaff/Hoechst clearly wish to avoid a repetition of this. As Dr. Jean-Michel Alexandre, president of the French government's Medical Sales Commission, is reported to have said:

> **"... (the) main drawback to the new drug (RU-486) is that it increases the risk of birth defects in babies who survive, and all women who take it would be virtually obliged to have another abortion if the pregnancy was not terminated the first time".**[702]

There are additional concerns about the less obvious effects of RU-486, particularly at the cellular level. Misgivings have been raised by bio-ethicist Mr Nick Tonti-Filippini.[703] He has drawn attention to the lasting effects of RU-486 on the tissues of the cervix and the uterus.[704] Both of these structures and their proper functioning are of a paramount importance to the viability of any future pregnancies.

As well, RU-486 crosses the blood-follicle barrier. In a study which involved 21 women, Cekan and co-workers were able to detect RU-486 in the follicular fluid after administration of a 100mg dose. It should be noted that this dose of 100mg is one-sixth (1/6th) the dose given to a woman undergoing the abortion procedure.[705] The obvious question is this: does a six- fold increase in dose from 100mg to 600mg, which is the 'abortion' dose, translate into a six-fold increase in the follicular fluid levels of RU-486, and a six-fold increase in the potential for damage? From the perspective of a woman's lifelong fertility, the presence of a teratogenic drug inside her ovaries is cause for grave concern. A woman is born with her life's supply of "eggs" . Her body does *not* create a new egg during each cycle; it merely brings one to maturity, ready for release. If her life's supply is damaged from exposure to RU-486, the damage may manifest itself in *any or all* of her future pregnancies. This point has been noted by Klein *et al:*

> "If a woman after RU 486 decides to become pregnant, does she need to worry about RU 486 residues and /or irreversible damage to that follicle and perhaps others too? And what about cycles disturbances? To our knowledge no long-term follow-up studies of women after RU 486/PG have been undertaken to evaluate later pregnancies and menstrual cycles .".[706]

9.3.11 FEMINIST RESPONSE TO RU-486/PG.

It is interesting to note the various objections raised to RU-486 by feminists, and the substance of their grievances.

Some women, such as Janice Raymond of the Massachusetts Institute of Technology, objected to the over-medicalisaton of women by the RU-486 procedure and the lack of privacy caused by the stringent controls on the drug's distribution. [707] A need for four visits over more than a week lend credence to this concern. Others objected to the inclusion of the prostaglandin as the final part of the abortion procedure. As previously mentioned, one of these prostaglandins (sulprostone) has been responsible for a number of fatalities.[708] [709]

Dr. Lynette Dumble considered that prostaglandins **"have the potential to have serious life threatening side-effects".** She further added that **"I think it (prostaglandins) is one of the most ill-conceived ideas to come out of medical science".**[710] In her co-authored book entitled *RU-486: Misconceptions, Myths and Morals,* Dr. Dumble criticised the use of synthetically made prostaglandins, because of the long half-life that they have in the body.[711]

'Half-life' is an important concept in pharmacology. It is the measure of the amount of time it takes for the blood level of a drug to fall back to *half* the peak level which was reached when a single dose of a drug has been given.[712] It takes 24 hours for 50% of an administered dose of gemeprost to be eliminated as inactive by-products in the urine,[713] whereas **"the half-life of natural occurring prostaglandins may be a mere fraction of a second"**.[714]

Whilst Dr Dumble was happy with the use of prostaglandins in life-threatening or debilitating health states, she saw no place for them in pregnancy terminations because, as she points out, pregnancy **"is obviously not an illness"**[715] and the **"exposure to synthetic PG during abortion procedures can be regarded as an immune insult "**.[716]

Furthermore, Klein, Dumble and Raymond opposed RU-486 on the basis of its capacity to cause birth deformities. They stated that: **"For us, nothing less than a zero incidence of developmental lesions** (in the embryo) **is acceptable"**.[717] It should be noted that these researchers fully support surgical abortion, a point unambiguously made in their book.

There is justified disquiet at the *ad hoc* manner in which the RU- 486/PG administration protocol has been developed. I have taken the following from Klein et al's book (referenced in the footnotes.) I highly recommend it for those seeking to broaden their knowledge on the topic of RU 486.

> **"In the beginning, there was:**
>
> **1.   RU 486**
> **Then, the researchers and clinicians added:**
>
> **2.   RU 486 + PG**
> **Then, the studies begin to cite:**
>
> **3.   RU 486 + PG + narcotic and other analgesics**
> **Then came the addition of :**

4.   RU 486 + PG + analgesics + pre-medication
Finally, we read of:

5.   RU 486 + PG + analgesics + pre-medication +
antibiotic"

This is a piecemeal approach to problem solving and is an example of poor poly-pharmacy. The escalating admixture of drugs is fraught with potentially worrying drug/drug interactions. Future events will reveal if this potential is actualised.

9.3.12 OTHER USES FOR RU-486.

As a response to criticisms from a variety of organisations and lobby-groups (feminists, pro-life advocates and scientists) attempts have been made by the supporters of RU-486 to apply a gloss of respectability to the drug by suggesting that RU-486 may have a number of medical applications other than that of being an abortifacient.

Dr Regelson, for example, writing in the *Journal of the American Medical Association* (1990), suggested that his research showed RU-486 had many treatment applications other than abortion:

> **"This clearly includes breast cancer, inoperable meningioma**
> **(brain tumour) and Cushing's disease ... (and)... its potential value,**
> **based on laboratory evidence and the experience with Cushing's**
> **Disease, in treating some forms of hypertension, diabetes,**
> **osteoporosis, obesity, and AIDS.".**[718]

Responding swiftly to this latter hypothesis, the international marketing director of Roussel, Ariel Mouttet said that it was: **" 'scandalous' to suggest that 486 could be used in the treatment of AIDS. Such claims only serve to raise the hopes of the sick 'and to make Roussel-Ulcaf look wicked'. ".**[719]

The biological reason for this rejection of RU-486 in AIDS treatment was that research had showed that **"...some suppression of the immune system may occur at clinically used doses.".**[720] AIDS sufferers require medication to bolster their immune system, not suppress it.

In support of the recommendation that RU- 486 might be suitable in cancer therapy, Dr Regelson cited a trial which reported that **"18%** (of patients) **showed significant measurable tumour regression".**[721] Closer scrutiny revealed that this claim was based upon only *one* trial of twenty-two women over a *three* months. Klein *et al* have expressed reserved uncertainty over the suitability of Dr Regelson's claim.[722]

The parameters of this study and the subsequent conclusions by Dr Regelson have also been called into question by Richard Glasow, Ph.D.[723] Dr Glasow drew attention to other studies which showed that RU-486 *stimulated* the growth of breast cancer cells in a test tube.[724] According to Dr Glasow: **"most breast cancers are oestrogen-related, not progesterone-related".**[725] RU-486 acts on progesterone receptors, not on oestrogen receptors, hence its proposed use would appear to be of debatable merit.

Powles and co-workers (1989) indirectly supported Dr Glasow's criticism of Dr Regelson's claim:

> **"Experimental evidence indicates that oestrogens are involved in carcinogenic promotion of mouse mammary tumours. In humans, epidemiological evidence supports the hypothesis that this mechanism may be important in the promotion of breast cancer.".**[726]

More evidence, of a direct and substantive nature, has suggested further that RU-486 is unsuitable in breast cancer treatment. Perrault and co-workers, writing in the *Journal of Clinical Oncology* (Oct, 1996) reported that only 3 out of 28 women with breast cancer responded favourably (a partial reduction in tumour size) when treated with RU-486. Half the women in the trial (fourteen) had their disease *progress* whilst on RU-486. As the authors of this report noted:

> **"We do not feel that mifepristone (RU-486) should be pursued as a single-agent treatment for breast cancer.".**[727]

The claim that RU-486 might have an application in the treatment of Cushings Disease (pituitary-dependent bilateral adrenal hyperplasia)[728] would seem to be based on inadequate evidence. Dr. Regelson depended upon two studies, with a total of only six patients to support his claim. One study went for *less* than one week. The second study was also rather limited. It involved only *one* patient (who had Cushing's syndrome as distinct from Cushings Disease)[729] The distinction between Cushing's Disease and Syndrome is important.[730] Other researchers have also indicated that Dr Regelson's claims may be erroneous. Nieman *et al* say that:

> **"Although RU 486 was an effective therapy in our patient with Cushing's syndrome due to ectopic ACTH secretion, control**(with RU-486) **may be difficult to achieve in patients with hypercortisolism of pituitary origin (Cushing's Disease).".**[731]

Of some interest is the mention of the Population Council on the front page of Dr Regelson's research paper on RU-486. Readers will recall that the Population Council is the developer of the heavily maligned Norplant®, and in late 1995 gained the licensing rights to RU-486 from Roussel-Uclaf.

9.3.13 THE IMAGE MANIPULATION OF RU-486.

One further aspect of the image manipulation of RU-486 requires mention; the emerging practice of *not* calling RU-486 an abortifacient. This trend is evident in an article in the *Lancet* (June, 1996). The author in question referred to RU-486 as a **"post-implantation menstruation-inducer(s)"**.[732] A similar creative aversion to naming medical actions appropriately was demonstrated in the following quote.

> **"Some patients who would be comfortable with barrier or hormonal contraceptives that block fertilization might firmly object on moral or ethical grounds to methods such as** *menstrual extraction or luteolytic agents (e.g., RU-486) that interrupt* **pregnancy after fertilization and uterine implantation."**[733] (emphasis added).

In this second citation, the author is clearly cognizant of the correct definition of 'pregnancy', yet has failed to apply the necessary terminology to its 'interruption'. A similar disinclination to use the term 'abortifacient' is manifested by the same writer when discussing IUDs. In the context of this devices' mechanism of action the author stated:

"The analysis of the evidence strongly suggests that the
contraceptive effectiveness of intrauterine contraceptive devices
is achieved by both a prefertilization spermicidal action and a
postfertilization inhibition of uterine implantation ."[734]

9.4   METHOTREXATE.

More recently, abortion providers have begun to use the anti-cancer
(chemotherapeutic) drug methotrexate (MTX), in conjunction with misoprostol
(a prostaglandin), to terminate a pregnancy. Methotrexate has a wide range of
anti-cancer activity affecting breast cancer, small cell lung cancer, ovarian
carcinoma, non-Hodgkin's lymphoma and squamous cell carcinoma of the head
and neck.[735] It is also prescribed for certain types of arthritis[736] due to its capacity
to suppress inflammation. Misoprostol is part of the abortion process because
it will generate forceful contractions of the uterus and hence the expulsion of the
dead pre-embryo from the uterus.

The use of an anti-cancer drug with such a diversity of applications may seem
illogical, since pregnancy is not a disease and the fertilized ovum is not a hostile
entity. To understand the reasoning behind the abortionists use of such a potent
chemical, a brief review of MTX will be beneficial.

Methotrexate is a chemotherapeutic drug classified as an antimetabolite,[737] which
means that MTX interferes with the formation of the pyrimidine ring, a precursor
to DNA & RNA.[738] RNA and DNA are the essential genetic components of cellular replication.

In the context of cancer therapy, MTX works effectively because a greater
proportion of cancer cells are undergoing cell cycle activity then the surrounding
normal cells. As a result, there is a faster 'take-up' rate of MTX by the cancer
cells. This works against the cancer cells because MTX is 'false cellular food';
the cancer cells cannot use MTX to generate RNA and DNA, the building
blocks of cellular regeneration. The inability to generate new RNA and DNA
leads to the death of cancer cells.

The same principles apply when MTX is used as an abortifacient. The cells of both the pre-embryo (or blastocyst) and, later, the embryo are rapidly developing and growing, which is **"characterized by a high DNA turnover rate"**.[739] This high demand for DNA means that the pre-embryo or embryo (see glossary) incorporates more MTX into its cellular structure than the slower growing maternal cells. One of the organs most affected by the uptake of MTX is the trophoblast, the structural portion of the blastocyst[740] which has nutritional functions. Because MTX interferes with the growth and development of the trophoblast,[741] it adversely impacts on the generation of nutrition. Because the drug **"is cytotoxic to the proliferative trophoblastic tissue,"**[742] it is also fatal for the pre-embryo or embryo.

It should be noted that I have used the term 'pre-embryo' to refer to that stage of pregnancy prior to implantation.

9.4.1 THE MTX ABORTION PROCEDURE.

The *New England Journal of Medicine* (1995) detailed a study conducted on 178 women 9 weeks pregnant or less, using intramuscular methotrexate and misoprostol vaginal tablets. At a practical level, this technique bears a striking resemblance to the protocol for RU486/misoprostol administration.

At the first visit, each patient received an intra-muscular (IM) injection of methotrexate ranging from 67mg to 110mg, depending on the woman's body weight. Patients returned 5-7 days later for intravaginal insertion of 800ug of misoprostol, held in place by a tampon. For pain or cramping each patient was given a prescription for paracetamol/codeine phosphate. Seven days after receiving the misoprostol, each patient returned for a manual pelvic examination and an intravaginal ultrasound.

Twenty- five of the 178 women in the study required a second intravaginal dose of misoprostol, since there was detectable foetal cardiac activity (the foetus was not dead). For 7 of this last group of 25 women, a surgical abortion was required due to the failure of the previous procedures,[743] an eventuality not unlike that of a 'failed' RU-486/misoprostol abortion. These results indicate that 14% of women (25 of 178) failed to abort at the first attempt, necessitating a second dose of the prostaglandin. Of this second group of 25, 28% (7 of 25) required a surgical abortion.

It is hard to imagine how these results could be interpreted as a positive health outcome for the women involved. Aside from the known dangers associated with the anaesthesia required for the surgical abortion and the problems of prostaglandins previously discussed, there is also the inherent danger of multiple exposure to MTX. The list of problems is extensive.

9.4.2 DANGERS ASSOCIATED WITH MTX.

As a potent chemotherapeutic drug, methotrexate is known to cause disorders of the blood system (leukopenia, thrombocytopenia and anaemia), aphasia (defective language function), paresis (partial paralysis), convulsions, colitis (inflammatory large bowel condition), toxic megacolon (gross enlargement of the bowel which may lead to death), nephrotoxicity (kidney damage), and stomatitis (inflammation of the mouth)[744 745 746] Ironically, methotrexate has also been shown to cause chromosomal damage to human bone marrow,[747] with the inference that this effect may be carcinogenic.

The research on this last point is inconclusive, and precisely because of this uncertainty it is all the more worrying. This sense of trepidation is reflected in the medical literature. The *Australian Prescription Products Guide* notes that:

> **"Methotrexate must be used only by physicians experienced in anti-metabolite chemotherapy... patients should be fully informed of the risks of fatal or severe toxic reactions involved with the administration of methotrexate and should be under the constant supervision of the physician... Deaths have been reported with the use of methotrexate in the treatment of psoriasis.".**[748]

Even the physicians promoting this technique are mindful of the attendant risks:

> **"There are important questions about the potential risks to the woman when a potent cytotoxic agent such as methotrexate is administered and about possible teratogenic consequences related to MTX or misoprostol should a pregnancy continue to the third trimester.".**[749]

Yet, inexplicably, they are enthusiastic about the method.

Some might suggest that these side-effects are not relevant for women using MTX because the women are using the drug only once or twice. Whilst it is true that the *time-exposure* is brief, *the dose-exposure* is precipitously high. In the abortion trials, women varyingly received 67-110 mg of MTX. This is between 9 and 15 times the recommended dose used on an arthritic patient, who might take 7.5 mg per week of methotrexate.[750]

In light of the grave potential and actual problems from prostaglandins and methotrexate, the relevant question to ask is how their use can be justified from a health perspective. The risks to women occasioned by these drugs are substantial in their nature, wide-reaching in their effect and frequently unpredictable. Given these harmful qualities, weighty questions pertaining to their prescribing to healthy women need addressing.

9.5 KEY POINTS.

1. RU- 486 is a potent anti-progesterone which causes serious birth defects when it fails to induce a chemical abortion.

2. The RU- 486 procedure is a two-drug cocktail (RU-486 and a prostaglandin) which is the result of an *ad hoc* process of trial and error, rather than of thoughtful application of medical principles.

3. RU- 486 has been fatal. It also has caused a number of cardiac problems. The list of contra-indications is extensive.

4. The use of prostaglandins has been assessed by experts as constituting an 'immune insult'. The side-effects of prostaglandins are many, severe and unpredictable.

5. Methotrexate, used as a substitute for RU-486, is a chemotherapeutic agent which is used also in arthritis. Its high dose use as an abortifacient is fraught with significant health and legal implications.

CHAPTER TEN.

10. HORMONE REPLACEMENT THERAPY.

"Hormone replacement therapy in older women is safe", says menopause guru, Sydney-based Professor Barry Wren of the Menopause Clinic at the Women's Hospital in Paddington.[751]

10.1   INTRODUCTION.

The purpose and direction of this chapter is similar to that on the pill: the provision of information which will allow women to make an informed choice. After a brief review of the symptomatology of menopause, I shall present the foremost research material on hormone replacement therapy, employing a time-line approach.

10.2   DEFINITION AND SYMPTOMS OF MENOPAUSE.

Menopause is medically defined as **"the physiological cessation of menses as a result of decreasing ovarian function".**[752] It is more commonly understood as referring to the time of the female climacteric[753], the transitional phase beginning prior to menopause and continuing after it, during which a woman passes from the reproductive stage of her life. The diagnosis is usually retrospective, made when there has been no menses for a year. Menopause can be natural, artificial or premature.[754]

The onset of the menopause is due to the decline in ovarian function and a subsequent drop in the oestrogen levels in a woman's body. It is varyingly stated as beginning at age 45 to 49, and going through to age 60.[755] This reduction in bodily production of oestrogen leads to some of the more unpleasant characteristics of this stage in a woman's life - namely the hot flushes which may vary in intensity and be intermingled with times of cold sweats, paresthiasias (prickling, itchy sensation in skin) and formication ("crawling" sensation within the skin).[756] Other symptoms include muscle cramps, headaches, gastro-intestinal upset, palpitations and atrophic vaginitis which may make intercourse painful and unappealing.

Doctors originally began prescribing artificial oestrogens because of these unpleasant hormonal- linked symptoms and the desire to alleviate them. Also, there was a perceived cardio-protective aspect to the use of postmenopausal oestrogen:

> **"Estrogens can cause changes in circulating lipids. They decrease concentrations of low-density lipoprotein cholesterol and increase those of high-density lipo-proteins. These changes may lower the risk of coronary artery disease and contribute to the lower incidence of myocardial infarction in premenopausal women. Use of estrogens in postmenopausal women has also been associated with a decreased incidence of coronary artery disease. However, the data is not uniformly supportive of this notion, and increased incidences of myocardial infarction and stroke have been observed in some studies.".[757]**

It is doubtful that HRT, and in particular oestrogen replacement therapy (ERT), would have been started primarily to alleviate or prevent post-menopausal osteoporosis, since as far back as 1964 it had been demonstrated that oestrogen used for this purpose was only marginally successful, and then for only a short time. Lafferty, for example, showed that **"the benefits of estrogen replacement, however, last only 9 to 14 months in spite of continued estrogen treatment "**. [758]

10.3   EARLY CONFLICTING STUDIES ON HRT: 1976-86.

Despite this positive but qualified assessment, the suspicion that HRT might in fact be of dubious benefit was expressed by the medical editorial team of Louis Goodman & Alfred Gilman as early as 1975:

"...indefinite systemic replacement in all menopausal patients, advocated by some, is certainly controversial and may introduce more undesirable effects than the symptomatic improvement warrants.". [759]

This view was a reasonable one, although it may have only been based upon a theoretical presumption. There was not a wealth of corroborative research in the early years to support it. In fact, research work into "undesirable effects" was sparse.

Upholding the views of Goodman & Gilman were:

"...the results of several case-control studies conducted in North America (which) had indicated a 4-6 fold increase in the risk of endometrial cancer in women receiving conjugated equine (derived from horse urine) oestrogens in the form of Premarin. (Smith *et al*, 1975; Ziel& Finkle 1975; Mack *et al*. 1976).". [760]

Also, Hoover (1976)[761] reported that breast cancer risks doubled with estrogen replacement therapy (ERT) but only reached significant levels after 15 years of use.

Contrary to these reports advising caution were a substantial number of reports released in the years 1980 to 1986 which **"failed to find evidence of any overall excess risk "**.[762] To explain this event it is of benefit to recall earlier discussions on latent period as canvassed in the chapters on breast and cervical cancer. Many years need to elapse before hormonal drugs cause evident cellular damage which is clinically detectable.

10.4   FIRMER DATA IN 1986.

In 1986, more consistent epidemiological trends regarding ERT began to emerge. A paper by Louise Brinton (1986) reported on a study of 1,960 post-menopausal breast cancer cases. Brinton found that:

"After appropriate adjustment, there was a significant increase

in risk (P<0.01) with extended exposure, with those reporting 20 or more years of use having a 50% excess of risk (compared to never-users). **Risk was further elevated among those using hormones 25 years or more (RR =1.7, CI 0.9-3),** (a 70% increase in the risk of breast cancer) **although this estimate was based on only 28 exposed cases. Further evidence for an effect of duration of use was derived when years of use was entered in the** (computer) **model as a continuous variable, where it showed a significant (P<0.001) effect on risk. This analysis also showed that the estimated multiplication of breast cancer risk was 1.02 for every year of menopausal hormone use."**[763] (A 2% p.a. increase in BC risk).

The demographic and sociological impact of this report was noted by the author, who said:

"**Thus, our findings indicate that if hormone use increases breast cancer risk, the risk is limited to relatively long-term users and is small, at least in comparison to the risks for** *oestrogen-related endometrial cancer.* **However, given the extensive population exposure to menopausal oestrogens and the frequency of breast cancer in the general population, even a slight excess risk associated with hormone use is cause for concern."** (emphasis added).[764]

I have highlighted endometrial cancer in this quote because it would appear that Louise Brinton   considered the risk of endometrial cancer to be an issue of greater clinical significance than the   singular focus on breast cancer. The researchers were suggesting that problems caused by ERT required a duality of focus: both breast *and* endometrial cancers, and the influence of ERT on both these disease states.

10.5   THE ROLE OF OESTROGEN.

A brief review of the physiological effects of oestrogen clearly highlights the logical basis for the concern with endometrial cancer. "**By a direct action, they** (oestrogens) **cause growth and development of the vagina, uterus and Fallopian** tubes...". Furthermore, under the influence of estrogen " **during the follicular (pre -ovulation) phase of the cycle, there is a proliferation of the vaginal and uterine mucosae** (surface tissue)... ". Conversely, a **"decline in estrogenic activity at the end of the cycle can bring about menstruation and its attendant phenomena.".**[765]

From this it can be seen that oestrogen prompts the cells of the endometrium to divide and grow, a fact confirmed by the R.J.B.King of the Imperial Cancer Research Fund, Surrey (U.K.): **"Oestrogen increases the proliferation of normal epithelial cells in both** (wo)**man and rodents.".**[766] The highly regarded British research team of T.J.A.Key and M.C.Pike (1988) also made the same point:

> **"The marked increase in risk associated with postmenopausal ERT shows that oestrogen alone is capable of increasing the risk of endometrial cancer. Since the only known effect of oestrogen on endometrial cells is to stimulate cell division, it appears very probable that oestrogen increases the risk of endometrial cancer by increasing the rate of cell division.".**[767]

And what of the role of oestrogen in *breast* tissue development? Whilst there are some unresolved issues concerning the precise nature of the hormonal interplay on breast tissue growth, it is clear from laboratory studies that oestrogen does cause increased cellular division. Key & Pike (1988) suggested three theories, discarding one,[768] whilst King (1991) suggested that:

> **"Given the conflicting data on estrogen and progestin effects on the proliferation of normal mammary epithelium, it is not possible to make firm conclusions but this reviewer feels that the balance of evidence favours a combined role of both classes of steroids.".**[769]

At this point there is merit in a comparison between the response of the two physiological structures (breast and endometrium) under the influence of oestrogen. In the natural (drug-free) physiological environment of the pre-menopausal woman the cellular division of the endometrium is rhythmically cyclical and regulated[770] (if fertilisation does not occur). Studies have shown that:

"... during normal menstrual cycles... the endometrial cell division is very low during days 1-4 of the menstrual cycle, then increases rapidly to a maximum and remains at about the same maximal rate until day 19; the rate then decreases sharply to the very low levels found on days 1-4 and remains at this level for the remainder of the cycle.".[771]

The increased cellular growth of breast tissue is also cyclical, although it occurs over a slightly delayed time-scale to that of the endometrium:

"...breast epithelial cell division rates are low during the follicular phase and high during the luteal phase, with a peak at days 23-25."[772] (see footnote[773]).

If this is the action of oestrogen on normal pre-menopausal physiology, why does ERT pose such a problem? Is medicine not merely mimicking for the post-menopausal woman what occurs naturally for the pre-menopausal woman?

The problem with post-menopausal ERT supplements is that there is no progesterone-like hormone present in the drug to counteract and balance the stimulatory cellular effects of oestrogen on endometrial tissue.[774] But why is progesterone, or a synthetic copy of it, necessary? The answer is that the cells of the endometrium receive a 'slow down' message from progesterone, the hormone which is produced shortly after mid-cycle ovulation by the corpus luteum (in the pre-menopausal woman). Progesterone is known to have an anti-oestrogenic effect upon these oestrogen- stimulated cells of the endometrium, [775] [776] which are in a mid-cycle proliferative (high growth) state. The biological mechanism by which progesterone effects this action is related to its reduction in the number of endometrial oestrogen 'receptors'.[777]

The addition of progesterone to ERT is referred to as 'opposed' HRT. This means that the stimulatory effects of oestrogen on cell growth are 'opposed' - or curtailed - by the presence of progesterone. Without the counter-balancing effects of progesterone there is the potential danger of oestrogen 'over-exposure' which may cause cellular activity to shift from order to disorder and become disorganised, desynchronised and uncontrolled. This is what we call cancer.[778] To negate this dangerous possibility, nature supplies progesterone to protect the endometrium. From a review of the medical literature there would appear to be universal agreement on the need to use 'opposed' HRT (for women with an intact uterus). It should be noted that there would appear to be less agreement about the beneficial 'opposing' effects of *progesterone* on breast tissue and hence breast cancer. In fact, the 'slow down' or 'opposing' role of progestagins on oestrogen-stimulated cellular breast tissue division is a matter of some medical debate.[779]

What dosage of progestagen should be given to act in an 'opposing' manner to ERT? This has been an area of some uncertainty. Clearly the female biochemistry has been able to produce the required levels of these two hormones, but the early research indicated that science misjudged the levels of progestagen needed.

Illustrative of this was a report by Kathryn Hunt (1987). Her research confirmed that 'unopposed' ERT was associated with a high risk of endometrial cancer. It also highlighted the inadequacy of the progestins dosages which women had been taking.

Her study involved 4,544 British women, who on average had been on ERT for 67 months (five and a half years). Of this number, 43% had been taking opposed ERT. She reported a 184% increase in the risk of endometrial cancer (RR 2.84, 95% CI 1.46-4.96) and a **"significantly increased"** risk of 59% for breast cancer (RR 1.59, 95 CI 1.18-2.1). The latter result was of sufficient gravity to cause Hunt and her fellow researchers to note that they were **"... worried about the high incidence of the disease"**.[780]

Three points emerged from this study. *First*, too few women had taken too little progestin to achieve a truly 'opposed' effect: hence the 184% increased risk of endometrial cancer. *Second*, in keeping with the uncertainty of the role of progesterone on oestrogen-stimulated breast tissue as set out by Key & Pike (1988) and King (1991) - see earlier footnote - Hunt's study reported a significant increased risk of breast cancer from poorly opposed ERT. *Third*, the improved cardio-vascular condition of women on unopposed ERT had been lost due to the presence of progestins in the formulations which 43% of the women had taken. The presence of the progestins, whilst inadequate to protect the endometrium from ERT, was still sufficient to obliterate the positive effects that oestrogens had on the lipid profile of pre and post-menopausal women.

This study indicated that because of a misjudgment over the levels of artificial 'progesterone' needed, women had fallen into a lose\lose situation. They had lost in the areas of endometrial and breast cancer, and had lost the cardio-protective effects of oestrogen-only therapy.

10.6   BENEFITS AND RISKS FROM H.R.T.

As Hunt noted, the promotion of ERT posed something of a conundrum. It was true that unopposed oestrogen protected against coronary disease (a benefit), but it also endangered a woman via increases in endometrial cancer. Other researchers have also noted this point:

> "... estrogen therapy after menopause relieves many menopausal side effects but it is known to increase the risk of cancer of the endometrium , the uterine lining.".[781]

In an attempt to reduce the risk of endometrial cancer, a progestin had been added to the formulation because of its anti-oestrogenic effects. Unfortunately it appeared to remove the beneficial effects of ERT on the cardio-vascular system. [782 783] In endeavouring to address one serious problem created by unopposed HRT - endometrial cancer - the new 'opposed' drug approach appears to have created extra problems in the cardio-vascular area.

Notwithstanding the disappointing results of opposed ERT which Hunt's study unveiled, there was, in the minds of many doctors, reason to hope that the combined HRT approach was still a valid medical option for the treatment of menopausal symptoms.

For example, the National Alliance of Breast Cancer Organisations (1989) said that:

> "The addition of progestin to the estrogen reduces the added uterine cancer risk, and it was hoped, would reduce the risk of breast cancer as well.".[784]

10.7   THE BERGVIST STUDY OF 1989.

Serious doubt was cast on the merits of the combined HRT approach by the 1989 report of Swedish researcher Leif Bergkvist. This study involved 23,244 women who had taken oestrogen or an oestrogen-progestin formulation to alleviate the symptoms of the menopause.[785]

The researchers found that for women *only* on estradiol (the most potent naturally occurring oestrogen) for six years or more, there was an 80% increase in the risk of breast cancer (RR 1.8 CI 0.7-4.6). Of more dramatic significance though was the finding, somewhat unexpected it must be said, that for women who had taken *both* oestrogen and progestin for six years or more, the risk of breast cancer was 340% higher than for women who had never taken HRT (RR 4.4 95% CI 0.9-22.4).

This result added another dimension to the conundrum referred to earlier. The addition of progestins to ERT reduces the incidence of uterine cancer, but Bergkvist's results indicated that it also *greatly* elevates the risks of breast cancer. This particular result fits with the 'oestrogen plus progestagen hypothesis' of Key & Pike (1988). The significance of these results should not be ignored, particularly when viewed in the light of what Dr Bergkvist's professional peers have said about his study.

Dr. I. Craig Henderson, for example, a breast cancer expert at Harvard Medical School and a National Alliance of Breast Cancer Organisations (NABCO) Medical Advisory Board Member, said that:

> **"... the findings make biological sense because progestins stimulate the growth of breast tissue. Dr. Henderson cited several other studies investigating the use of progestin alone as a contraceptive pill which already had indicated an increased risk of breast cancer.".**[786]

Dr Henderson also referred to Dr Bergkvist's study as **"a landmark"**.[787]

In part, Dr Henderson's remarks answer some of the earlier scepticism on the role of progestins on breast tissue: they do have a stimulatory effect.

Another noted expert, Dr. Malcolm Pike, Chairman of the Department of Preventive Medicine at the University of Southern California Medical School in Los Angeles, said that ERT alone did confer some benefits against heart disease but these gains had to be evaluated against the increased risk of breast cancer. Dr. Marc Lippman, Director of Georgetown's Lombardi Cancer Center and also a NABCO Medical Advisory Board member, added, **"Progestins will protect the uterus, but I am personally unenthusiastic about their use."**.[788]

Further comment came from Dr. Elizabeth Barrett-Connor of the University of California, San Diego, who pointed out that whilst there was some protective gains from endometrial cancer, the increased risk of breast cancer was a serious issue, since **"uterine cancer is less common and less lethal than breast cancer"**.[789]

What Dr Barrett-Connor called into question is the wisdom of adding progestins to ERT to reduce the oestrogen-generated endometrial cancer, given that the price paid for a reduction in endometrial cancer is an increase in the breast cancer risk rates. This is an odious choice, particularly when the disease that is being made worse, breast cancer, is more common and more lethal than the endometrial cancer which the patient is seeking to avoid.

10.8   THE NURSES' STUDY OF 1995.

In June 1995 a major work was published in the prestigious *New England Journal of Medicine* by Dr Graham Colditz. This report is commonly known as the Nurses' Study. It is the most extensive and authoritative epidemiological analysis yet done on the health implications of HRT. The study began in 1976 and involved 725,550 person-years of follow-up investigation of the nurses enrolled as study subjects. Dr Colditz was seeking answers to questions about the safety of estrogen plus progestins, the risks of progestins alone, and the variations in risk associated with various ages groups of patients:

> **"We observed an elevated risk of invasive breast cancer among postmenopausal women who were currently taking estrogen alone or both estrogen and progestin…"**

furthermore,

> **"...our data ... suggest that the use of hormones at older ages after menopause may have a particularly deleterious effect on the risk of breast cancer.".**[790]

The use of the terms 'particularly deleterious' is powerful language not normally evident in medical journals. Describing a drug therapy as 'particularly deleterious' indicated an unshakeable certainty of mind on the part of the researchers. Their phraseology is a type of medical 'code' language designed to express absolute sureness, mingled with a measure of shock, but without recourse to the more emotive, over-worked cliches of newspaper or television journalism. From a review of the Nurses' Report, this approach by the researchers would seem justified.

Dr Colditz found that the risk of breast cancer was highest for the oldest women who had taken HRT. For women 65-69, the relative risk was 69% higher (RR 1.69) than that for women of the same age who had not taken HRT. For women 60-64 years, the increased risk was 42% (RR 1.42), for women 55-59 the risk was 41% higher (RR 1.41), and for women 50-54 years, the risk was 46% (RR 1.46). Further:

> **"The risk of breast cancer increased significantly only among women currently using hormone therapy who had used such therapy for five or more years.".**[791]

Dr Colditz found that the addition of progestin (a contentious topic of many years standing) did *not* increase the risk of breast cancer:

> **"For each stage of menopause, the relative risk of breast cancer was at least as high for women taking estrogen plus progestin as for those taking** (unopposed) **estrogen alone.".**[792]

Significantly, though, the addition of progestin did not decrease the breast cancer risks.

Readers may have observed that this particular finding from Dr Colditz is different from that of Dr. Bergkvist, who noted that combined therapy has a higher incidence of breast cancer than oestrogen alone. What can be made of this apparent conflict?

The answer is linked to the concept of *latent period* discussed earlier. As Dr Colditz (1995) noted, in America "**... widespread use of progestins is a recent phenomena,** (therefore) **we were unable to examine associations with risk according to the dose or duration of progestin use.".**[793] Hence insufficient time had elapsed for the true impact of progestins to express itself via an increase in breast cancer when compared to oestrogen-only users. In support of the relevance of the latent period, Dr Bergkvist (1989) noted that in Sweden, "**combination therapy has become more widely used in recent years.".** Therefore, in Sweden, the latent period might have allowed for the proper and fulsome expression of the deleterious, additive impact of progestins *and* oestrogens on breast tissue.

Despite this difference in results, the finding from Dr Colditz and his concluding comments are clear, sharp, and deserving of careful attention:

> "**The significant increase in the risks of breast cancer and of death due to breast cancer among postmenopausal women over 55 who are currently taking hormones and who have used this therapy for five years or more suggests that the risks and benefits of hormone therapy among older women should be carefully assessed.".**[794]

Interestingly, this cautionary view from Colditz has been reflected by other researchers who also see breast cancer as the 'risk' part of the 'risk-benefit' equation which a practitioner must assess prior to prescribing any medication.[795] [796]

Finally, it is instructive to convert the statistical concept of relative risk to a more person-centred assessment of risk. A woman contemplating the use of HRT needs to known what her absolute risk of breast cancer from HRT is. Colditz has provided this more meaningful assessment in a *Letter* to the *New England Journal of Medicine* (1995):

> "**For a 60-year-old woman who has never used hormones after menopause, for example, the risk of receiving a diagnosis of breast cancer during the next five years is 1.8 percent. If she has taken hormones for five years and continues to take them, the risk is 3 percent. Alternatively for every 80 women taking hormones for five years from the age of 60 to 65, 1** (one) **will receive a diagnosis of breast cancer.".**[797]

10.9   HEALTH TRADE-OFFS WITH HRT.

Two more results reported by Dr Colditz are deserving of consideration, as they are germane to the promotion of HRT. For example, the conclusions of earlier studies by Lafferty (1964), had cast doubt upon the bone-density benefits of HRT; Dr Colditz (1995) confirmed the veracity of this earlier cautious view:

> **"... short-term estrogen therapy - for up to seven years - in the decade after menopause *cannot* be expected to protect against osteoporotic fractures many years later."**[798] (emphasis added).

In a follow-up paper by Dr Golditz (1996), he advanced the argument against ERT as a presumed solution to the problem of postmenopausal hip fracture:

> **"The discussion of risks and benefits of the use of postmenopausal estrogen therapy typically includes consideration of breast cancer, heart disease and hip fracture. Recent data indicate that to obtain protection from hip fractures, women must take replacement hormone therapy into their 80s, as half of all hip fractures occur in women after age 80 and protection is lost within 7 years after stopping use of postmenopausal hormones."**.[799]

From this statement it is clear that any bone density benefits gained from ERT do not persist into later life if therapy is stopped. This finding has substantial medical implications because it suggests that the trade-off between a short-term gain in bone strength has to be carefully measured against a demonstrable increased risk of breast cancer.

Similarly, Dr Colditz (1996) sounded a note of caution with regard to the reduced risk of heart disease which may be derived from HRT. He also offered a variety of alternate approaches to address this problem, and that of postmenopausal hip fracture:

> **"The reduction in risk of heart disease seen among postmenopausal women is greatest for women who are currently**

taking postmenopausal hormones. The reduction in risk after stopping therapy is attenuated. Age is a key issue in considering the trade-offs. **We have reported that** *the adverse effects of estrogen is greater among older women and that the reduction in risk of heart disease is less among older women.* **This raises the question, "Should breast cancer be the price we pay for reduced risk of heart disease and fracture?" I believe that the answer is no. Alternate approaches to preventing heart disease are available (including not smoking, increasing physical activity, avoiding weight gain, and taking aspirin and vitamin E), but this is not so for breast cancer.**[800] (emphasis added).

The success of alternate, non-drug therapies suggested by Colditz had also been advocated by pharmacologists Goodman and Gilman (1990) as the better course of treatment for the majority of women:

> **"... since only 35%** (one third) **of menopausal patients develop significant osteoporosis and because exercise and increased intake of calcium is also effective, the routine use of estrogen is difficult to justify.".**[801]

Other researchers have also noted the positive impact of non- pharmaceutical interventions, such as diet and exercise, on osteoporosis in postmenopausal women, depending on when the therapy is initiated.[802 803]

If these facts were known by women, they may not be willing to accept the attendant risk. My own clinical experience indicates that many women are not aware of these risks and, when appraised of them, decline to use HRT, opting instead for the aforementioned alternate treatments.

Finally, and of much consolation for women who have been on HRT and have subsequently ceased the treatment, is the finding by Dr Colditz (1995) that the cancer risks wane over time. For those women who have taken HRT for less than 5 years, or have not taken HRT for more than two years, the risk of breast cancer is effectively the same as for women who have never taken HRT. [804] Time removed the risks associated with HRT.

10.10 THE RISK OF VENOUS THROMBOEMBOLISM (VTE) AND HRT.

As the reader will have noticed, research quoted thus far has highlighted the frequency with which HRT is promoted because of its capacity to reduce the incidence of heart disease. Whilst some contemporary research has suggested that this claim may still be valid,[805] reports in the *Lancet* and the *British Medical Journal* during 1996 and 1997 indicated that the prevalence of HRT-induced venous thromboembolisms (blood clots) and pulmonary embolism (PE - arterial lung clot) may tarnish the overall appeal of HRT from a cardiovascular perspective.

In October 1996, the *Lancet* carried an editorial on the findings from three research papers which investigated the role of HRT in venous thromboembolisms (VTE) and its related disease, pulmonary embolism (PE). [806] Commenting on that research, the editorial noted that whilst textbooks had previously advocated there was little risk of VTE from HRT, **"revisions about risk of venous thrombosis can be expected in new editions of textbooks.".**[807] The following are the salient conclusions from these three papers:

•   The risk of venous thromboembolism (VTE) was 260% greater in users of oestrogen-only HRT compared to non-users (RR 3.6, 95% CI 1.6-7.8).[808]

•   The risk of VTE increased with an increasing dose of oestrogen taken. The risks of VTE were 110%, 230% and 590% greater for 0.325mg, 0.625mg and 1.25mg use of oestrogen compared to non-users.[809]

•   The risk of VTE appeared to be **"highest amongst short-term current users.".**[810]

•   The risk of pulmonary embolism (PE) - a lung clot - was 110% greater for current users of postmenopausal hormones. Past use showed no associated risk of PE (RR 2.1 95% CI 1.2-3.8).[811]

These findings must be given thoughtful consideration. In particular, there is a question mark over the suitability of using ERT as a symptomatic short course therapy since the risk of VTE was highest at the start of the therapy. [812] As well, **"prescribing for purely preventive purposes** (of osteoporosis), **without clinical indications, should be underpinned by strong evidence of benefit.".**[813]

Confirming the findings published in the *Lancet* was a report in the *British Medical Journal* in March 1997. Briefly, this report noted that the odds ratio (a measure of increased risk) of VTE was 110% higher for users of HRT compared to non-users. This increased risk was only evident during the first year of use of HRT. Interestingly, the greatest risk for this group of women was during the first six months of use; during this time there was a 360% greater risk of VTE. The authors calculated that this increased risk would result in an additional one to two cases of VTE per 10,000 women per year.[814]

Further doubts regarding the possible cardio-protective effects of HRT were voiced in a review paper from Hemminki and McPherson (*Br Med J.,* 19th July, 1997). After the authors combined the results of 22 previously published trials, totalling 4,124 women, they concluded that the results from these studies **"do not support the notion that postmenopausal hormone therapy prevents cardiovascular events.".**[815]

The interim results of the Heart and Estrogen-Progestin Replacement Study (HERS) also indicate that the use of HRT is associated with an increased, not decreased incidence of venous thromboembolisms.[816] This notable study is due to conclude in mid 1998, with a final report soon thereafter.

As was the case with the pill and breast or cervical cancer, there is the ever-present question of 'how', at a cellular level, does HRT precipitate such serious health consequences as blood clots. A letter by Lowe, Rumley and co-workers (*Lancet ,*May 1997) addressed this fundamental issue. The authors suggested that activated protein-C (APC) resistance may be **"a common mechanism"** which linked risks factors such as HRT use to the formation of blood clots.[817] To recall, APC is a natural anticoagulant defence mechanism. If APC's effects are nullified by the use of HRT, the anticoagulant effect of APC is reduced. Blood coagulation, in the form of a DVT, is the manifest result.

10.11   NEW PHARMACEUTICAL ALTERNATIVES TO HRT IN THE MENOPAUSE.

With such a large body of research indicating major health-related problems with HRT, it is pleasing to report that there are non-hormonal drug therapies available for the prevention and/or the treatment of menopausal osteoporosis which is resistant to a diet and exercise program. The newest of these therapies is a drug known as a alendronate (Fosamax™).

Alendronate is classified as an aminobisphosphonate, a class of drugs which does not act on the female hormonal system.[818] It is preferentially taken up by the bone at sites where there is active bone turnover[819] and it acts to preserve or increase bone mass.[820] The medical literature has indicated that alendronate is superior in effect to other drugs which belong to the same drug class. **"As an inhibitor of bone resorption** (a process leading to osteoporosis)[821] [822] **alendronate is 200 to 1000 times more potent than etidronate or tiludronate.".**[823] The latter two drugs are earlier 'versions' of alendronate.

Clinical trials conducted to assess the efficacy of alendronate have been most encouraging. Liberman and co-workers (*NEJM,* 1995) reported an 8.8% improvement in bone mineral density (BMD) of the spine, 5.9% improvement in the femoral neck, 7.8% in the trochanter (pelvic end of the femur) and 2.5% in total body mass. They also reported a 48% reduction in the proportion of new cases of vertebral fracture.[824] This study was conducted over three years, using varying doses of 5,10 and 20 mg of alendronate.

Similarly, Adami and co-workers (*Bone* 1995) reported that at the end of a 2-year trial, which involved 286 postmenopausal women of Italian ethnicity, doses of 10 or 20 mg daily increased bone mass by 5.2% and 7.3% at the lumbar spine, 3.8% and 4.6% at the femoral neck, and 7.1% and 7.5% at the trochanter.[825]

A report in the *New England Journal of Medicine* (1995) by Sambrook also noted an 8% increase in lumbar bone density. This was achieved after 3 years of therapy with alendronate.[826] Similar positive results were announced by Karpf and co-workers in 1997. They analysed previously published data and concluded there was approximately a 30% reduction in the incidence of nonvertebral (non-spinal) fractures at various body sites, including the hip and wrist.[827]

Whilst these results convey a positive medical message, alendronate can only claim to be a valid treatment alternative if the improvements in bone density compare favourably with those attainted by HRT. What then is the magnitude of improvement in bone density from HRT?

One indicative study appeared in the *Journal of the American Medical Association* (1996) which reported a 3.5% to 5% gain in spinal BMD and a 1.7% increase in BMD in the hip with 3 years use of various HRT combinations.[828] Also supportive of HRT use in osteoporosis was the work from Eiken and co-workers (1996) who reported that *10 years* use of HRT increased lumbar (spinal) bone mineral density by 14.5% when compared to non-users. Also, femoral bone mineral content was **"20.3% higher in women who had received HRT than in those who had not received therapy at the end of the 10 year follow-up...These results confirm that long-term HRT exerts a continuous effect against bone loss in postmenopausal women.".**[829]

The results from Eiken (*Bone,* 1996) would appear superior to those cited for alendronate, and therefore authenticate the view that HRT is the premium drug therapy. Yet there are two problems with this 'claim'.

First, readers will recall that Colditz (1995) found an increased risk of breast cancer with only *five* or more years use of HRT. Thus, the gain in lumbar bone density reported by Eiken, whilst greater than that seen in the alendronate studies, was evident only after 10 years of HRT use. This BMD gain may have come at a high price. A pertinent question to keep in mind is whether this excess 'exposure time' to carcinogenic hormones was justified by the gains seen in bone strength?

Second, whilst of some broad clinical merit, the comparison of HRT and alendronate results from disassociated studies is less revealing than the results obtained from studies which compare the two osteoporosis drug therapies directly. In my view, study results obtained by this second direct method have greater medical integrity and patient applicability.

One such directly comparative study, not yet finalised, was published in August 1996 by Hocking and associates. The details of this study are set out in the end-notes.[830] Briefly, this study compared two groups of healthy postmenopausal women aged 45-59 years. The 1609 study subjects were divided into three groups, one took an estrogen/progestin combination, another received 2.5 or 5mg alendronate, the third received a placebo. At the end of 2 years of this 6 year study, bone mineral density (BMD) changes for the spine, hip and total body were measured and compared to the measurements prior to study commencement.

The best results were obtained from 5mg alendronate and the estrogen/progestin combination of 17-β-estradiol (1-2mg per day) and norethisterone (0.1mg per day). Alendronate 5mg improved BMD by 3.46% and the estrogen/progestin combination improved BMD by 5.14%. Possible drug-related side effects occurred in 2% of alendronate treated subjects and 11.8% of estrogen/progestin treated subjects. Given that these are interim results only, and the study will be 6 years in length, the choice between the two drug therapies is one of risks and benefits. HRT improved BMD by 1.6% more than alendronate but had nearly a 10% higher incidence of side-effects.[831] As well, the total length of the study, of six years, means that estrogen/progestin patients will move into the breast cancer 'at-risk' time-frame previously reported by Colditz (*NEJM*, 1995).

The decision to select either HRT and alendronate was made more difficult for both the clinician and patient with the April 1997 announcement that HRT:

> "... should increase the life expectancy of most women, with gains up to 41 months (a 15 per cent for women at greatest risk of CHD and lowest for breast cancer)... Approximately half the gains in life expectancy anticipated from lifelong therapy accrue after 10 years of treatment, and 75 per cent of gains accrue after 20 years.".[832]

Prior to this announcement it was the view of some researchers that:

> "... treatment with bisphosphonates may be an acceptable alternative to ovarian hormone therapy in increasing bone mass and decreasing fractures associated with osteoporosis. Compared with estrogens, biphosphonates are bone-tissue specific, have equal or greater antiresorptive effects and have few side-effects and no known risk for carcinogenesis.".[833]

Whilst the previously mentioned increase in life expectancy is positive news, it is relevant to highlight that it took 10 years use of HRT to acquire the first 20 months of this increased longevity. Thus the prior reference to the 'at-risk' time-frame is again pertinent. As Colditz has pointed out on another occasion,

> "The key question is not whether a woman who has ever used hormones has an increased risk of breast cancer, but rather how long a woman can use hormones before the risk is appreciably

elevated and how rapidly any excess risk decreases after she stops using hormones.".[834]

Until the final results from Hosking (*J Bone Miner Res,* 1996) are published four years hence, a definitive decision on the relative merits of the two competing drug therapies may have to wait. Given the dubious recent history of H.R.T., opting for alendronate, coupled with a diet designed to reduce cardio-vascular risk factors such as high cholesterol levels, plus the use of calcium supplements, and participation in age-appropriate exercise such as aqua-aerobics to aid in weight regulation and increase bone, muscle and ligament strength, would seem the more prudent course to take.

10.12 THE SOCIAL COST AND MEDICAL COSTS OF OSTEOPOROSIS.

The medical evidence has indicated that osteoporosis has a staggering impact on both individual suffering and also the cost to the national health budget. In Australia, it has been estimated that the median cost of hospital-treated fractures was $10,511 per event. The direct cost for the national health budget was $779 million.[835]

The situation in America is equally distressing. The medical literature has reported that there are almost 1.3 million fractures per year, with an estimated cost approaching $10 billion per year.[836] Moreover, these costs are expected to double in the next 25 years.[837] Thus there is a compelling need for remedial therapies that are both safe and have the public's confidence.

10.13 THE BENEFITS OF MENOPAUSE.

Clearly menopause should not be viewed as a disease state which arrives around age 50 and necessitates the unquestioning, almost sanguine instigation of hormonal therapy. Indeed other cultures, for example India, celebrate menopause as a time of freedom.[838] Menopause is a *natural* event in a woman's life, signifying change rather than deterioration.

Adding scientific authority to the cultural norms of Asian women has been the work of Key and Pike (1988) who concluded that there is a **"protective effect of**

menopause on breast cancer risk...".[839]   They amply justify this conclusion:

> **"The** (beneficial) **effect of menopause can be seen most clearly by looking at the age-incidence curve for breast cancer. When the logarithm of age is plotted against the logarithm of incidence the resultant 'curve' is approximately two straight lines: the increase in incidence with age is much steeper during the premenopausal period than after the menopause. This indicates that the hormonal pattern of premenopausal women** (cyclic production of relatively large amounts of oestradiol [E2] -the female oestrogen- and progesterone [Pg]) **causes a greater rate of increase in breast cancer than the hormonal pattern in postmenopausal women (constant low E2 and very low Pg).".**[840] (my clarifications)

A graphical adaptation of the above quote is set out in the following diagram. It is adapted from a log-log graph presented by Pike, Spicer and co-workers (*Epidemiologic Reviews,*1993).[841]

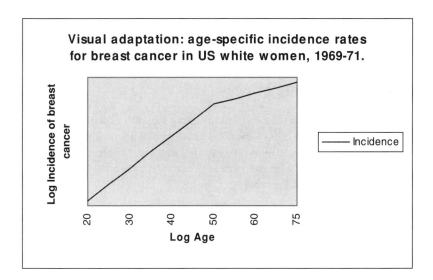

Explaining this graph, Pike (1993) and co-workers said:

> "Breast cancer incidence continues to increase with age but ...
> there is a distinct slowing of the rate of increase at around age
> 50, i.e., around the average age of menopause. This slowed rate of
> increase continues from about age 50 on. The important etiologic
> elements for breast cancer thus appear to be present in pre-
> menopausal women and to be sharply reduced following the
> menopause.".[842]

Pike (1993) noted that this observation was a **"profoundly important conclusion** (which) **has been verified by direct epidemiologic study"**.[843] The obvious
question is: 'What are these important "etiologic elements for breast cancer"
which present before but not after the menopause?.'

Pike (1993) addressed this issue thus:

> "The clear, undisputed protective effect of menopause, however,
> shows that if ovarian hormone levels are drastically reduced,
> breast cancer is reduced.".[844]

From this it can be seen that the absence of naturally produced estrogen and
progesterone during the menopause is associated with a reduction in the risk of
breast cancer. Conversely, **"postmenopausal women on estrogen replacement
therapy have twice the normal annual rate of incidence** (of breast cancer) **."**.[845]

A similar view was expressed by Rosner (1994).

> "The decrease in the rate of tissue aging seen after menopause
> is consistent with the observation that, at a given age, women who
> are premenopausal, and thus exposed to higher levels of endo-
> genous female hormones, are at greater risk than postmeno-
> pausal women of the same age.".[846]

Further validation for the views of Key (1988), Pike (1993) and Rosner (1994) was
forthcoming from Dr. Graham Colditz (1995), who reported that both an **"early
age at menarche and late menopause increase the risk of breast cancer"**.[847]

The significance of these two co-factors for post-menopausal breast cancer rates must not be overlooked. Early menarche will expose a young woman's breast tissue to more years of naturally produced hormones than that of a woman who began menstruation at the 'average' age. Similarly, the late onset of menopause means that a woman's breast tissue is exposed to the effects of naturally produced hormones for longer than that of a woman who entered the menopause at an 'average' age.

Similar findings have been reported by T.J.Key (1995) of the Imperial Cancer Research Fund, Oxford. Whilst acknowledging that the role of hormones on breast tissue in non-pregnant women is not as well understood as their effects on the endometrium, Key could still state that:

> "... **both oestrogen and progestins appear to stimulate mitosis** (cell division). **Breast cancer risk increases with early menarche, late menopause and oestrogen replacement therapy, probably due to increased exposure of the breast to oestrogen and/or progesterone.**",[848]

A more recent paper by Dr Colditz (1996) separately analysed these two predictive factors. First he reported that:

> "**For every year of decline in age at menarche** (the younger menstruation began), **the rate of breast cancer among women increases by 20 cases per 100,000 women per years.**".[849]

Second, Dr Colditz reported on his own research which showed that, **"after adjusting for other breast cancer risk factors, the increase in risk of breast cancer with each year of delay in age at menopause was 1.03."**.[850] This means that for each year of delay *before* a woman enters menopause, her breast cancer risk *rises* by 3% per annum. Other researchers cited by Dr Colditz uncovered similar trends. For example, a 32 % reduction in breast cancer risk was reported for women entering menopause at age 35-39 compared to women with natural menopause at age 45-54.[851]

Work by Ewertz (*Eur J Surg,*1996) of Denmark is in harmony with that of Key (1993,1995) and Colditz (1996). Specifically, **"the age-specific incidence of female breast cancer suggests that the menopause has a *protective* effect."**[852] (emphasis added).

Based upon the preceding evidence it would seem that the promotion of various forms of HRT to healthy women deprives these same women of what may otherwise have been a healthier future. This makes it very difficult to understand the remark of Prof. Wren at the beginning of this chapter.

10.14 KEY POINTS.

1. Diet and exercise are sufficient preventative treatment for osteoporosis for two thirds of women.

2. Only one third of women may require HRT to treat or prevent osteoporosis.

3. A natural menopause is safer than a menopause with HRT.

4. ERT and HRT are associated with a greater risk of breast and endometrial cancer, as well as VTE.

5. Cancer rates increase with age for women on HRT.

6. Risks incurred from previous use of HRT wane over time.

7. Improvements in bone density from HRT are lost within 7 years after stopping postmenopausal HRT.

8. The use of HRT to reduce the risk of heart disease is questionable, in part because of the increased risk of breast cancer, and also because positive results can be achieved solely by life-style modifications.

9. Non-hormonal drug therapies now exist which successfully treat osteoporosis, without the fear of cancer or blood clots.

CHAPTER ELEVEN.

11.   INFORMED CONSENT & PATIENT SOVEREIGNTY.

"It is a government requirement that all information supplied by pharmaceutical companies about their products be approved by the Therapeutic Goods Administration."[853]

11.1   INTRODUCTION.

The whole of this book has had as its focus the question of patient sovereignty. This is a legal term which has been described as the **"the provision of information sufficient to allow a patient to make informed decisions about treatment(s)".**[854] It is also a relatively new term which has been coined to reflect the shift in the legal definition of 'duty of care' away from what a doctor may do to what a patient has a right to be told (*Rogers v Whitaker* 1992,175 CLR 479).[855]   Female drug therapies are examples in which patient sovereignty and informed consent exist more in name than in observance.

This final chapter will analyse the processes by which drug information is collated, vetted and disseminated to those in the medical and health care professions, the media, and most importantly, to women, the consumers of sexual and reproductive medicines. Particular attention will be focused on the role of Australian Government health instrumentalities in this process: a pivotal reference point in understanding the mechanisms involved in the generation of drug information. To underscore current deficiencies in this process, examples will be presented to substantiate the view that, currently, the provision of accurate *and* contemporary drug information in the province of female sexual and reproductive health is seriously inadequate.

As a related issue, this chapter also discusses certain problems in the presentation and interpretation of research reports. Specifically, I will highlight problems emanating from scientific review papers, as well as the frequent practice of 'pooled data' analysis. Statistical concepts such as 'overall results' and 'category-specific results' will also be explained - a benefit for both the lay and medical reader - since problems of interpretation and understanding arise in these areas as well. Discussion of such statistical methods and their application or understanding is not a tedious digression; rather, it highlights the way in which the profitable flow of drug information from the original source of scientific investigation can be impeded. The result, as we shall see, is that the consumer of medicines is deprived of vital drug information germane to the informed decision making process. Also, a brief word will be said on the relevance of drug/animal studies to humans.

Finally, some comment must be made on the role of the media in drug information dissemination, the need for specialist medical journalists, and examples of certain lapses in judgement by the media which have resulted in a diminished level of informed public debate, a resultant loss of patient sovereignty over drug information, and an undermining of the decision-making process.

11.2   PI AND CPI LEAFLETS.

The starting point for all officially approved drug information in Australia is when a pharmaceutical company submits data on the drug for which it seeks approval, together with a draft version of the attendant product information (PI). These two sets of data are submitted to the Government department known as the Therapeutic Goods Administration (TGA) for evaluation. The TGA could reasonably be equated in role and responsibility to the American Food and Drug Authority (FDA). The TGA is advised by a committee of experts known as the Australian Drug Evaluation Committee (ADEC). The role of ADEC is multifaceted. It assesses the veracity of drug information given to it by pharmaceutical manufacturers who are seeking to have a drug licensed for distribution or, alternately, to have the list of approved indications for a drug altered. Further, it reviews pre-existing approved product information (PI) in the light of any new revelations from ongoing clinical use of a currently prescribed drug. ADEC also has the authority to make 'recommendations' to the TGA if the approved product information (PI) requires variation as a result of newly discovered adverse drug reactions reported in the medical literature. A manufacturer may appeal a recommendation of ADEC, but ultimately, the TGA has the 'final legal word'. With the pronouncement of the 'final word' by the TGA, the approved product information (PI) becomes a legal document which cannot be altered in any way without TGA approval. Once approval is given, all printed and spoken words on a drug *must* be based on the approved PI.

The approved PI is published in such texts as *MIMS Annual* and the *Australian Prescription Products Guide* (*APPG*):

> **"It is a government requirement that all information supplied by pharmaceutical companies about their products be approved by the Therapeutic Goods Administration. At the present time (Nov 1995) this does not apply to long established products, many of the traditional remedies supplied OTC or alternate medicine products...The policy adopted by the APPG, is that product information approved by the TGA is reproduced in full with just sufficient editing to provide relatively standard format.".**[856]

It is upon the contents of the PI in these books that many doctors, pharmacists and nurses make clinical decisions. The approved PI is the principle source of drug information for these health-care professionals.

As well, the approved PI is the primary source of information for consumers, albeit translated into a more 'user-friendly' style of writing known as a consumer product information leaflet (CPI). This 'lay' presentation does not mean that the consumer product information (CPI) leaflet represents a variation of the approved PI. Indeed, by law, changes in content or context from that of the approved PI are *not* permitted in the CPI. The CPI leaflet must be an accurate distillation of the PI, without omissions or inclusions that have not been approved by the TGA . The CPI shall not be inconsistent with the PI. No divergence from this protocol is permitted.

The provision of the CPI leaflet is a relatively new legal requirement in Australia. This law states that all new drugs approved for prescribing after January 1, 1993, must contain the relevant approved CPI. For drugs which pre-existed the legislation, the inclusion of a CPI is not required until 2001. Many drugs in this latter 'old' category, including the majority of formulations of the pill, contain a package insert of information derived from the approved PI, with all the attendant legal requirements associated with the PI. This leaflet may simply be called a 'package insert'.

CPI leaflets are given out by a pharmacist at the time of dispensing and therefore act as a principal source of drug information for the patient. CPI leaflets act to inform or deform the decision-making process commensurate with the level of accurate, contemporary information they contain. The nexus between the government-approved PI, the CPI leaflet and informed decision making is thus of critical importance.

To summarize: there are two main avenues by which consumers receive drug information: first, via a health care professional's use of such texts as *MIMS* or the *Australian Prescription Products Guide* when answering questions from a patient, and second, via patient receipt of CPI leaflets at the time of dispensing from the pharmacist.

11.2.1 CPI ON THE PILL.

In the author's opinion, the two following examples of deficient or erroneous product information (PI) highlight the extent to which a woman's perception of the medical reality of the pill can be distorted, since it is from the approved PI that the pill CPI leaflets are 'generated'.

The 1996 and 1997 approved product information (PI) for Triphasil® 28 & 21, Biphasil® 28 & 21 , Nordette® 28 & 21, Nordiol 28®, Nordette® 50/28 (Wyeth Pharmaceuticals) and Trifeme® (Ayerst Pharmaceuticals), stated:

> **"Long-term continuous administration of either synthetic or natural oestrogen in certain animal species increases the frequency of carcinoma of the breast, cervix, vagina, and liver. At present, there is no confirmed evidence from human studies which would indicate that an increased risk of cancer is associated with oral contraceptives. Close clinical surveillance is nevertheless essential in all women taking these drugs."**[857] [858]

As well, the 1996 and 1997 approved product information (PI) for Microgynon® 30 ED, Levlen ED®, Logynon ED®, Triquilar® ED & 21 (Schering AG,Germany) stated:

> **"Oestrogens administered long-term to certain animal species increase the frequency of carcinoma of the breast, cervix, vagina**

and liver. Certain other progestogens increase the incidence of mammary nodules, benign and malignant, in dogs, and of endometrial carcinoma in monkeys.".[859 860]

Bearing in mind the aforementioned derivative link between the approved PI and the CPI (or its antecedent, the patient information package insert), it is instructive to reflect upon the CPI leaflets for these same products All the pill formulations made by Ayerst/Wyeth and Schering (and listed in the two following endnotes) contain patient leaflets which are identical on the question of carcinogenicity:

"Although some components of oral contraceptives have been associated with the development of cancer when given continuously to certain animals, there is no evidence that they have such an effect in humans.".[861 862]

It can be seen that these pill CPI leaflets accurately present the information in the approved PI. Thus the requirements of the legislation are fulfilled. Simultaneously however these CPI leaflets are, in the author's opinion misleading in view of the scientific evidence.

First, they tend to imply that the data acquired from animal studies have no health bearing for women. This is a nonsense which is addressed more fully later in this chapter. Second, it wrongly informs the reader that no scientific evidence exists to substantiate a link between "some components of oral contraceptives" and cancer.

In light of the preceding chapters it is difficult to understand how a CPI leaflet could be officially authorized for publication when it contains such an inaccurate assessment of the last thirty years of medical research. It is a statement at stark variance with the medical facts. The amount of research which must have been ignored by ADEC is evident from this and the preceding chapters. As a reflection of the medical research, Wyeth-Ayerst's and Schering's CPI statements, assessed by ADEC and approved by the TGA, are *non sequiturs par excellence*. Researchers whose work can only have been ignored in the formulation of the approved PI and the CPI documents — Olsson, Ranstam, Brinton, Pike, Henderson, Ursin, Beral, Chilvers, Key, King, Brock, Hunt, Vessey, La Vecchia, Meirik, Rookus, Whittlemore, Gray—[863] are numerous.

Paradoxically, in the same Schering CPI leaflet there is the reassuring advice that: **"the information contained in it is continually being brought up to date."**.[864] In my view this statement implies (a) that the publication at the time was an accurate document and (b) the manufacturers are assiduously endeavouring to maintain this position. Yet we have already seen in this book that information given to women about female drug therapies is anything but up-to-date. It would be more accurate in my view to describe this information as selective in content and prejudicial to good health.

The TGA, were it to apply more rigorous standards, would ensure that these publications not only meet statutory legal requirements, but are also accurate and reliable documents *devoid of error*. This it has not done in the case of the Ayerst/Wyeth and Schering material. In the interests of public health, a regulatory body must ensure that there is a candid presentation of all the relevant information, including what is known, what is uncertain and what is doubtful or debatable.

Currently the PI material or CPI leaflets do not score well from any of these perspectives. In addition, the poor quality of the PI & CPI statements casts doubt on the calibre of the material submitted to the TGA by pharmaceutical manufacturers in the initial instance.

11.2.2 ANIMAL STUDIES AND THE RELIABILITY OF APPROVED INFORMATION.

In view of adverse references to animal studies in the pill CPI and other researcher material,[865] it is important that some comments on this subject be made. There is a convincing level of agreement amongst research experts on the merits of using animal studies as an indicative guide to a drug's potential to harm humans. The American and Australian 'Drugs in Pregnancy' guidelines (see appendices 4 and 5) are clearly predicated on the sure knowledge that animal studies can be relied upon to assess the embryotoxicity and teratogenicity of any given drug. It is against this background that a critical appraisal of the approved product information (PI) can be made.

The approved product information (PI) for Trioden® ED, Femoden® ED, Minulet® and Triminulet® - all of which contain gestodene - states, under the heading of carcinogenesis and mutagenesis, that:

"Pre-clinical studies revealed an increased incidence of mammary and hepatic (liver) **tumours in gestodene-treated rats. The reason for such increases is unknown. The relationship of this finding to the development of similar tumours in women using gestodene has not been established.".**[866]

A number of questions arise from this statement. First, why were rats used as 'test models' if the finding could not be relied upon to have a certain and pre-defined relevance to humans? Second, if the results from rats could not be extrapolated from one species to another, why were the tests not done on animals which would yield meaningful data? Third, why are animal studies held to be valid and meaningful in some circumstances— i.e., when treating medical diseases such as endometriosis[867]— but deemed purposeless if the drug is the pill?

The TGA's endorsement of this statement for Trioden® ED, Femoden® ED, Minulet® and Triminulet® as a scientifically valid conclusion to animal studies reflects a coy uncertainty which is inconsistent with the 'expert committee' status of ADEC, the TGA's advisory body. This style of opaque inconclusiveness has the effect of casting doubt on the validity of animal studies as an authentic branch of medical research, and the veracity of information acquired by these studies.

The whole process of drug-evaluation tests is both baffling and bizarre. What can doctors, pharmacists, the media and women realistically conclude from reading information like the above? That rats are at risk but women aren't? Or that rats are at risk and so are women, but we don't know why? Or that rats aren't at risk but women are? If clarity is a virtue in the dissemination of medical information, then this material is an example of an unacceptable standard. One wonders if this sort of standard would be tolerated in any other area of medicine.

Those who approved this product information on animal studies would gain substantially from acquainting themselves with a selection of research papers on the important topic of animal research, especially that of R.J.B. King, M.Sc., Ph.D., D.Sc., of the Imperial Cancer Research Fund, Human Breast Biology Group, University of Surrey (United Kingdom). On animal research broadly, King stated: **"The relevance of experimental studies in rodents to man is often questioned but, in this author's opinion, a case has been established for their**

inclusion.".[868]

Alternatively, an earlier work by J. T. Casagrande and co-workers in the area of ovarian cancer would be instructive. These researchers noted that animal studies in rats and mice **"support"** a key hypothesis about the cause of ovarian cancer in infertile women.[869] Other research papers by many other scientists also testify to the validity of extrapolating from animal studies and applying their findings to human gynaecology.[870 871 872 873 874]

11.2.3 APPROVED INFORMATION ON FERTILITY DRUGS.

It is not just the various forms of patient information material for the pill which are deficient in their medical content. The patient information on fertility drugs also deserves remedial review in at least two major areas.

First, neither the approved product information (PI) or a patient information brochure, *'Clomid - A Guide for Women',* published by Marion Merrell Dow (1993),[875] explicitly makes mention of Clomid's potential to work against conception. This side-effect of a fertility drug may surprise some, since it is in conflict with the *raison d'etre* of the drug therapy. Yet the international medical literature documents this consequence. The mechanism by which clomiphene works *against* conception is two-fold:

> **"1. UNFAVOURABLE CERVICAL MUCUS, defined as a decrease in the quality or quantity of cervical mucus, may result from the use of CLOMIPHENE (Randall & Templeton, 1991).** *These effects may be related to treatment failure in some patients.*

and further:

> **2. ANTIESTROGENIC EFFECTS of CLOMIPHENE on the uterus may include the absence of an increase in uterine volume and an inhibition of endometrial thickening, both of which are processes that would normally occur during the follicular phase. These antiestrogenic effects have been observed in normally ovulating study subjects in comparison with untreated ovulatory cycles, and** *these effects could be related to treatment failure in some patients* **(Eden et al, 1989)."**[876] (Italics only added).

Put more simply, clomiphene (Clomid®) may cause (a) detrimental changes to the cervical mucus needed to assist fertilization, and (b) structural alterations to the cellular nature of the endometrium, making implantation problematical. On this first point the Clomid booklet merely notes, whilst instructing the reader on the mucus observation method of fertility monitoring that **"Clomid can alter the characteristics of cervical mucus in some women."**[877] Informing a woman that Clomid may interfere with her 'reading' of the changes in cervical mucus does not equate with the greater imperative of informing her that these drug-induced changes may act as an impediment to conception. The Clomid booklet is silent on point (b).

The second deficiency to be found in some of the approved product inform-ation (PI) of fertility drugs (the primary source of information for doctors and pharmacists) is the less than universal recognition that fertility drugs have been linked to a number of fatalities (see chapter eight). As previously mentioned, one of the adverse consequences of fertility drugs is their capacity to cause gross enlargement of the ovaries, known as ovarian hyperstimulation synd-rome (OHSS), **"a common complication"**, which has been reported as the secondary cause of more than one fatality.[878] The approved product inform-ation for Clomid®, Pregnyl®, and Pergonal® notes that OHSS can occur but fails to then inform the reader of the nexus between OHSS and documented fatalities. There is no inference that these products were specifically respon-sible for the reported fatalities — in fact the *Lancet* (1995) paper only refers to IVF treatments — nonetheless, since the common thread between the drugs named above and the fatalities was the occurrence of OHSS, a woman contemplating IVF treatments would make a more informed decision if she was aware of this significant health implication.

Only the approved product information for Profasi®,[879] Humegon®,[880] Metrodin® [881] and APL Injections® [882] informs the reader that the drug can ca-use OHSS and that OHSS is serious, may be occasionally life-threatening and is sometimes fatal. Indeed the PI for Metrodin® is commendably candid: it sets out the 3 grades of OHSS as determined by the WHO Technical Report Series No.514. This style of product information represents a standard of health care deserving of imitation.

The overriding concern with some of the approved product information and the Clomid 'booklet' is that they circumvent two issues which are indispensable to a woman's capacity for informed decision-making: *Does it work?* and *Is it safe?* Women need this information so that they can weigh it, first, against the other significant problems with fertility drugs which *are* listed in both the approved literature and the patient booklet, and, second, against the pregnancy rate of clomiphene therapy, which is only 21%.[883]

To omit discussion of such fundamental issues makes the patient's judgment a meaningless operation, since the decision is not based on all the facts. It is an understatement to observe that the welfare of women would be best served if a greater level of frankness were evident in these publications.

11.2.4   CPI ON HORMONE REPLACEMENT THERAPY.

A review of the CPI leaflets for a variety of HRT products reveals that there are a number of shortcomings in the information contained within the packets of many of the products which have been on the market for some years. The same cannot be said of the newer products. On occasion they are encyclopedic in their attention to detail: a positive advancement for women's health.

In my opinion, the CPI leaflet for Provelle® (last officially reviewed on 10th October 1995), Menoprem®, (last approved by the Department of Health on 20th December 1995), Premarin® (last revised on 17 January 1996) and Menorest® (updated on 7th February 1995) are not contemporary in terms of their comprehensive and appropriate reflection of recent cancer research.

For example, these CPI leaflets do not explain why some women on oestrogen replacement therapy (those who have *not* had a hysterectomy) should also take a progestagen supplement. As was discussed in Chapter Ten, these women need a progestagen to protect the uterus from endometrial cancer associated with 'unopposed' oestrogen therapy. The Menorest®, Premarin ®, Provelle® and Menoprem® CPI leaflets make only unspecific reference to the need for a progestagen to protect the uterus. But from what? The answer 'uterine cancer' is forthcoming in the Estraderm®, Trisequens®, Climen®, Climara® and Ogen® CPI leaflets. Indeed, on this point all five CPI leaflets are commendably candid.

When informing women of the risks of breast cancer from HRT the same complement cannot be bestowed on *any* of the CPI leaflets listed above, with the exception of Trisequens® (which was last officially reviewed in May 1993).

It informs its readers that **"Cancer of the breast or lining of the womb, blood clots and changes in liver function have been reported with hormone replacement therapy.".**[884] With the exception of Trisequens®, all other CPI leaflets have failed to note the significant findings of either Bergkvist (1989) or Colditz (June, 1995) on breast cancer.

One caveat must apply to my favourable opinion of the Trisequens® CPI leaflet. Immediately following the above quote is the statement: **"Trisequens and Trisequens Forte are not likely to increase the risk significantly of any of these conditions.".**[885] In my view this statement is without scientific or logical foundation. For these reasons this sentence should be removed, as it can only act to confuse and undermine the process of informed decision making by women.

It may be argued that the work by Colditz (1995) was published after the last review date of many of the CPI leaflets—hence the absence of all reference to his research. This, in my opinion, is a spurious defence. If the purpose of the CPI leaflet is to educate and inform women, then the deficient CPI leaflets should have been updated *when* the Colditz study was published. As previously pointed out, the Colditz study was the most comprehensive and lengthy study of the health impact of HRT to date. It merits suitable acknowledgment.

An excuse predicated on the inadequate availability of pertinent epidemiological data cannot be proffered in the case of the research of Bergkvist (1989). To recall: this study found a 340% risk increase of breast cancer for HRT users when compared to never-users. Of course the risks revealed by this study can be ignored, as they have been by most CPI authors, but only at the expense of the informed consent of all women unfamiliar with Bergkvist's findings. A decrease in health is the price women will pay for the exclusion of this vital medical information.

All the aforementioned CPI leaflets more than adequately explain many of the unpleasant side-effects women might experience from HRT, and they all strongly advise against a woman using the product if there is a history of *any* breast irregularity: lumps, cysts, nodes or abnormal mammograms. Yet it is puzzling that only one CPI leaflet makes reference either directly or obliquely to HRT's potential as a *cause* of breast cancer. It is as though the comprehensive research by Bergkvist and Colditz had never taken place.

Of the aforementioned CPI leaflets, the Estraderm® leaflet most comprehensively informs its readers that there are many unanswered questions and unproven benefits with regard to HRT and osteoporosis:

> **"We know that taking oestrogens after the menopause slows down bone loss and reduces bone thinning but we do not know what the long term effects are in terms of preventing fractures. Bone strength is helped by proper diet and exercise.".**[886]

If the Estraderm® CPI were to incorporate the findings from Colditz and Bergkvist, or if the Trisequens® CPI were to incorporate more material on the doubtful long-term merits of HRT in osteoporosis, and delete the sentence which exempts itself as a potential carcinogenic/thrombotic/liver-damaging agent, then these CPI leaflets would be models for other leaflet providers. Alternately, if Climen®, Climara® and Ogen® incorporated a recognition of the role of HRT in breast cancer, they too would be models worthy of imitation, particularly because of the all-encompassing list of side-effects, precautions and contraindications they contain.

The least informative leaflet is that of Menorest®. It only lists headache or dizziness, local skin reactions, nausea, breast tenderness or enlargement and irregular vaginal bleeding as side-effects. Unlike the other CPI's, it fails to mention vaginal thrush infections, weight gain, visual impairment, intolerance to contact lenses, retention of fluid or cystitis-like symptoms. These significant omissions impede informed decision-making by women—hence this CPI requires a serious and comprehensive re-evaluation. The previously mentioned legal implications for manufacturers who do not attend to these issues may be substantial.

11.3   FAMILY PLANNING ASSOCIATION MATERIAL.

Another source of misinformation, which could not have been published without T.G.A. approval, is a glossy 'Q & A' booklet prepared by the *Family Planning Association (NSW)* and presented by Wyeth Aust. Pty/Ltd:

"Q. Does the pill cause certain cancers?

A. There is no evidence at the present time that the pill can cause any cancer in a woman's body.

The largest study investigating any link between the pill and breast cancer is being carried out in the United States. It has not shown any increased risk of breast cancer from pill taking before 25 years of age, even if there is a late age for first pregnancy.".[887]

The FPA's statement is at variance with a vast quantity of contemporary and historical evidence which affirms the link between OCs and breast cancer (see chapter two). Thus, the F.P.A. booklet does much to undermine the authority and prestige of those who prepared it, and little to advance the cause of informed decision-making on the part of women.

Aside from the carcinogenic capacity of the pill which has been ignored, this booklet also conflicts with a large body of reputable research on break-through ovulation (see Van der Vange 1988, Corson 1993, and chapter one for discussion of this concept).

Q. "How does the pill work?

A. "When taken every day according to the instructions, the pill prevents the body producing hormones which normally stimulate the ovary to release an egg. Therefore, no egg is released from the ovary.".[888]

Is this error important? According to *holistic pharmaceutical practice* (also known as holistic health care), it is. Holistic theory states that medical care should be all-encompassing and mindful of the total person, including their **"physical, emotional, social, economic and spiritual needs"**[889] and not just those of a medical nature. The FPA booklet inadequately attends to this philosophical basis of medical practice.

The principles which underpin holistic pharmaceutical care have been the substance of an article by Ross Evans, a correspondent to *Pharmacy Connection*, the official journal of the Ontario College of Pharmacists (1995). Mr Evans discussed holistic pharmaceutical care in the context of the inaccurate

use of the term 'contraception' as applied to the 'morning-after' pill. His central
message is equally applicable to all areas of female drug therapy:

> "... pharmaceutical care of the 90s should be concerned with the
> overall wellbeing of the patient...(therefore) the name emergency
> 'contraception' is misleading and potentially deleterious to the
> pharmaceutical care of the patient. An emergency 'contracept-
> ion' patient may be subject to prolonged psychological and
> emotional trauma if they understand the Yuzpe (post-coital)
> regimen as a contraceptive method that prevents conception, then
> discover that it in fact is an abortifacient that prevents contin-
> ued development of an already fertilized ovum... Educating the
> patient on pharmaceutical matters is to enable the patient to ma-
> ke knowledgeable decisions ...
>
> Is misleading our patients not an example of poor pharmaceut-
> ical care ...? Why were potentially ethical implications not
> included when they can play a major role in a particular patient's
> care? This could be especially valuable to the pharmacist who
> has no convictions against any early abortive attempts but
> encounters a patient who does.".[890]

11.3.1   MORE MISLEADING MEDICAL INFORMATION.

The erroneous nature of the FPA material is not an isolated example of unreliable
presentation of medical information. Publications from Organon Pharmaceuticals,
the manufacturers of Marvelon®, and a 'Q & A' booklet from Schering Pty. Ltd.
are cases in point. What makes these two examples unique is that they are
unmistakably glossy, marketing brochures. The Organon material is aimed at
doctors, whilst the Schering material is written for patients. Both are ancillary to
the legally required PI and CPI leaflets, but nonetheless they would still require
approval from the TGA. In their defence it might be suggested that they exist to
enhance their respective audiences' understanding of their associated drugs.
This is a laudable ideal, were it not for the errors contained therein. Consider the
following:

Organon's literature states that 60ug per day of desogestrel, the progestin component of Marvelon®,"is sufficient to achieve 100% ovulation inhibition".[891]

At face value this claim would have much significance for certain groups of women, notably - but not exclusively - those of a Judeo-Christian or Islamic tradition. These and other women's groups could well have a moral objection to the abortifacient nature of the currently prescribed oral 'contraceptives'. Hence, they might see some merit in a drug which is promoted on the basis of its capacity to completely stop ovulation. If ovulation is always stopped, then fertilization cannot take place and there is no possibility for a pill-induced abortion to occur. If the Organon claim were accurate, Marvelon® would appear to have a clear moral and marketing advantage, since the drug does not possess an interceptive/early abortive capacity.

Regretfully, the claim from Organon is in my view scientifically unsupportable. The company has based its boast upon the flimsiest of research outcomes: the complete suppression of ovulation proclaimed by Organon was achieved with the dose of 60ug of desogestrel in only *one* women and in only *one* cycle.[892] A reading of the original scientific paper will show that Organon selectively quoted out of context and presented the data inaccurately. I see no scientific basis which would imply that this individual result can have any relevance to every woman.

The universalisation of a single test result in one woman is an invalid extra-polation of unjustifiable proportions. The result from this one trial could have occurred entirely by chance and have had nothing to do with the ingestion of desogestrel, a point originally made by Prof. Rahwan of Ohio University, Dept of Pharmacology & Toxicology (private correspondence).

Another unacceptable approach to information dissemination (and holistic pharmaceutical care) is adopted by Schering Pty Ltd, the manufacturers of Trioden® and Femoden®. In a booklet entitled *'Modern Oral Contraceptives - Your Questions Answered'* and dated Jan '95 we were presented with the following:

Q. "Are there any side-effects"

A. "The pill is one of the most thoroughly tested and widely prescribed prescription medicines... However, some women should not use the pill (for example those who suffer from certain forms of cancer).".[893]

As a statement of the obvious, this quote is commendable: cancer-promoting drugs should not be administered to cancer sufferers! But as a statement which properly reflects the pill's carcinogenic capacity in women who don't *currently* suffer from cancer, it is from an educative perspective devoid of any meaning. Healthy women need to know if their health is at risk.

11.4   DOUBLE STANDARDS IN PUBLIC HEALTH: TOBACCO, THE PILL AND TOXIC SHOCK SYDROME.

Yet the role of government goes beyond the validation and approval of PI and CPI. There is now a demand from all levels in the community for a more pro-active approach to public health. This is exemplified by the universal accept-ance of the important role of preventative medicine in both lowering costs and improving health outcomes. Government response to tobacco related disease and toxic shock syndrome (TSS) are but two examples which can be cited. Sadly, a response to the risks of the pill is yet to be seen.

Government response to the risks of tobacco consumption has taken a wide and far-reaching approach. Advertising of cigarette smoking is no longer permitted in the media, either directly via advertisements or indirectly via sporting events tagged with the name of a tobacco manufacturer. Cigarette manufacturers are legally compelled to print large warnings on the packet containing the cigar-ettes, informing the user that smoking is detrimental to health, or will affect the unborn child, or will reduce a person's fitness. Beyond this, society further seeks to protect its youth by imposing heavy fines on retailers who are guilty of selling cigarettes to persons under 16 years of age. As well, there are distance restrictions on shop signs promoting cigarettes if a shop is in proximity to a school.

Clearly, society rightly perceives that marketing dangerous products to a 'young' market is both morally reprehensible and physically injurious. The risks to the health of teenagers takes precedence over all other considerations including financial ones. Added to this are the growing number of restrictions on smoking in airplanes and restaurants specifically because of the risks associated with passive smoking.

The basis for such public health policies against tobacco includes the following list of serious health risks:

11.4.1 HEALTH RISKS RELATED TO SMOKING.

•   The risk of developing fatal prostate cancer is **34%** higher in smokers versus non-smokers.[894]

•   The risk of developing lung cancer due to passive smoking (inhaling airborne smoke) is **24%** higher than for persons not exposed to environmental tobacco smoke.This data was classified as **"strong and consistent evidence."**.[895]

•   The risk of developing lung cancer from cigar or pipe smoking is **160%-480%** greater than for non-smokers. The risk due to cigarette smoking varies from a low of **130%** (1-9 cigarettes per day) to **510%** (30-39 cigarettes per day). [896]

•   The risk of foetal limb deformities is **26%** increased for babies of mothers who smoked whilst pregnant.[897]

•   The risk of developing breast cancer is **26%** greater for smokers than for non-smokers.[898]

These percentages stand in stark comparison to the significantly higher percentage increase risks of consuming the pill. Some of these risks include:

11.4.2 HEALTH RISKS RELATED TO THE PILL.

•   The risk of breast cancer for young women is **200% - 480%** higher than for non-pill users.[899] [900]

•   The risk of cervical cancer for women aged less than 20 years is **280%** greater; for women aged 20-24 years is **70%** greater, and for women aged 25-29 years is **40%** greater when compared to non-users.[901]

•   The risk of DVT from third-generation progestagen versions of the pill is **600% - 900%** higher compared to non-users of the pill.[902]

- The incidence of major neonatal malformations is **26%** greater in off-spring prenatally exposed to female sex hormones.[903]

Whilst these figures present a convincing case to support the view that the pill is substantially riskier than smoking, there is scant evidence to suggest that the laudable health warnings on cigarette packs, such as "Smoking when pregnant will harm your baby", "smoking causes lung cancer" or "smoking reduces your fitness", will be mirrored by health pronouncements on the outside of packets of the pill alluding to that product's carcinogenic or thrombo-embolic characte-ristics. Until medical warnings are printed on the external facing of the pill packet, criticism of the Australian Department of Health's policy in this matter is both necessary and valid. Many women's lives continue to be placed at risk whilst these warnings are absent.

One of the most striking facts to emerge from the research on the pill, as we ha-ve seen, has been the marked susceptibility of young pill users to its ill effects, particularly breast cancer. The younger women are when they start taking the pill, the larger the tumours and the worse the prognosis. For these reasons their situation deserves a special and separate response from government, specifi-cally on what is disseminated in the CPI leaflets and other approved informat-ion sources.

The laudable approach to cigarette smoking is not an isolated example of right-minded paternalism. The swift reactions of health ministers to the deaths in 1995 of three young women from tampon-induced TSS reveals a similarly respon-sible attitude towards the dissemination of essential information to those entit-led to it. The then Minister for Family Services, Senator Rosemary Crowly, ord-ered an inquiry into the quality of materials incorporated into tampons.[904] The then Australian Minister for Health, Dr Carmen Lawrence, intimated that a required warning may be printed on tampon packets to inform women of the health risks of this product.

Yet when it comes to the health implications of the pill for women, this same vigilance and care are not being exercised. In fact, both would appear to have been jettisoned. The duality in health policy leads one to conclude that informed choice and longevity for women are expendable extras. Some risks just have to be lived with and died for.

This poses a poignant question: will those in government who failed to appropriately warn of the risks of the pill during the years when so many studies advised caution be around to hold the hands of those women who present with pill-induced breast or cervical cancer twenty years hence? Must we wait until health costs begin to spiral before recognition is made of the human cost?

11.5   CONVENTIONS OF SCIENTIFIC REPORTING.

Yet another impediment to the flow of accurate drug information exists within research papers themselves once they are published in medical journals. These journals are read by other researchers, and a wide range of health care professionals and journalists, all of whom may face four problems in evaluating the material before them.

The *first* way in which unwitting deception can occur is through the selective manner in which a number of related research documents on a particular topic are collated into a review paper, with the intention of bringing the reader up-to-date on research. What is included or excluded in a review paper is a matter of professional judgement on the part of the 'review' author. In an ideal world, contentious or 'politically' damaging data would be included as a mark of res-pect for the truth, yet there have been instances where the results published in the original paper were not as fully represented in the review paper as they should have been. (See Schlesselman, chapter three, and the exclusion of pap-ers favouring a long latent period for the pill).

The *second* way is linked to the first: the interpretation a review author places on papers summarized. The same Schlesselman review paper highlights this point:

> **"Some investigators suggest that long-term latent effects can explain the 'negative' results. A number of reports have addressed this issue directly, none of which supports a long-term latency hypothesis.".**[905]

One of the papers cited as *not* supporting the long latency period was that of McPherson, Vessey *et al.* (*Br J Cancer,*1987). My reading of McPherson's paper does not accord with the views of Schlesselman. Consider the following quote from the original McPherson paper which Schlesselman suggests does not support a long-term latency hypothesis:

> "The data also suggest (but not strongly) a latent period of at
> least ten years for E-O (ethinyloestradiol) pills between long te-
> rm early exposure and an increased risk of breast cancer diagno-
> sis."[906] further: "... latency could plausibly be related to the app-
> arent discrepancies in published epidemiological results." [907]
> finally: "The notion of a latency efficacy is consistent with the
> known epidemiology of breast cancer and with the observed eff-
> ect of radiation and diethylstilboestrol exposure.".[908]

Within 'review papers' there is a *third* possibility of unwitting deception for
the reader. This can occur via the practice of 'pooled data'. The 'pooling' of
data in a review paper occurs when the 'review' author (s) blend or combine the
statistical results from a number of different research centres. Pooling data can
result in significant adverse findings from one centre being offset, diminished or
even neutralised by favourable findings from another centre. Thus, 'pooling'
data unwittingly obscures key differences in data.

Dr Paul's paper of 1989,[909] for example, reported a 360% greater risk of breast
cancer for New Zealand women who had used Depo-Provera (DMPA) for 2
years or more prior to age 25. (RR 4.6; CI 1.5-15.1).Yet in a pooled analysis review
paper in 1995 (*JAMA*),[910] this result from Dr Paul was not mentioned in the
'Results' section of the paper, and only in a diminished form when combined
data from New Zealand, Mexico, Kenya and Thailand was presented in Table 5
of the results.[911] Thus the implications of the New Zealand study, and the inherent
health warnings it contained, were obscured at the expense of proper informed
consent. From this example of 'pooled data' it can be seen that if studies are
analysed in this way, women's ready access to 'the full picture' is seriously
hampered.

A similar criticism could be made of the review paper published in the *Lancet*
(1996). After pooling the data from 54 research papers, the *Lancet* (1996) paper
concluded that for current users of the pill there is a small increase in the risk of
breast cancer of 24% (RR 1.15-1.33).[912] Yet one of the studies included in this
review paper, and whose data was 'pooled' was that of Meirik, Lund, Adami,
Bergstrom *et al* (1986). These researchers had previously reported that: **"The
relative risk of breast cancer after 12 or more years of OC use was 2.2"**.[913]

This represents a 120% increase in risk. This example shows that the 'pooling' of the Meirik data in the *Lancet* (1996) paper had the effect of diminishingt the gravity of Meirik's original report. Another example of research work which was pooled in the same *Lancet* (1996) paper was that of Rookus, van Leeuwen *et al* (1994). They had previously reported a 110% increased risk of breast cancer for women under 36 years with 4 or more years of pill use (when compared to women under 36 with shorter pill use).[914] Again this contrasts with the pooled figure of only 24% as reported by the *Lancet* (1996). One final example of the impact of 'pooling' data must be cited because of the implications for young women's health.

It will be recalled from chapter three that Olsson, Moller & Ranstam (1989) had reported on a study which had involved women in Southern Sweden. They noted that: **"... the odds ratio for women starting OC use before 20 years of age was 5.8.".**[915] This translated into a 480% increased risk of breast cancer for women aged less than 20 who had used the pill. Yet in the *Lancet* (1996) paper, which included this study from Southern Sweden, the 'pooled' data reported that the relative risk increase of breast cancer for women aged less than 20 years was only 22% (Table 2b, p. 1715). Again it can be seen that when original research data is pooled with data from other research centres and presented in a review paper, the net effect is a diminution in the gravity of the primary research findings.

A similar reduction in the relative risk of breast cancer was reported by a variety of other papers whose data were 'pooled'. These are reported in the attached footnote.[916]

Review papers and the associated practice of 'pooled data' are a principle source of information for primary health care professionals such as doctors, pharmacists and nurses. Time for continuing education for these busy health care professionals must compete with the demands of running a practice, a pharmacy and/or shift work. Review papers and their ilk *seem* the ideal way for these professionals to keep abreast of all the recent research, since restraints preclude the opportunity to examine all research in its original published form. Yet unless the summaries provided in reviews and similar documents are accurate, professionals unwittingly run the risk of harming their patients by making clinical decisions not based on *all* the research data.

Great care is required when reading a review paper summarizing the main points from a number of original research documents. Facts printed in the summary or the review may be right, but they may not be all the facts. Only the complete original research document will suffice to provide an accurate account of research findings.

The *final* aspect deserving of mention — and one that is equally relevant to original research publications *or* review papers — are the terms 'overall' results and 'category-specific' results used by researchers.

In the medical literature the normative practice for presenting research data is to first report the 'overall' result, which frequently appears in the 'summary' or 'abstract' at the beginning of the paper, and then analyse the data in greater detail in the body of the research paper according to 'category-specific' criteria. We have encountered this latter concept earlier, most notably in chapters two and three. To recall: 'category-specific' sub-groups of women might be defined by age, marital status, age at first pregnancy, years of use of a drug etc. In practice, an 'overall' result, reported without intent to deceive, may greatly differ in significance from a 'category-specific' result.

Typical of 'overall' reporting in a medical article is a statement by Dr Paul (*BMJ*, 1989, p.759), who noted in her study on DMPA (Depo-Provera) use in New Zealand: **"Overall, the relative risk of breast cancer associated with duration of use was 1.0.".**

A result of 1 means that there was no increased risk from DMPA. The difficulty is that this 'overall' result alone, *without an additional category-specific breakdown of information,* might be misleading.

Indeed, without reference to the 'category-specific' risks from DMPA (or any other drug), problems connected with drug use can easily vanish. An 'overall' safe result of 1.0, in any research paper, can come about if, for instance, the negative (dangerous) results obtained from young women are added to the positive (safe) results obtained from older women. Since the two results can nullify each other, a 'no increased risk' result for Depo-Provera is the outcome. Hence the need for the reader to be cognizant of the 'category-specific' results.

In her article on DMPA (*BMJ*, 1989), Dr Paul first noted the 'overall' safe result of tests carried out using Depo-Provera and then proceeded to explain the relative risks for various sub-categories of women according to age at first use, age at diagnosis, length of use, and parity. For example, Dr Paul drew attention to the significant risks for younger women; to recall, young women using DMPA had a 360% increased risk of breast cancer. From this it can be seen that if the 'overall' result were all that were read or reported, then one could easily conclude that DMPA was safe.

11.6 THE MEDIA.

11.6.1 AN OVERVIEW.

For many people who lead busy lives, the luxury of having large portions of time to sit and diligently read through scholarly medical journals rarely exists. These persons frequently rely on varied media outlets to provide health and medical information in brief 'grabs'. The media is well suited to this task because of its ubiquitous nature. Magazines, newspapers, TV programs and radio broadcasts regularly carry news items pertaining to new drug discoveries, notification of drug recalls, advice on diet, healthy living and a variety of allied topics. The steady flow of drug and health information represents a positive discharge of the media's social responsibility (exemplified below in two brief excerpts).

Unfortunately, there are troublesome areas for journalists in their quest for greater levels of accuracy. To highlight central problem areas in journalism, this chapter examines an eclectic range of typical selections from British and American tabloids and national broadsheets, glossy Australian women's magazines, professional medical magazines, and a snippet from a radio interview with the developer of RU-486, Prof. E Baulieu. I also refer to a form of 'media' deception which is uniquely disturbing: misinformation purveyed in the *Letters to the Editor* pages of respected daily newspapers. To illustrate what can happen in this area, I shall describe an incident in which I was personally involved in 1995.

11.6.2 EXAMPLES.

First, as an example of how the mass media can 'massage' public opinion, it is instructive to note the recurring tactics of the pro-female-drug-therapy lobby. In my view, whenever 'bad' news about the pill is made public, protestations are heard about minimal risk,[917] the need for further peer review,[918] and the importance of more studies to clarify the issue; or else the excuse is made that the pill is better than being pregnant.[919] Since the use of these drugs has obvious 'political' ramifications, the drugs themselves are tirelessly promoted in the media at every opportunity, even if feigned uncertainty regarding the link between the pill and cancer is the approach employed.[920]

Polly Toynbee, writing in defence of the pill during the blood-clotting controversy of October 1995, is typical of its defenders when she says that: **"It is quite wrong to think Mother Nature knows best. In matters of women's fertility, she is the enemy.".**[921] This statement suggests that a woman's biochemistry is her own worst enemy, representing a perverse variation of the cliche 'I looked for the enemy without and found the enemy within'.

Some feminist writers have offered a more reflective, less strident view of the pill's bad press. British writer Mary Ann Sieghart, for example, says of the same press reports:

> **"... stories such as today's touch a raw nerve in millions of women. Contraception is not just a bore and a chore, it is a low grade but continuous worry in our lives ... feeling like a rodent in a laboratory is not a very comfortable way to live.".**[922]

Another journalist, the Australian writer Emma-Kate Symons, has also written critically of the pill:

> **"As the 'pill generation' reaches middle age, medical evidence is mounting towards a higher risk of breast and cervical cancer among oral contraceptive users of any age. More than a dozen studies published over the past 10 years highlight a connection between the contraceptive pill and cancer. In some studies pill users have been shown to be between 200 and 500 per cent more likely to develop breast and cervical cancer, with those below the age of 24 appearing more vulnerable.".**[923]

Sadly, however, in most instances of media reporting on the pill, breast cancer is rarely mentioned. In the glossy magazines which so many women read, the frequent omission of 'politically incorrect' facts is striking. Why this occurs is beyond the scope of this book, but that it does is undeniable. Consider the following example of one journalist's coy hesitancy in reaching conclusions which, one would have thought, are starkly self-evident. That these conclusions are not enunciated may well have tragic consequences for the women who read this magazine.

The May 1994 edition of the now defunct *Ita,* an expensive, up-market lifestyle magazine, carried a story entitled *"Breast cancer, women's health enemy No. 1 "*. The journalist first informed the readership that: **"We don't understand the causes but we know some of the high risk factors.".**[924] If by 'we' the author meant 'my professional acquaintances and I', then this statement might have been accurate. Unfortunately, because of the contextual nature of the statement, in particular the many doctors quoted, 'we' unwittingly suggested 'we the informed medical and journalistic community'. This is a most unfortunate and inaccurate implication.

Then readers were informed that:

> **"Studies point to a strong link between breast cancer and the long amount of time that women are exposed to oestrogen and support the theory that the female sex hormone is the major stimulus of cell proliferation.".**[925]

So what factors *increase* a woman's exposure to oestrogen and the 'strong link' between it and breast cancer? The journalist rightly noted that **"women who menstruate early, have their first baby late in life, don't breast-feed and have menopause late are more at risk.".**[926]

Yet nowhere in this article of seven pages was the reader informed that the greatest single source of avoidable oestrogen is in the pill. The word 'pill' was never mentioned: a stark omission.

Another illustrative case of poorly informed journalism occurred in the May (1991) issue of the mass circulation, glossy magazine *Australian Women's Weekly,* which stated that **"There is no controversy about the efficacy or safety of RU-486... no complications and no major side effects.".**[927] This statement was made despite the widely reported death of a French woman from an RU-486 induced abortion,[928] the **"lack of independent research on RU-486/PG"**[929] and **" a mere 17 months of animal research on rabbits, rats and monkeys**(which) **was**

deemed sufficient to judge RU–486 promising and 'safe' enough to warrant clinical trials in women.".[930]

In my view, this is not the only occasion when the *Australian Women's Weekly* has presented material to its readers which is demonstrably at variance with the facts. In the February 1997 edition, in a feature article entitled *"Contraception: what's new, what works"* the safety of the third- generation pill was discussed.

After briefly canvassing the October 1995 decision from the British Committee on Safety of Medicines (CSM), discussed in Chapter four, the *Women's Weekly* quoted a professor from Sydney's Royal Hospital for Women thus:

> **"Subsequent work has shown that there is absolutely no truth in the suggesting that the new progestogens carry any different risk whatsoever from the previous progestogens that were in the Pill.".**[931]

To recall from chapter four, Vandenbroucke (*Lancet,*1995) reached a conclusion on the role of third- generation progestogens which is fully opposed to the view expressed in the *Weekly:*

> **"When we come to look back on the history of oral contraception it is certain that the decrease in the dose of ethinyloestra-diol** (the oestrogen component of the pill) **will be seen to have contributed to a reduced thrombotic risk, especially for arterial disease. However, the use of a third-generation progestagen does seem to have led to an unexpected and yet unexplained return of a higher risk of venous thrombosis.".**[932]

Likewise, Spitzer (*BMJ,*1996) also wrote in an unequivocal manner on this topic:

> **"... probability of death due to venous thromboembolism for women using third-generation products is about 20 per million users per year, for women using second generation products it is about 14 per million users per year, and for non-users it is five per million per year.".**[933]

Spritzer referred to this increased risk as "**modest**" but nonetheless recommended that it be taken "**seriously**".

The journalists responsible might well claim that they were merely reporting on the government-approved literature or quoting the assessment of an 'expert'. But since these magazines are, directly or indirectly, a major source of information for many women, there is a need for independent journalists to evaluate current medical research for themselves without having to rely on statements from 'experts' or government bureaucracies.

Often, as has been seen, journalists who cover health issues in the popular media appear to have an understanding of statistical terminology, research methodologies, pharmacology and physiology which is not sound enough to ensure proper public understanding of these key issues. As issues related to drug use become more complex, the need for journalists to report on health matters with appropriate thoroughness and accuracy is becoming more pressing.

The visit to Australia in 1991 of Prof. Baulieu, the co-inventor of RU-486, further underscored the need for specialist medical journalism. At the time, few journalists challenged the then accepted view that this drug was a positive reproductive health option. One notable exception was Anne Delaney of A.B.C. Radio, whose precise questioning so infuriated Prof. Baulieu that he abruptly terminated the interview.[934]

Unfortunately, deficient reporting is also found in professional magazines which exist to educate their readership, and hence the public. One such example is the *Australian Journal of Pharmacy* (*AJP*), the leading and longest-running monthly magazine for pharmacists. It typically carries an admixture of political and legal comment, feature articles on recently launched pharmaceutical products, and a monthly update supplement to the *APPG*. Whilst the content is pharmaceutical, the style is more appropriate to a glossy magazine, complete with double page advertisements for drugs. In February, 1996, the *AJP* concluded a story on women's health and HRT thus:

> **"As HRT develops there will certainly be more options for menopausal women and the choices for HRT should be up to the woman. If a woman is mentally, physically or sexually active it is likely she will need some form of HRT...".[935]**

Ironically, one might suggest that based upon these three criteria, only the mentally compromised, paralysed and the celibate would *not* need HRT. Indeed, if pharmacists took this journalist's opinion seriously, many women would consequently receive inaccurate advice (see chapter ten).

A medical magazine, similar in style to the *AJP* and supplied only to doctors can also be cited for containing 'educational' articles of doubtful clinical benefit or suitability. *The essentials*™, designed for **"the committed doctor"**—the doctor **"who is interested in people and has no intention of losing touch"**,[936] carried a story in the Autumn 1996 edition entitled "The pill - debunking the myths. Easy, safe and effective birth control.". The interviewee was Dr Edith Weisberg, Director of NSW Family Planning. Dr Weisberg was quoted as saying that:

> **"Many women mistakenly believe it's unnatural or unsafe to take the pill on a long term basis, but the fact is, the modern pill is probably the most thoroughly tested pharmaceutically product on the market ... You can take the pill until you're 50, then stop for six months to see if menopause has occurred.".**[937]

At no stage was the medical practitioner reading *The essentials*™ informed of any adverse research on the pill. Not a single journal article from the *Lancet*, the *British Medical Journal*, the *Journal of the American Medical Association*, the *American Journal of Epidemiology*, the *American Journal of Obstetrics and Gynaecology*, or many other respected research publication outlets referenced by the journalist. This disregard for, or ignorance of, the many medical research papers which support a more measured appraisal of the pill's safety is inexplicable. Doctors, and hence their patients, are deserving of a much higher level of informed medical writing.

11.6.3   THE 'DR. LINCOLN' AFFAIR.

A more worrying instance of poor scientific reporting in the media occurred in 1995 when a Dr.R.Lincoln responded to a letter co-signed by a group of doctors and pharmacists of which I was a part. We were alarmed at the under-reporting by the 'lay' media of significant new research which had detailed a strong link between the pill, and an increase in both breast and cervical cancer rates in women. Our group tried to alert women to these contemporary studies via our correspondence to *The Australian*. Dr. Lincoln sought to refute our concerns with a letter in which she claimed that the research to which we referred was unreliable.

Whilst this incident, along with other media reports is mentioned principally because it took place via the pages of a national daily, it is nevertheless quite different in nature from those other reports, referred to earlier, by journalists without medical training. In this latter instance the author not only claimed to be a doctor but also a medical researcher with intimate knowledge of the research in question. It would be good to be able to assume that an editor of a major national broadsheet would only need to check the identity of the author and not the veracity of her comments. However, from what follows it will be seen that it is clearly not possible to assume this any longer.

Normally, the place for a serious airing of such grievances is the letters page of the *Lancet*, where the original scientific reports first appeared. Why Dr. Lincoln instead chose a national daily broadsheet to criticise research scientists from the University of Southern California and the Netherlands Cancer Institute is as much a mystery as it is inappropriate. The potential for misinformation would have been reduced had her comments been confined to the *Lancet*.

The following is: (1) the original published letter co-signed by a number of doctors and pharmacists, (2) the refutation of that letter by Dr Rosemary Lincoln of London, (3) the refutation by the principal researchers in America and the Netherlands, both of whom stated that, contrary to her published claims, Dr Lincoln was *not* associated with either of the two pill/cancer studies.

THE AUSTRALIAN
February 7 1995
LETTERS TO THE EDITOR

Once-over-lightly reporting on pill
Last week saw the release of new forms of low dose oral contraceptives onto the Australian market. While some mild and transient side-effects have been mentioned (*The Australian*, 31/1/95) major issues pertaining to women's health go unreported. We wish to register our concern that substantial evidence linking the use of oral contraceptives with cervical and breast cancer is receiving scant mention in the media.

For example, the authors of "Oral contraceptive Use and

Adenocarcinoma of the Cervix" state unequivocally that, "ever use (as distinct from never use) of oral contraceptives was associated with twice as great a risk of adenocarcinoma of the cervix. The highest risk (a four-fold increase) was observed for oral contraceptive use for more than 12 years" (*Lancet*. 1994:344;1390-94)

The research also highlighted that short term users of oral contraceptives did not escape risks; " Women who had used oral contraceptives for 1-6 months had an odds-ratio of 2.9"(ie the risk of adenocarcinoma was increased 2.9 times over never users).

Research on breast cancer is equally worrying. In "Oral contraceptives and risk of breast cancer in women aged 20-54 years" (*Lancet*, 1994;344:844-851) M Rockus and co-workers stated: "We conclude that four or more years of oral contraceptive use, especially if partly before age 20, is associated with an increased risk of breast cancer developing at an early age. There is limited evidence that the risk disappears as the cohort of young OC users ages, but this issue needs confirmation."

Women's health is one of the major medical issues of the '90s. We believe that women ought to be able to make their choices, fully conscious of the serious risks associated with oral contraceptives.

Drs Andrew Foong, Kevin Hume, Catherine and Richard Lennon, Roberta Augimeri, Roshni Geresis, and John Wilks B.Pharm MPS, John Gordon B.Pharm MPS, and John Carabetta B.Pharm. MPS

THE AUSTRALIAN
February 17 1995
LETTERS TO THE EDITOR
Conflicting reports about the pill

Since visiting Australia I have noticed conflicting information about the oral contraceptive pill. In response to an article in *The Sunday Age* (5/2) on a new pill, I would say in clarification that it is not instant and is not a dramatic development in oral contraception. Most women on oral contraception take the combined pill which contains oestrogen and progestogen.

The pill described in *The Sunday Age* contains a progestogen called gestodene. Although very few risks (if any) have been attributed to the progestogen component, gestodene is more "lipid friendly" than some other progestogens and therefore gives a normal blood fat profile, which is good news.

In response to a *Letter to the Editor* in your paper on 7/2, the risk benefit ratio of the pill has to be considered by any woman choosing a method of contraception.

The pill gives maximum efficiency in contraception, thus avoiding the risks of termination of pregnancy or perhaps the stress to the mother and family with coping with an unwanted pregnancy. It also eliminates the risks which occur during pregnancy and childbirth. There are non-contraceptive benefits such as the relief of many menstrual problems and a reduction of cancer of the ovaries by 50 per cent.

Having myself been involved in the data collection for the *Lancet* studies mentioned, I accept their importance, but I would point out that it is very difficult to make allowances for the change in lifestyle which the security of the pill made possible. Earlier sexual activity, an increase in the number of partners and non-use of barrier methods of contraception (condoms and caps) also all have effects on the cervix. People do not always like to reveal their sexual lives!. The pill has been with us for 30 years and fortunately so far there has not been an explosive increase in breast cancer and so, hopefully, there is no marked increase in the risk for most women.

Dr Rosemary Lincoln
Member, Faculty of Family Planning and Reproductive Health, London

THE REFUTATIONS.
Letter one.

Giske Ursin, M.D., Ph.D.
University of Southern California School of Medicine
Department of Preventive Medicine
1420 San Pablo Street, PMB B-308
Los Angeles, CA 90033-9987

Dear Mr Wilks,

Enclosed is a list of the different Ocs used in our study.

Neither Dr Peters nor I have ever heard of Dr Rosemary Lincoln; she was definitely not involved in the data collection of our study. We had detailed information about a woman's sexual and contraceptive history (see reprint which is in the mail), and did not have the problems she is referring to.

As for OC's and sexual practices, both are risk factors for adenocarcinoma of the cervix (see paper). We in addition found that women who had never used barrier contraceptive methods were at even higher risk if they had used Ocs.

Sincerely,

Giske Ursin, M.D., Ph.D.
Fellow.

Letter two.

The Netherlands Cancer Institute
Amsterdam, 13 March, 1995

Dear Mr Wilks,

Since we do not know of any dr. Lincoln, having been involved in our study as a scientist, interviewer, study assistant or what-soever, we have checked in our data whether a mrs. Lincoln has been interviewed for our study. This was not the case. Since we collected OC information from women as well as physicians, we checked whether she has been approached to provide us with this kind of information as a general practitioner or gynecologist for one of our participants. This also was not the case. We collected all our data ourselves and no other institutes have been involved than listed in our Lancet article.

She definitely never approached us for some sort of collaboration. So, we can clearly state that she has not been involved in our study.

Sincerely,
Mattis Rookus, Phd.
epidemiologist. *(sic)*

These letters raise two considerations.

First, it is one thing to criticise a major report for perceived shortcomings. Such criticism constitutes part of the healthy process of even-handed peer review. But what should not be acceptable is criticism which misrepresents the state of medical knowledge.

Second, how can doctors be expected to make accurate decisions about the safety of a widely-used drug like the pill if the data they rely upon is misquoted by persons holding positions of authority and prestige? Misinformation seriously undermines the basis of clinical decision making, specifically the inherent trust which clinicians must give to legitimately conducted and reported medical research. It also exposes both well-intentioned journalists and the ordinary reading public to inaccurate information about matters affecting their individual well-being and the common good.

The Australian did subsequently grant us right of reply in which we were able to clarify Dr. Lincoln's lack of involvement in and knowledge of the cited research. However, it is unclear whether such action has been sufficient to remove confusion in the minds of health care professionals and the general public.

11.7   FINAL STATEMENTS.

It is reasonable, logical, and consistent with the material reviewed in this book to suggest that it is not always possible for women to trust advice which uses the word 'safe' to describe female hormonal drug therapies. Research summarised in this book has demonstrated the considerable and sometimes fatal risks which are attached to all such drugs, risks which are too rarely weighed against the expected benefits and possible alternatives. So who should be taking responsibility for this failure?

The predominate need for improvement lies with the government-approved product information. Whilst pharmaceutical manufacturers may not be compelled by law to report the full range of disadvantageous studies on their products, they certainly have a moral responsibility to ensure that consumers of their products are better informed than they have been to date.

On the whole, medical research is diligently conducted and reliable. However, the reporting of research findings outside the primary document, as we have seen, is not always true to the original. A great deal needs to be done to ensure that women are more reliably informed about issues affecting their health than they have been to date in many existing CPI leaflets.

With regard to the deficiencies in reporting by the mass media, it is much less likely that misleading articles could or would be published if government-approved production information accurately and fulsomely reflected medical research. Whilst incomplete drug information does emanate from pharmacies and surgeries, it does so because of the unacceptable weaknesses in the approved product information.

There is a marked lag between what research scientists know and public policy formulation about the drugs cited in this book, most particularly their effect on young women. A similar lag occurred when public policy failed to keep pace with the research findings connecting cigarette smoking with lung cancer and solar radiation with skin cancer. In the case of the former, litigation has provided the impetus for change, whilst in the case of the latter, a public education campaign has been spectacularly successful. Whilst litigation may, in the future, highlight the risks of female hormonal drugs, there is nonetheless an immediate imperative to establish a public education program to ensure that all women possess accurate information about their bodies and their health in this area.

The days of treating women "like a rodent in a laboratory" should be quickly brought to an end. "Patient sovereignty" must come to mean something outside legal textbooks; for every woman it must become a practical reality.

12. APPENDICIES.

12.1 APPENDIX ONE: THE ABORTIFACIENT CAPACITY OF THE PROGESTERONE ONLY PILL.

The medical literature reported that Micronor®, a progesterone-only pill, has "an average pregnancy rate of 2.54 per 100 woman years"[938] Clearly there is a discrepancy between a pregnancy rate of on 2.54 per 100 women and an ovulation rate, as suggested by Dr E Weisberg- of 4 in 10 (or 40 per 100) woman This discrepancy supports the view that there is an abortifacient aspect to the mini-pill.

12.2 APPENDIX TWO - PILL FORMULATIONS BY BRAND AND TYPE. [939]

PROGESTERONE ONLY PILL FORMULATIONS

BRAND NAME	COMPOSITION
Microlut®	Levonorgestrel 30mcg, 28 tablets.
Microval®	As above.
Depo-Provera®	Medroxyprogesterone 150mg/1ml.
Micronor®	Norethisterone 350mcg, 28 tablets.
Locilan®	As above.
Noriday®	As above.

COMBINED FORMULATIONS - FIXED

BRAND NAME	COMPOSITION
Ovulen 0.5/50®	Ethynodiol 500mcg & ethinyloestradiol 50mcg, 21 tablets.
Ovulen 1/50®	As above for drugs, 1mg and 50mcg respectively.
Microgynon 50 21	Levonorgestrel 125mcg & ethinyloestradiol 50mcg, 21 tablets.
Microgynon 50ED	As above plus 7 sugar tablets.
Nordette 50®	As above.
Microgynon 30®	Levonorgestrel 150mcg & Ethinyloestradiol 30mcg, 21 tablets.
Nordette 21®	Levonorgestrel 150mcg & Ethinyloestradiol 30mcg, 21 tablets.
Levlen ED®	As above plus 7 sugar tablets.
Monofeme 28®	As above.
Microgynon ED®	As above
Nordette 28®	As above

Nordiol 21®	Levonorgestrel 250mcg & ethinyloestradiol 50mcg, 21 tablets.
Nordiol 28®	As above plus 7 sugar tablets.
Brevinor®	Norethisterone 500mcg & ethinyloestradiol 35mcg, 21 tablets.
Norimin 28®	As above plus 7 sugar tablets
Brevinor 28®	As above
Brevinor-1®	Norethisterone 1mg & ethinyloestradiol 35mcg, 21 tablets.
Norimin-1 28®	As above plus 7 sugar tablets.
Brevinor-1 28®	As above.
Norinyl-1®	Norethisterone 1mg & mestranol 1mg, 21 tablets
Norinyl-1/28®	As above plus sugar tablets
Marvelon®	Desogestrel 150mcg & ethinyloestradiol 30mcg, 21 tablets & 7 sugar tablets.
Minulet 28®	Gestodene 175mcg, ethinyloestradiol 30mcg, 21 tablets & 7 sugar tablets.
Femodene®	As above.

COMBINED FORMULATIONS - SEQUENTIAL

BRAND NAME	COMPOSITION
Biphasil 21®	Levonorgestrel 50mcg & ethinyloestradiol 50mcg 11 tabs, 125mcg & 50mcg respectively in next 10 tabs.
Biphasil 28®	As above plus 7 sugar tablets.
Sequilar ED®	As above.
Triphasil®	Levonorgestrel 50mcg & ethinyloestradiol 30mcg - 6 tabs, 5 tablets of 75mcg & 40mcg respectively, and 10 tabs of 125mcg & 30mcg respectively.
Triquilar®	As above.
Logynon ED®	As above plus 7 sugar tabs

Trifeme 28®	As above.
Triphasil 28®	As above.
Triquilar ED®	As above.
Synphasic 28®	Norethisterone 0.5mg, ethinyloestradiol 35mcg- 7 tabs then 9 tabs of 1mg & 35mcg respectively, then 5 tabs of 0.5mg and 35 mcg, then 7 sugar tabs.
Improvil 28 Day®	As above.
Triminulet 28®	Gestodene 50mcg & ethinyloestradiol 30mcg -6 tabs then 5 tabs of 70mcg & 40mcg respectively, then 10 tabs of 100mcg & 30mcg respectively, then 7 sugar tablets.

12.3   APPENDIX THREE: STAGES OF DEVELOPMENT OF CERVICAL CANCER. [940][941]

"There is now evidence of a continuum of disease from cervical dysplasia to carcinoma-in-situ to invasive cancer.".[942]

Diagrammatically, the development of cervical cancer can be represented thus:

Cervical dysplasia (abnormal development) → **carcinoma-in-situ** (pre-malignant, not invading the basement membrane, but showing cytological characteristics of invasive cancer; also known as pre-invasive cancer or intraepithelial carcinoma [943]) →**invasive cancer.**

85% of cervical cancers arise from the squamous epithelial lining of the vagina. The pre-cursor condition of invasive cervical cancer is known as cervical intraepithelial neoplasia (CIN), of which there are three grades.

CIN 1 = mild dysplasia
CIN 2 = moderate dysplasia
CIN 3 = severe dysplasia or carcinoma-in-situ → invasive cancer.

The remaining 15% of cervical cancers are from the columnar epithelium lining of the cervical canal. These are called adenocarcinomas. There are 3 precursor lesions leading to invasive adenocarcinoma
1. Glandular atypia
2. Glandular dysplasia
3. Adenocarcinoma-in-situ (ACIS)

NB. Squamous epithelial carcinoma and adenocarcinoma may occur together or follow each other.

12.4   APPENDIX FOUR - CLASSIFICATION OF DRUGS IN PREGNANCY: AUSTRALIA.

Australian Drug Evaluation Committee Pregnancy Category Definitions.[944]

A - Drugs which have been taken by a large number of pregnant women and women of childbearing age without any proven increase in the frequency of malformations or other direct or indirect harmful effects on the fetus having been observed.

B - Drugs which have been taken by only a limited number of pregnant women and women of childbearing age, without an increase in the frequency of malformation or other direct or indirect harmful effects on the human fetus having been observed. As experience of effects of drugs in this category in humans is limited, results of toxicological studies to date (including reproduction studies in animals) are indicated by allocation to one of three subgroups:

B1 - Studies in animals * have not shown evidence of an increased occurrence of fetal damage.

B2 - Studies in animals * are inadequate or may be lacking, but available data show no evidence of an increased occurrence of fetal damage.

B3 - Studies in animals * have shown evidence of an increased occurrence of fetal damage, the significance of which is considered uncertain in humans.

C - Drugs which, owing to their pharmacological effects, have caused or may be suspected of causing, harmful effects on the human fetus or neonate without causing malformations. These effects may be reversible. Accompanying texts should be consulted for further details.

D - Drugs which have caused, are suspected to have caused, or may be expected to cause, an increased incidence of human fetal malformations or irreversible damage. These drugs may also have adverse pharmacological effects Accompanying texts should be consulted for further details.

X - Drugs that have such a high risk of causing permanent damage to the fetus that they should not be used in pregnancy or when there is a possibility of pregnancy.

*Animal studies submitted in support of new drug applications must conform to New Drug Form Guidelines.

In addition, labelling for drugs with a recognized use during labor or delivery, whether or not the use is stated in the INDICATIONS section of the labelling (eg, analgesics), describes the available information about the effect of the drug on the mother and fetus.

CONCLUSION:
These categories are guidelines intended to assist health-care professionals prevent potential fetal adversities. Even if placed in the lowest risk category (Category A), a drug should not be used during pregnancy unless clearly indicated.

12.5   APPENDIX FIVE: CLASSIFICATION OF DRUGS IN PREGNANCY:AMERICA

PREGNANCY RISK CATEGORIES
US Food and Drug Authority (FDA) Pregnancy Category Definitions

A - Controlled studies in women fail to demonstrate a risk to the fetus in the first trimester, and the possibility of fetal harm appears remote.

B - Animal studies do not indicate a risk to the fetus and there are no controlled human studies, or animal studies do show an adverse effect on the fetus but well-controlled studies in pregnant women have failed to demonstrate a risk to the fetus.

C - Studies have shown that the drug exerts animal teratogenic or embryocidal effects, but there are no controlled studies in women, or no studies are available in either animals or women.

D - Positive evidence of human fetal risk exists, but benefits in certain situations (eg, life-threatening situations or serious diseases for which safer drugs cannot be used or are ineffective) may make use of the drug acceptable despite its risks.

X - Studies in animals or humans have demonstrated fetal abnormalities or there is evidence of fetal risk based on human experience, or both, and the risk clearly outweighs any possible benefit.

12.6 APPENDIX SIX: ABORTION OF UNDECTED PREGNANCY.

Ovulations per 100-women years.

Number of ovulations x 1200 (months)
_____

Number of women observed x number of months observed

6 x 1200
_____

70 x 6 months = 7200/420 = 17.14 ovulations per 100 women years.

Given that we have the failure rate for the pill - the Pearl index - which measure the number of women who present with a confirmed pregnancy, and also a measure of the number of women who ovulate per 100 women-years, it is possible to calculate a theoretical maximum abortifacient rate for the pill. This is done by simply subtracting the Pearl Index (being the lesser number) from the ovulation Index (being the greater number) to give us the abortion of undetected pregnancy rate (AUP) rate.

Ovulation Index - Pearl Index = AUP rate.

12.7 APPENDIX SEVEN: BREAST CANCER RATES IN N.S.W (AUST).

NEW SOUTH WALES CENTRAL CANCER REGISTRY.
Age-standardised incidence rate of breast cancerper 100,000 women. NSW, 1972-1994

YEAR	INCIDENCE	YEAR	INCIDENCE
1972	50.28	1984	58.46
1973	51.10	1985	57.69
1974	56.26	1986	60.33
1975	52.27	1987	64.36
1976	55.63	1988	65.62
1977	53.28	1989	64.66
1978	52.63	1990	66.11
1979	54.03	1991	73.83
1980	55.53	1992	67.37
1981	55.13	1993	74.83
1982	54.02	1994	80.98
1983	55.05		

NEW SOUTH WALES CENTRAL CANCER REGISTRY
Age-specific incidence rate of breast cancer per 100,000 women. NSW

YR.	AGE-BRACKET						
	20-4	25-9	30-4	35-9	40-4	45-9	50-4
1972	0.53	3.3	24.6	34.6	88.9	132.4	129.3
1982	2.2	6.1	23.8	52.5	102.0	122.5	127.5
1993	3.0	7.9	22.2	56.5	124.6	180.1	218.4

YR.	AGE-BRACKET						
	55-9	60-4	65-9	70-4	75-9	80-4	85+
1972	142.8	152.3	180.9	220.0	243.2	254.1	269.5
1982	162.8	189.4	204.1	190.7	244.7	230.2	253.4
1993	227.3	264.6	304.4	286.3	266.2	266.4	300.8

13. GLOSSARY.

To avoid unnecessary footnotes, the following definitions are taken from Mosby's Medical, Nursing & Allied Health Dictionary (3rd Edition) [945] , except those ending in *, indicating they were taken from Mosby's Medical Encyclopedia CD for Windows 1995 Ver. 1 In my view these two products are superior resources for the student, casual reader or health care professional.

Abort - (L *ab* away from, *oriri* to be born), to terminate a pregnancy before the fetus has developed enough to live ex utero (outside the uterus).

Abortifacient - an agent that causes abortion.

Adenocarcinoma - (Gk *aden* pertaining to a gland + *karkinos* crab, *oma* a combining form meaning a "tumour"), any one of a large group of malignant, epithelial cell tumours of the glands. Specific tumours are diagnosed and named by cytological identification of the tissue affected; for example, an adenocarcinoma of the uterine cervix is characterised by tumour cells resembling the glandular epithelium of the cervix.

Adenosquamous - (*aden* + L *squama* scale), of or pertaining to scales of a gland.

Aetiology - (Gk *aitia* cause, *logos* science), the study of all factors that may be involved in the development of a disease. (NB This is the English spelling. The American rendition omits the 'A'.

Antigen - (Gk *anti* a combining form meaning 'against or over against' + *genein* to produce), a substance... which causes the formation of an antibody and reacts specifically with that antibody.

Anovulatory - (Gk *a*, a combining form meaning 'without, not' + L. *Ovum* egg), menstruation bleeding that occurs even though ovulation has not taken place.

Aplasia - (Gk *a, plassein* not to form), developmental failure resulting in the absence of an organ or tissue.

Atypia - (Gk *a, typos* not type), a condition of being irregular or not standard.

Blastocyst - (Gk *blastos* germ + *kystis* bag), the embryonic form that follows the morula in human development. It is a spheric mass of cells having a central, fluid-filled cavity (blastocele) surrounded by two layers of cells. The outer layer (trophoblast) later forms the placenta; the inner layer (embryoblast) later forms the embryo. Implantation in the wall of the uterus occurs at this stage, on approximately the eight day after fertilization.

Camptomelic syndrome - (Gk *kamptos* bent, *daktylos* finger), a congenital anomaly characterized by bending of one or more limbs, causing permanent bowing or curving of affected area.

Cancer - (L, crab) a neoplasm characterized by the uncontrolled growth of anaplastic (malignant) cells that tend to invade surrounding tissue and to metastasize (spread) to distant body sites.

Carcinoma - (Gk *karkinos* crab , *oma* tumour), a malignant epithelial neoplasm that tends to invade surrounding tissue and to metatasize to distant regions of the body.

Carcinoma - in- situ. - (Gk *karkinos , oma;* L, *situs* location), a premalignant neoplasm that has not invaded the basement membrane but shows cytological characteristics of invasive cancer. Such neoplastic changes in stratified squamous or glandular epithelium are frequently seen on the uterine cervix.....cervical carcinoma-in-situ is treated successfully by various methods, including cryosurgery, electrocautery, and simple hysterectomy.

Cerebrovascular accident (CVA) - an abnormal condition of the blood vessels of the brain characterized by occulsion by an embolus or cerebrovascular hemorrhage, resulting in ischemia of the brain tissue normally perfused by the damaged vessels.

Choreoathetosis - (Chorea Gk *choreia* dance), a condition characterised by involuntary, purposeless, rapid motions, as flexing and extending the fingers, raising and lowering the shoulders, or grimacing + (athetosis Gk *athetos* not fixed), a neuromuscular condition characterised by slow, writhing, continuous and involuntary movements of the extremities, as seen in some forms of cerebral palsy and in motor disorders resulting from lesions in the basal ganglia.

CIN - cervical intra-epithelial neoplasia, (see appendix 3) and [946] .

Conception - (L *concipere* to take together), the beginning of pregnancy, usually taken to be the instant that a sperm enters an ovum and forms a viable zygote; the act or process of fertilization.

Contraception - (L *contra* against + *concipere*), a process or technique for the prevention of pregnancy by means of a medication, device, or method that blocks or alters one or more of the processes of reproduction in such a way that sexual union can occur without impregnation (to make pregnant).

Double-blind study - an experiment made to test the effect of a treatment or drug. Groups of experimental and control subjects are used in which neither the subjects nor the investigators know which treatment is being given to which group. In a double-blind test of a new drug, the drug may be identified to the investigators only by a code. *

Dysplasia - (Gk *dys* bad + *plassein* to form), any abnormal development of tissues or organs.

Embolus - (Gk *embolus* plug), a piece of thrombus that circulates in the blood-stream until it becomes lodged in a vessel.

Embolism - an abnormal circulatory condition in which a embolus travels through the bloodstream and becomes lodged on a vessel wall.

Embryo - (Gk *en* in, *bryein* to grow), the stage of prenatal development between the time of implantation of the fertilized ovum (about two weeks after conception) until the end of the seventh or eight week.

Endocrine - (Gk *endo* within + *krinein* to secrete), pertaining to a process in which a group of cells secrete into the blood or lymph circulation a substance that has a specific effect on tissues in another part of the body.

Endocrinology - (Gk *endo* within + *krinein* to secrete , *logos* science), the study of the anatomy, physiology, and pathology of the endocrine system and the treatment of endocrine problems.

Epidemiology - (Gk *epi* on, upon + *demos* people + *logos* people), the study of the occurrence, distribution, and causes of disease in humankind.

Epithelium - (Gk *epi* + *thele* nipple), the covering of the internal and external organs of the body, including the blood vessels. It consists of cells bound together by connective material and varies in the number of layers and the kinds of cells.

Exogenous- (Gk *exo* outside + *genein* to produce), originating outside the body.

Factor V - a blood-clotting factor that occurs in normal plasma but is lacking in patients with a blood-clotting disease (parahemophilia). It is needed to change prothrombin rapidly to thrombin (see below).*

Fertilization - (L *fertilis* fruitful), the union of male and female gametes to form a zygote from which the embryo develops.

Foetus - (L fruitful), the human being in utero after the embryonic period and the beginning of the development of the major structural features, usually from the eighth week after fertilization until birth.

Gamete - (Gk marriage partner), a mature male or female sex cell that is capable of functioning in fertilization.

Gravid - (L *gravida* pregnant), pregnant; carrying fertilized eggs or a foetus.

Hemorrhage - (Gk *haima* blood + *rhegynynei* to break forth), a loss of a large amount of blood in a short period of time, either externally or internally.

Hemiplegia - impairment to the movement of the limbs on the side of the body.

Heterozygous - having two different genes at the same place on matched chromosomes. An individual who is heterozygous for a particular trait has inherited a gene for that trait from one parent and the alternative gene from the other parent. A person heterozygous for a genetic disease caused by a dominant gene, as Huntington's chorea, will show the disease. An individual heterozygous for a hereditary disorder produced by a recessive gene, as sickle cell anemia, will not show the disease, or will have a milder form of it. The offspring of a heterozygous carrier of a genetic disorder have a 50% chance of inheriting the gene dominant for the trait. *

Homozygous -having two identical genes at the same place on matched chromosomes. An individual who is homozygous for a particular characteristic has inherited from each parent one of two identical genes for that characteristic. A person homozygous for a genetic disease caused by a pair of recessive genes, as sickle cell anemia, shows the disorder, and his or her offspring have a 100% chance of inheriting the gene for the disease. *

Hormone - (Gk *hormaien*), a complex chemical substance produced in one part or organ of the body that initiates or regulates the activity of an organ or a group of cells in another of the body.

Hydrocephalus - (Gk *hydor* pertaining to water or hydrogen + *kephale* head), a pathologic condition characterized by an abnormal accumulation of cerebrospinal fluid, usually under pressure, within the cranial vault and subsequent dilation of the ventricles.

Hypospadias - (Gk *hypo* under +*spadon* a split), an inherited defect in which the urinary opening is on the underside of the penis. Incontinence does not occur because nothing else is defective. Surgical correction is performed as necessary for cosmetic, urological, or reproductive purposes. A corresponding defect in women is rare but recognized by the location of the urinary opening in the vagina. *

Implantation - the process involving the attachment, penetration and embedding of the blastocyst in the lining of the uterine wall during the early stages of prenatal development, In humans, the process occurs over a period of a few days, beginning about the seventh or eighth day after fertilization.
NB. This definition accords with the traditional view that a woman is pregnant from the moment of fertilisation, *not* from the moment of implantation, as some have sought to contend.

Ischaemic - (Gk *ischein* to hold back, *haima* blood), decreased blood supply to a body organ or part, often marked by pain and organ dysfunction, as in ischaemic heart disease. Some causes of ischemia are arterial embolism, atherosclerosis, thrombosis, and vasoconstriction.

Menarche - (L *memsis* month; Gk *archaios* from the beginning), the first menstruation and the commencement of cyclic menstrual function.

Meningomyelocele - a saclike bump, or rupture, of either the brain or spinal membranes (meninges) through a defect in the skull or the spinal column. It forms a lump (hernial cyst) that is filled with fluid from the brain and the spine. It does not contain nerve tissue. The defect is called a cranial meningocele or spinal meningocele, depending on where it is. It can be easily repaired by surgery.*

Mitosis - (Gk *mitos* thread), a type of cell division that occurs in somatic cells and results in the formation of two genetically identical daughter cells.

Morula - (L *morulus* blackberry), a solid, spherical mass of cells resulting from the cleavage of the fertilized ovum in the early stages of embryonic development. It represents an intermediate stage between the zygote and the blastocyst and consists of blastomeres that are uniform in size, shape, and physiologic capabilities.

Mutagenesis - the induction or occurrence of a genetic mutation. See also teratogenesis.

Myocardial infarction- (Gk *mys* muscle, *karkia* heart; L *infarcire* to stuff), an occulsion - blockage - of a coronary artery, caused by atherosclerosis or an embolus resulting from a necrotic (dead) area in the vasculature myocardium.

Neoplasia - (Gk *neos* new *plasma* formation), any abnormal growth of new tissue, benign or malignant. Also called tumour.

Nulligravidas - (L *nullus* not one + *gravida* pregnant), a woman who has never been pregnant.

Nulliparous - (*nullus* + *parere* to bear), a woman who has not delivered of a viable infant.

Oncogene - (Gk *onkos* swelling + *genein* to produce), a potential cancer-inducing gene.

Oncogenic - (Gk *ongos* + *genesis* origin), the process of initiating and promoting the development of a neoplasm through the action of a biologic, chemical, or physical agent.

Papilla - (L *papillae* nipple, a small nipple-shaped projection.

Papillomavirus - (papilla + *Gk oma* tumour + L *virus* poison), the virus that causes warts in humans.

Parity - (L *parere*)- to give birth.

Placebo - an inactive substance given as if it were a real dose of a needed drug. The substance may be a salt-water solution, distilled water, or sugar, or a less-than-effective dose of a harmless substance, as a vitamin that dissolves in water. Placebos are used in drug studies to compare the effects of the inactive substance with those of an experimental drug. They are also given for patients who cannot be given a drug they may want or who do not need that drug. Placebo treatment is useful in some cases, and side effects often occur as they would from the actual drug. The benefit to the patient of a placebo may sometimes outweigh the ethical, moral, and legal problems raised by giving it. *

Pregnancy - (L *praegnans* childbearing), the gestational process, comprising the growth and development within a woman of a new individual from conception through the embryonic and fetal periods to birth. Pregnancy lasts approximately 266 days from the day of fertilization.

Progestin - (Gk *pro* first, or in front of + L *gestare* to bear) 1. Progesterone 2. Any of a group of hormones, natural or synthetic, secreted by the corpus luteum, placenta, or adrenal cortex that has a progesterone-like effect.

Progestogen - any natural or synthetic progestational hormone. Also spelt progestagen. Also called progestin.

Pulmonary - (L *pulmoneus* relating to the lungs), of or pertaining to the lungs or respiratory system.

Pulmonary embolism (PE) - the blockage of a pulmonary artery by foreign matter such as fat, air, tumour tissue, or a thrombus that usually arises from a peripheral vein.

Relative risk (RR) - an assessment of the degree or incidence of adverse effects that may be expected in the *presence* of a particular factor or event as compared with the expected adverse effects in the *absence* of the factor or event.

Squamous cell - (L *squama* scale + *cella* storeroom), a flat, scale-like epithelial cell.

Squamous cell carcinoma - (L *squama* scale : *cella* storeroom), a slow-growing, malignant tumour (also called neoplasm) of squamous epithelium.

Somatic cells - any of the cells of the body tissue that have the diploid number of chromosomes as distinguished from germ (sex) cells, which contain the haploid (half) number.

Steroid- (Gk *stereos* solid + *eidos* form), any of a large number of hormonal substances with a similar basic chemical structure, produced mainly in the adrenal cortex (kidneys) and gonads (sex organs).

Stroke- see cerebrovascular accident.

Teratogen - (Gk *teras* monster + *genein* to produce), any substance, agent, or process that interferes with normal pre-natal development, causing the formation of one or more developmental abnormalities in the fetus.

Teratogenesis - the development of physical defects in the embryo.

Teratological - (Gk *teras* monster + *logos* science), the study of the causes and effects of congenital malformations and developmental abnormalities. (In the context of this book, the suspected cause is the drug under discussion)

Tetralogy of Fallot - an inborn heart problem that is made up of four defects: lung narrowing (pulmonic stenosis), a defect in the dividing wall of the lower chamber of the heart (ventricular septal defect), malposition of the aorta so that it arises from the septal defect or the right ventricle. The main symptoms in the infant are bluish skin due to too-little hemoglobin (cyanosis) and lack of oxygen (hypoxia), usually during crying, difficulty in feeding, failure to gain weight, and poor development. In older children a typical squatting position and clubbing of the fingers and toes are evident. *

Thrombin - an enzyme formed in plasma during the clotting process from prothrombin, calcium, and thromboplastin. Thrombin causes fibrinogen to change to fibrin, essential in the formation of a clot.*

Thrombus - (Gk *thrombos* lump), a collection of platelets, fibrin, clotting factors stuck onto the interior wall of a vein or artery, sometimes causing a blockage.

Thrombosis - an abnormal condition in which thrombus develop within a blood vessel of the body.

Thromboembolism - (Gk *thrombos* + *embolos* plug), a condition in which a blood vessel is blocked by an embolus carried in the bloodstream from the site of formation of the clot.

Tumour - also called neoplasm.

Tumourogenesis - the process of starting and helping the growth of a tumor.

Women-years - (in statistics) 1 year in the reproductive life of a sexually active woman; a unit which represents 12 months of exposure to the risk of pregnancy.

Zygote - (Gk *zygon* yoke), the developing ovum from the time it is fertilized until, as a blastocyst, it is implanted in the uterus.

14. ENDNOTES

1. White, M. Dr. (1985), *"The Pill: the Gap between Promise and Performance"* Published by Responsible Society Research and Education Trust, Wicken, Milton Keyes, Bucks, MK196BU, England.

CHAPTER ONE.

2. Grimes DA, Godwin AJ, Rubin A, Smith JA, Lacarra M. Ovulation and follicular development associated with three low-dose oral contraceptives: a randomized controlled trial. *Obstet Gynae,* 1994;83:(1) p.31

3. Harper C, Ellerton C. Knowledge and perceptions of emergency contraceptive pills among a college-age population: a qualitative approach. *Fam Plan Perspectivies,* 1995;27:149-154. This article does not explicitly define 'conception' however the entire tenor of the text is predicated on the erroneous presumption that conception is synonymous with implantation, not fertilization.

4. *Ibid.*, p.149

5. Ellertson C, Winikoff B, Armstrong E, Camp S, Senanayake P. Expanding access to emergency contraception in developing countries. *Stud Fam Plan*, 1995;26,(5).p251.

6. "For >20 years the 'morning after' pill has been prescribed to women as a means of controlling pregnancy". in Grou F, Rodrigues I. The morning-after pill- How long after? *Am J Obstet Gynecol,* 1994;171:6:p.1529. The paper then proceeds to argue that the primary *modus operandi* of the 'morning after' pill is via its effects upon the endometrium. " This mode of action could explain the majority of cases where pregnancies are prevented by the morning-after pill". *op.cit.*, p.1532. Clearly the authors predicate their argument upon the presumption that pregnancy does not begin until implantation.

7. (Editorial) "Emergency contraception is not abortion." in *Lancet,* 1995; 345:1381-1382 (Editorial)

8. Ellerton, *op.cit.,* p.p. 251-263

9. Weisberg E, Fraser IS, Carrick SE, Wilde FM. Emergency contraception-general practitioner knowledge, attitude and practices in New South Wales. *Med J Aust*, 1995;162:136-138. This article is also based upon the supposition that pregnancy doesn't start until after implantation.

10. Rahwan R. (Letter), *Lancet.*1995;346:252. This definition has been

accepted by the US Supreme Court (Webster *vs* Reproductive Services, July 3, 1989).

11.   *Mosby's Medical, Nursing and Allied Health Dictionary.* 3rd Edition 1990 N. Darlene Como (Ed) p.610

12.   *Ibid,* p.954

13.   Dwyer Prof. J., *The Courier.* (The Inner Western Suburbs Newspaper, Publishing Address 170 Bourke Rd Alexandria 2015 NSW Aust) 2.1.96

14.   Llewellyn-Jones D. *Everywomen.* 2nd Edition 1978. Faber and Faber, London. p.8.

15.   *Mosby's, op.cit.,* p. 301

16.   Rahwan, Prof. R, *Contraceptives, Interceptives and Abortifacients.* Division of Pharmacology, College of Pharmacy, The Ohio State University, Columbus, Ohia 43210. 1995. p.7

17.   *Butterworth's Medical Dictionary* 2nd Ed. 1978 MacDonald Critchley (ed). "Conception- 1. The act of becoming pregnant. 2. The fertilization of the ovum by a spermatozoon and the beginning of the growth of the embryo." "Pregnancy - the state of being with child; the condition from conception to delivery of the conceptus." "Pregnant - being with child."

18.   *Gould's Medical Dictionary* 4th Ed.1979. McGraw-Hill Book Co. "Conception - the fertilization of the ovum by the spermatozoon.". "Conceptus - that which is conceived: an embryo or fetus." "Pregnancy - the condition of being pregnant: the state of a woman or any female mammal from conception to parturition..." "Pregnant - having potential offspring (fertilized ovum...)."

19.   *Stedman's Medical Dictionary* 26th Ed. 1995. Williams & Wilkins (Pub). "Conception - act of conceiving, or becoming pregnant; fertilization of the oocyte (ovum) by a spermatozoon to a viable zygote." " Pregnancy - the condition of a female after conception until the birth of the baby."

20.   *Harrup's Dictionary of Medicine and Health* Ist Ed. 1988. London. "Conception - moment and process of the fertilization of an ovum (egg cell) by a sperm, following sexual intercourse. The result is the formation of a zygote (a combined cell with 23 pairs of chromosomes in its nucleus), representing the beginning of pregnancy." "Pregnancy - begins with conception, when an ovum is fertilized by a sperm..."

21.   *Mellon's Illustrated Medical Dictionary* 3rd Ed. (1993) New York. "Conception- the fertilization of an ovum or the act of becoming pregnant." "Conceptus - the product of conception. Also called embryo." "Pregnancy - the period of time between conception and birth of the off-spring." "Pregnant- carrying a developing offspring within the body."

22. *Oxford Concise Medical Dictionary* 4th Ed. 1994. "Conception - the start of pregnancy, when a male germ cell (sperm) fertilizes a female germ cell (ovum) in the Fallopian tube." "Pregnancy - the period during which a woman carries a developing fetus, normally in the uterus."

23. *Pearce's Medical and Nursing Dictionary and Encyclopedia.* 15th Ed. 1983. p.99. Faber & Faber. "Conception - the union of the male and female reproductive elements, i.e. the ovum and the spermatozoon."

24. *Australian Prescription Products Guide (APPG).* 25th Ed 1996. Australian Pharmaceutical Publishing Company Ltd, 40 Burwood Rd, Hawthorn, Victoria, 3122, Australia. Microval (Wyeth Pharmaceuticals) p.1531

25. "... ovulation is almost always prevented when the agents are used in the usual way." *Goodman & Gilman's The Pharmacological Basis of Therapeutics.* Pergammon Press, Inc. Maxwell House, Fairview Press, Elmsford, New York 10523, U.S.A. 8th Ed p.1405 NB 'Almost' clearly means that suppression is not absolute.

26. *Micromedex* (Clinical Computerised Information System) Vol. 86. Triquilar ED monograph

27. "These findings indicate that ovarian suppression is far from complete with the low dose OC." in Van der Vange, N . Ovarian activity during low dose oral contraceptives. In: Chamberlain G, (Ed.) *Contemporary Obstetrics and Gynaecology.* Butterworths, London. 1988 p.323.

28. Rahwan, 1995, *op.cit.,* p.9

29. "Progestogens act to transform a proliferate uterine endometrium into a more differentiated, secretory one." *Micromedex,* Depo-Provera Monograph ,Vol 85.

30. "It seems unlikely that implantation would be possible in the altered endometrium developed under the influence of most of the suppressants [of ovulation]." *Goodman & Gilman's, op.cit.,* p.1405

31. "Integrins are a family of heterodimeric cell adhesion molecules composed of a and b subunits that have been implicated in a number of diverse physiological processes, including a role in fertilization and embryo implantation... Three different integrins (a1b1, a4b1 and avb3) exhibit cycle-dependent patterns of expression in endometrial epithelium...the avb3 integrin has emerged as a reliable marker of normal fertility." Somkuti SG, Sun JS, Yowell CW, Fritz MA, Lessey BA. The effect of oral contraceptive pills on markers of endometrial receptivity *Fertilty and Sterility.* 1996;65. p.484. (NB. The a & b are meant to be the Greek letters alpha and beta, but these could not be created via PageMaker.)

32.   "Oral contraceptives have a number of complementary actions at the hypothalmic, tubal, and cervical levels. They also have characteristic effects on endometrial morphology, including diminished thickness, narrow, widely spaced glands, and precidual changes in the stroma. The functional significance of these morphological effects is presumed to be an endometrium that is *unreceptive to an implanting embryo*. The changes in integrin expression we observed in the endometrium of OC users lend credence to this notion. Compared with patterns observed in fertile controls, expression of the a4b1 subtype is increased, whereas that of avb3 is diminished. These changes are consistent with an unreceptive endometrium and likely reflect the influence of continuos exposure to pharmacologic levels of contraceptive steroids." *Ibid.*, p.487.(My emphasis).

33.   Rahwan, 1995, *op.cit.,* pp.7-8

34.   See AMA: *Drug Evaluation Subscriptions.* AMA Dept of Drugs, Chicago, IL. 1991. and Balin H, Newton RE, Howtz AE et al. Pharmacophysiologic and clinical aspects of oral contraceptives. *Semin Drug Treatment.* 1973;3:121-142. and Morris JM. Mechanisms involved in progesterone contraception and oestrogen interception. *Am J Ob Gynae.* 1973;117:167. In *Micromedex* Vol 87.

35.   Somkuti, *loc.cit.*

36.   Rahwan, 1995, *op.cit.,* pp.8 & 10

37.   Van der Vange N. *op. cit.*, p. 323.

38.   Grimes DA, Godwin AJ, Rubin A, Smith JA, Lacarra M., *op.cit.,* p.34

39.   Rahwan, *op.cit.,* pp.7-8

40.   Vessey MP, Lawless M, Yeates D, McPherson K. Progestogen-only contraception. Findings in a large prospective study with special reference to effectiveness. *Br J Fam Planning.* 1985;10:p.119

41.   Weisberg E. Oral Contraceptives- fine tuning clinical use. *Patient Management.* July 1988.p. 33

42.   Sparrow MJ. Pregnancies in reliable pill takers. *New Zealand Medical Journal.* 1989:102 p.576

43.   That pregnancy does occur on the pill implicitly means that the endometrium is not *always* adversely altered.

44.   Vessey, *op.cit.,* p.119. Table 4. In this study, 20% of the women who became pregnant on the mini-pill had NOT missed any tablets. Therefore, even with regular daily doses, the endometrium was able to accept and

sustain the fertilized ovum.

45. Rahwan, *op.cit.,* pp.8-9

46. "The mini-pill finds its major indications as an interceptive...", *Ibid.*, p.34

47. "The generic reference to the combination pill as an oral 'contraceptive', therefore, is less than accurate", *Ibid.,* p. 26

48. *Ibid.*, p.17

49. *Ibid.*

50. *Ibid.*, p.34

51. *Ibid.,* p.17

52. Sweet M., The Contraceptive Revolution - still a bitter pill. *The Sydney Morning Herald.* March 13, 1995.

53. Llewellyn-Jones, *op.cit.*, p.104

54. Sparrow, *loc.cit.*

55. Weisberg, *op.cit.,* p.33.

56. Vessey, *op.cit.*, p.117

57. Sparrow, *loc.cit.*

58. Weisberg E. OCs and community failure rate. *Current Therapeutics.* 1994 (Sept)51-52

59. Khoo SK. Contraceptive efficacy of the Pill. *Med J Aust.* 1989;150. p.548

60. Weisberg, *Current Therapeutics. op.cit.,* In this particular article , Dr. Weisberg initially uses women years as the index when referring to theoretical-effectiveness, then switches to % measures in the next sentence when referring to use-effectiveness. As a matter of logic I presume that the 3% and 6% figures mean 3 or 6 pregnancies per 100-women years.

61. Sparrow, *loc.cit.*

62. *Merck Manual* 15th Ed, Robert Berkow (Editor) Merck Research Laboratories, Merck & Co.,Inc.Rahway, N.J.1987. p.1736

63. Sparrow, *loc.cit.*

64. Baciewicz AM.Oral Contraceptive Drug Interactions (Review). *Therapeutic Drug Monitoring.* 1985;7:26- 35. Raven Press. New York

65. see appendix 2.

66. Van der Vange, *loc.cit.*

67. *Ibid,* pp.315- 326

68. Corson S, Contraceptive efficacy of a monophasic oral contraceptive containing desogestrel. *Am J Obstet Gynecol.* 1993;168:1017-20

69. Grimes, *loc.cit.*

70. In this study there was an ovulation rate of 26.7 per 100 women years. ie (4 ovulations x 1200mths)/(30 women x 6 months).

71.   Grimes, *op.cit.*, p.33

72.   Llewellyn-Jones, *op.cit.*, p.116

73.   Rahwan, *op.cit.*, p.8

74.   "Even if ovulation were not prevented, it is easy to imagine that the contraceptive agents could interfere with impregnation [implantation] by their direct effect upon the genital tract [endometrium]" *Goodman & Gilman's* 8th Ed., *op. cit.*, p.1405

75.   Rahwan, *op.cit.*, p.37

76.   McCrystal P. What kind of prescription? *Chemist & Druggist.* 1995; Feb 25:304

77.   Sparrow, *loc.cit.*,

78.   Weisberg, *Patient Management, op.cit.*, p.33

79.   Sparrow, *op.cit.*, p.576

80.   *Goodman & Gilman's* 8th Ed., *op.cit.*, p.1405

81.   Rahwan, *op.cit.*, pp. 8-9

82.   Weisberg, *loc.cit.*

83.   See appendix one.

CHAPTER TWO.

84.   Women sue over Pill risks. *The Daily Telegraph-Mirror* (Sydney, Aust.) 13.4.95, p. 22

85.   Tyler E.T. Current status of oral contraception. *JAMA.* 1964;187:562-565. Pincus G, Garcia CR. Studies on vaginal, cervical and uterine histology. *Metabolism* (Suppl) 1965;14:344-347. Weid GL, Davis ME, Frank R, *et al.*, Statistical evaluation of the effect of hormonal contraceptives on the cytologic smear pattern. *Obstet Gynecol.* 1966;27:327-334. Miller DF. The effect of hormonal contraceptive therapy on a community and effects on cytopathology of the cervix. *Am J Obstet Gynecol.* 1973;115:978-982 in Peritz E, Ramcharan S., The incidence of cervical cancer and duration of oral contraceptive use. *Am J Epidemiol.* 1977;6: 462

86.   Worth AJ, Boyes DA. A case control study into the possible effects of birth control pills on pre-clinical carcinoma of the cervix. *J Obstet Gynae Br C'wealth.* 1972;75: 673-79 in Peritz E. *loc.cit.*

87.   Meland MR, Flehinger BJ. Early incidence rates of precancerous cervical lesions in women using contraceptives. *Gynecol. Oncol.* 1973;1:290-8 in Peritz E. *loc.cit.*

88.   Boyce JG, Lu T, Nelson JH, Fruchter RG. Oral contraceptives and cervical carcinoma. *Am J Obstet Gynec.* 1977; 128: 761-66 in Peritz E. *loc.cit.*

89. Peritz, *loc.cit.*
90. *Ibid.,* p.463
91. Ory HW, *et al.,* A Preliminary analysis of oral contraceptive use and risk of developing premalignant lesions of the uterine cervix. In: Garratini S, Berendes HW, eds *Pharmacology of steroid contraceptive drugs.* New York, Raven Press 1977 211-24. in Brinton LA. Oral contraceptives and cervical neoplasia. *Contraception.* 1991;43:(6). p. 584. Table 2.
92. Peritz, *op.cit.,* p.468
93. Brinton LA. Oral contraceptives and cervical neoplasia. *Contraception.* 1991;43:(6). p.582
94. Peirtz, *op.cit.,* p.468
95. Vessey MP, McPherson K, Lawless M, Yeates, D. Neoplasia of the Cervix uteri and contraception: A possible adverse effect of the pill. *Lancet.* 1983; Oct 22, pp., 932-933
96. *Ibid.,* p.933
97. *Ibid.*
98. *Ibid.,* p.934
99. Beral V, Hannaford P, Kay C. Oral contraceptive use malignancies of the Genital Tract. *Lancet.* 1988,Dec10, pp.1331-1332
100. *Ibid.,* p.1332
101. *Ibid.,* p.1334
102. Schlesselman JJ. Cancer of the breast and reproductive tract in relation to use of oral contraceptives. *Contraception.* 1989;40(1): p.1
103. Brock KE, Berry G, Brinton LA, *et al.,*Sexual, reproductive and contraceptive risk factors for carcinoma-in-situ of the uterine cervix in Sydney. *The Medical Journal of Australia.* 1989;15: p.125
104. *Ibid.*
105. *Ibid.*
106. *Ibid.,* p.129
107. *Mosby's, op.cit.,* p.1011
108. Brinton LA, Reeves WC,*et. al.*, Oral contraceptive use and risk of invasive cervical cancer. *International Journal of Epidemiology.* 1990; 19(1): 4-11, MEDLINE ABSTRACT (Ma)
109. Rodriguez-Contreras R, *et al*., Oral contraceptives and cancer of the cervix uteri. Analysis of the strength of the association. *Revista de Sanidad e higiene Publica.* 1991;65(1): 25-38. Ma
110. Brinton, *op.cit.,* p. 581
111. *Ibid.*

112. *Ibid.*
113. *Ibid.,* p.589
114. Gram IT, Macaluso M, Stalsberg H. Oral contraceptive use and the incidence of cervical intraepithelial neoplasia. *American Journal of Obstetrics and Gynaecology.* 1992;167(1):p.40.
115. *Ibid.,* pp.42-43
116. *Ibid.,* p.40
117. *Ibid.,* p.42
118. Delgado-Rodriguez M, *et al.,* Oral contraceptives and cancer of the cervix uteri. A Meta-analysis. *Acta Obstetricia et Gynecologia Scandinavica.* 1992;71(5):368-76, (Ma)
119. Kjaer SK, *et al.,* Case-control study of risk factors for cervical squamous-cell neoplasia in Denmark. 111. Role of oral contraceptive use. *Cancer Causes and Control.* 1993;4(6):513-9,(Ma)
120. Kohler U, Wuttke P. Results of a case-control study of the current effect of various factors of cervical cancer risk. 2. Contraceptive behaviour and the smoking factor. *Zentralblatt fur gynakologie.* 1994;116(7): 405-9, (Ma)
121. *Merck Manual* 16th Ed., *op.cit.,* p.1824
122. Ursin G, Peters R K, Henderson BE, d'Ablaing G, Monroe, KR, Pike MC. Oral contraceptive use and adenocarcinoma of cervix. *Lancet.* 1994; 344; 1390-1394
123. Kohler, *loc.cit.*
124. Schlesselman, *op.cit.,* p.19
125. New South Wales (Aust) Cancer Council March 1996 - Private correspondence.
126. Ursin, *op.cit.,* p.1390 (OR 4.4 p=0.04, one sided p for trend, CI 1.8-10.8)
127. *Ibid.*
128. *Ibid.,* p.1391
129. Brisson J, *et al.,* Risk Factors for Cervical Intraepithelial Neoplasia: Differences between Low-and High-Grade Lesions. *American Journal of Epidemiology.* 1994; 140:700-710.
130. Z. Ye, Thomas DB, Ray RM, *et. al.,* Combined Oral Contraceptives and Risk of Cervical Cancer in situ. *International Journal of Epidemiology.* 1995;24:19-26
131. Thomas DB, Ray RM . Oral contraceptives and invasive adenocarcinomas and adenosquamous carcinomas of the uterine cervix. *Am J Epid.* 1996;144:p.284. Table 2

132. Zondervan KT, *et al.,* Oral contraceptives and cervical cancer — further findings from the Oxford Family Planning Association contraceptive study. *Br J Cancer.* 1996 (May); 73:10, 1291

133. *Ibid.,* p.1296

134. *Ibid.,* p.1292

135. Schlesselman JJ. Net effect of oral contraceptive use on the risk of cancer in women in the United States. *Obstet Gynecol.* 1995;85:5 Pt 1, 793-801 Ma

136. *Ibid.,* p.793

137. *Merck Manual,* 16th Ed., p.1824

138. Arsmtrong B. Human papillomavirus and cervical cancer. *Lancet.* 1988: April 2.p.756

139. *Ibid.*

140. *Merck Manual,* 16th Ed., p.270

141. *Ibid.*

142. *Merck Manual* 16th Ed., p.271

143. Isselbacher *et al., Harrison's Principles of Internal Medicine.* 1994.13th Ed. Ch. 150. p. 801

144. *Merck Manual, op.cit.,* p.1824

145. Chang, AR. Hormonal contraceptives, human papillomavirus and cervical cancer; some observation from a colposcopy clinic. *Aust New Zeal Obstet Gynec.*1989;29:329-331 in Dunn, H.P. *The Doctor and the Christian Marriage.* Alba House, New York. 1992 p.68

146. Hildesheim A, Reeves WC, Brinton LA, Lavery C, Brenes M, De La Guardia ME, Godoy J, Rawls WE. Association of oral contraceptive use and human papillomaviruses in invasive cervical cancers. *International Journal of Cancer.*1990; 45(5):860-4. (Ma)

147. Pater A, Bayatpour M, Pater MM. Oncogenic transformation by human papillomavirus type 16 deoxyribonucleic acid in the presence of progesterone or progestins from oral contraceptives. *Am J Obstet Gynecol.*1990 Apr; 162:4,1099-103 (Ma)

148. Brinton, *op.cit.,* p.581

149. *Ibid.,* p.589

150. *Mosby's Dictionary, op. cit.,* p.873

151. Gitsch G, Kain C. Reinthaller A, Tatra G, Breitenecker G. Oral contraceptives and human papilloma virus infection in cervical lesions (meeting abstract). *Nineteenth European Congress of Cytology.* June 17-20, 1991, Turku, Finland, p 21

152. Brinton, *op.cit.*, p.581.
153. Gitsch G , Kainz C, Studnicka M, Reinthaller A, Tatra G, Breitenecker G.. Oral contraceptives and human papillomavirus infection in cervical intraepithelial neoplasia. *Arch Gynae & Obstet.* 1992;252(1): p.27 N.B. (test for trend: unadjusted P-value <0.02).
154. *Ibid.*, p.27.
155. *Ibid.*, pp.28-29.
156. *Ibid.*, p.29.
157. Brisson J, Morin C , Fortier M, *et al. American Journal of Epidemiology.* Risk factors for cervical intraepithelial neoplasia: differences between low- and high- grade lesions. 1994;140:(8).p.700 (p>0.0001: 95% CI 5.1-15.0)
158. Cox JT. Epidemiology of cervical intraepithelial neoplasia: the role of human papillomavirus. *Baillieres Clin Obstet Gynaecol.*1995;9:1,1-37 Ma
159. *Ibid.*
160. Bosch FX, Manos MM, MuAnoz N, Sherman M, Jansen AM, Peto J, Schiffman MH, Moreno V, Kurman R, Shah KV. Prevalence of human papillomavirus in cervical cancer: a worldwide perspective. International biological study on cervical cancer (IBSCC) Study Group. *J Natl Cancer Inst.*1995 (June7);87:,796-802 Ma
161. Ho GY, Burk RD, Klein S, Kadish AS, Chang CJ, Palan P, Basu J, Tachezy R, Lewis R, Romney S. Resistant genital human papillomavirus infection as a risk factor for persistent cervical dysplasia. *J Natl Cancer Inst.* 1995; 87:18, p.1365
162. Park TW, Fujiwara H, Wright TC. Molecular biology of cervical cancer and its precursors. *Cancer.*1995;76:10(Suppl),1902-13 Ma
163. "Cervical dysplasia, also referred to as squamous intraepithelial lesion (SIL) in cytology or cervical intraepithelial neoplasia (CIN) in histopathology, is thought to have the potential to advance in progressive stages to cervical cancer." in Ho GY, *Ibid.*
164. Thomas DB, Ray RM, Pardthaisong T, Chutivongse, Koetsawang S, Silpisornkosol S, *et al.,* Prostitution, condom use, and invasive squamous cell cervical cancer in Thailand. *AJE.* 1996;143:p.779.
165. This study was conducted in Thailand, where "female premarital sexual relations were rare...". *Ibid.,* p.784.,
166. Chen Y-H, Huang L-H, Chen T-M. Differential effects of progestins and estrogens on long control regions of human papillomavirus types 16 and

18. *Biochemical and Biophysical Research Communications.* 1996;224: p.654

167. *Ibid.,* p.657

168. *Ibid.,* p.652

169. *Ibid.*

170. Soussi T. The p53 tumour suppressor gene: a model for molecular epidemiology of human cancer. *Mol Med Today.*1996;1:32-7 Ma

171. Memorial Sloan-Kettering Cancer Center. Scientists Link Smoking, p53 and bladder cancer. 1996 http://.mskcc.org/document/cn950801.htm

172. *Ibid.*

173. Soussi T, *loc.cit.*

174. The role of differing pill formulations in breast cancer must not be underestimated. The variable manner in which artificial hormones interact with cells has now been shown to be intimately linked to the precise molecular structure of the particular hormonal composition of the pill. In my view, this greatly assists our understanding of how the pill causes various cancers, and other serious health problems. By altering the structure of the natural hormonal molecule, pharmaceutical companies give back to women a hormone which behaves differently to that which her body produces. By adding or removing certain portions of the natural molecule, the 'strength' with which the artificial molecules attaches to a cell (via a receptor) is also altered. These changed binding characteristic cause different behavioural patterns within cells, and many of these new patterns of cellular behaviour are clearly deleterious.

175. "A series of estrogens and progestins were examined for their effects on HPV16 or 18 gene expression. HeLa cells were transfected with p16CAT (chlorampenicol acetyltransferase) or p18CAT for 24 hours, followed by estrogens or progestins treatment for 72 hours. Pregnenolone, 17a-hydroxy-progesterone, cyproterone acetate, ethynodiol diacetate and norethynodrel at 10 to the minus 7 M showed an over 2-fold increase in CAT activity in p16CAT-infected HeLa cells. On the other hand, these progestins did not enhance CAT activity in p18CAT-transfected HeLa cells. Accordingly, all progestins except ethisterone and D(-) norgestrel were able to stimulate HPV16-LCR, but not HPV18-LCR (long control region). Similar to progestins, differential transactivation of HPV-16LCR and, less significantly, HPV18-LCR by estrogens was observed in HeLa cells. In addition to estriol and 17-b-estradiol, tamoxifen, an anti-estrogen, was also up-regulated by HPV16 gene expression through LCR in HeLa

cells. Effects of these progestins and estrogens on HPV16 LCR were dose dependent... According to structure-activity relationship (SAR) concept, introduction or substitution of functional groups may tremendously change solubility, stability and activity of the main structure. Hormone-dependent transactivation of HPV 16 was compared among a series of progestins and estrogens bearing a variety of functional groups. Progestins can be classified based on the positions of C21 or C19. Compounds derived from pregnenolone backbone (C21 derivatives) enhance HPV 16 gene expression in the order as follows: pregnenolone=cyproterone=17 a-hydroxy-progesterone>6- a methyl-17a-hydroxy-progesterone acetate>progesterone. Compounds derived from 19-nortestosterone (C19 derivatives), except D(-) norgestrel and ethisterone, also enhanced HPV 16 gene expression. Methyl group on C10 or ethyl group on C13 of 19-nortestosterone backbone may have hindrance effect on interaction with progesterone receptors, while (a) number of hydroxy groups on C16 and C17 of estrogens may be important for hormone-receptor interaction.". in Chen, *Ibid.,* pp.653-54

176.   Kenney JAW. Risk factors associated with genital HPV infection. *Cancer Nurse.* 1996 (Oct);19:5, p.353
177.   *A.P.P.G.,* Biphasil 21 Monograph (Wyeth Pharmaceuticals), p.489. 1996
178.   Women sue over Pill risks. *The Daily Telegraph-Mirror* (Sydney, Aust.) 13.4.95, p 22

CHAPTER THREE.

179.   *APPG.* Trifeme Monograph Vol. 2 1996. p.2346
180.   Schlesselman, *op.cit.,* pp.1-38.
181.   Vessey, *British Medical Journal.* 1972, *op.cit.,* p.723
182.   Vessey, *Lancet.*1975, *op.cit.,* pp.942-943.
183.   Boston Collaborative Drug Surveillance Programme. *Lancet*;1973:1:p.1399
184.   *Goodman and Gilman's The Pharmacological Basis of Therapeutics,* 5th Ed. Macmillan Pub. Co. N.Y.1975 p.1447
185.   Vessey MP, Doll R, Jones K, McPherson K, Yeates D. An epidemiological study of oral contraceptives and breast cancer. *Br Med J* 1979;1:p.1757
186.   Vessey MP, McPherson K, Yeates D, Doll R. Oral contraceptive use and abortion before first term pregnancy in relation to breast cancer risk. *Br J Cancer.* 1982;45:p.327

187. *Mosby's Dictionary, op. cit.*, p. 678 (paraphrased)
188. *Merck Manual,* 15th Ed., *op. cit.*, p.26.
189. *Ibid.*, p.1209
190. Vessey, *Br Med J.* 1972, *op.cit.*, pp.722-723
191. This proposition was put by Vessey to explain why their results showed that: "there is no suggestion that the use of oral contraceptives is related in any way to the risk of breast cancer in women up to 45 years of age." in Vessey, *Lancet.* 1975, *op.cit.*, p. 943
192. Beral V, Colwell L. Randomised trial of high doses of stilboestrol and ethisterone in pregnancy: long-term follow-up of mothers. *Br Med J.* 1980; 281:p.1098
193. McPherson K, Neil A, Vessey M.P, Doll R. Oral contraceptives and breast cancer. *Lancet.* 1983; ii:p.1415.
194. Shapiro S., Oral contraceptives - time to take stock. *N Eng J Med.* 1986; 315; 7; 450-451
195. McPherson K, Vessey M.P, Neil A, Doll R, Jones L & Roberts M. Early oral contraceptive use and breast cancer: Results of another case-control study. *Br J Cancer.* 1987;56:p.658-659
196. Olsson H, *et al.* Early oral contraceptive use and breast in Southern Sweden. *Proc Annu Meet Am Soc Clin Oncol.* 8:A367,1989 Ma
197. *Goodman and Gilman. op.cit.,* 5th Ed, p.1447
198. *Goodman and Gilman's The Pharmacological Basis of Therapeutics,* 8th Ed. Pergamom Press 1990, p.1407
199. Hume K. The Pill and other potions in perspective. *Healthcare Bioethics Perspectives.* 27.7.1991 (Seminar paper).
200. *Ibid.*
201. King RJB. Biology of female sex hormone action in relation to contraceptive agents and neoplasia. *Contraception.* Imperial Cancer Research Fund. University of Surrey. 1991;43:(6) p.533
202. CancerNet News - Oral Contraceptives and Risk for Breast Cancer in Young Women- National Cancer Institute August 1995. *Internet address - http://oncolink.upenn.edu/cancer_new/*
203. Schlesselman, *op.cit.,* p.3
204. *Ibid.*, p.9
205. *Mosby's Dictionary, op.cit.,* p.432
206. Pike M.C, Henderson BE, Krailo MD, Duke A. Breast cancer in young women and use of oral contraceptives:possible modifying effect of formulation and age at use. *Lancet.*1983;ii:p.929

207. Shapiro, *op.cit.*, p.450.
208. *Merck Manual*, 15th Ed. p.2365
209. Vessey, *Br Med J.* 1979, *op.cit.*, p.1760
210. Pike, *op.cit.*, p.928. Table V.
211. McPherson K, Neil A, Vessey MP, Doll R. Oral contraceptives and breast cancer. *Lancet* (Letter) 1983; Dec 17th:
212. *Ibid.*
213. Meirik O, Adami H-O, Christoffersen T, Lund E, Bergstrom R, Bergsjo P. Oral Contraceptive use and Breast Cancer in Young Women. *Lancet.* 1986;2; p.653
214. *Ibid.*, p.650
215. Stadel BV, Schlesselman JJ. Oral contraceptives and breast cancer. *Lancet.* 1986;ii:922-3
216. Chilvers C, *et al.*, Oral contraceptive use and breast cancer risk in young women. *Lancet.* 1989: 6th May; 973-982
217. Miller DR, Rosenberg L, *et al.* Breast Cancer before age 45 and oral contraceptive use: new findings. *American Journal of Epidemiology.* 1989;129(2):269-80, Ma
218. Romieu I, *et al.*, Oral contraceptives and breast cancer. Review and meta-analysis. *Cancer.* 1990;66(11): 2253-63, Ma
219. Weinstein AL, *et al.*, Breast cancer risk and oral contraceptive use: results from a large case-control study. *Epidemiology.* 1991;2(5):353-8, Ma
220. Olsson H, Borg A, Ferno M, Moller TR, Ranstam J. Early oral contraceptive use and premenopausal breast cancer - a review of studies performed in Southern Sweden. *Cancer Detection and Prevention.* 1991;15(4):p.267
221. *Ibid.*, p.267, Table 2.
222. Rookus M A, E van Leeuwen. Oral contraceptives and risk of breast cancer in women aged 20-54 years. *Lancet* 1994; 334; p.849
223. *Ibid.*, p.850
224. Pike, *op.cit.*, p.926
225. Olsson H & ML, Moller TR, Ranstam J, Holm P. Oral contraceptive use and breast cancer in young women in Sweden. *Lancet.* (Letter) 1985. March 30. 748-49.
226. Shapiro, *op.cit.*, p.450
227. Meirik, *op.cit.*, p.650
228. Chilvers C, McPherson K, Peto J, Pike MC, Vessey MP. Oral contraceptive use and breast cancer risk in young women. *Lancet.* 1989 6th May p.980

229. Olsson H. Oral contraceptives and breast cancer. A review. *Acta Oncologica.* 1989;28(6):849-63, Ma

230. Olsson H, Moller TR, Ranstam J. Early oral contraceptive use and breast cancer among premenopausal women: Final report from a study in Southern Sweden. *Journal of the National Cancer Institute.* 1989; 81(12):1000-4.

231. Shapiro, *op.cit.,* p.450

232. Johnson JH. Weighing the evidence on the pill and breast cancer. *Family Planning Perspectives.* 1989 ; 21(2):89-92, Ma

233. Anonymous. Oral contraceptive use and breast cancer risk in young. UK National Case-control study group. *Lancet:*1989;1(8645):973-82. Ma

234. Olsson H, Ranstam MA, Baldetrop, Ewres SB, Ferno M, Killander D, Sigurdsson H. Proliferation and DNA ploidy in malignant tumours in relation to early oral contraception use and early abortions. *Cancer.*1991; 67(5) 1285-90,

235. Olsson H, Borg A, Ferno M, Moller TR, Ranstam J. *op.cit.,* p.265

236. Sweet M. Mystery as rarer types of cancer gain ground. *Sydney Morning Herald (Aust).* May 17, 1997, p. 5.

237. Ranstam JP. Oral contraceptives and breast cancer. *Diss Abstr Int(C).* 1992;53(4):705, Ma

238. *Ibid.*

239. Wingo PA, Lee NC, *et al.,* Age-specific differences in the relationship between oral contraceptive use and breast cancer. *Cancer.* 1993;71(4 Suppl): 1506-17.

240. Rookus M A, E van Leeuwen. Oral contraceptives and risk of breast cancer in women aged 20-54 years. *The Lancet* 1994; 334; 884-851.

241. Olsson H, *et al.,* Proliferation and DNA ploidy in malignant tumours in relation to early oral contraception use and early abortions. *Cancer.* 1991;67(5): 1285-90

242. *Ibid.*

243. Palmer JR, Rosenberg L, Rao RS, Strom BL et. al., Oral contraceptive use and breast cancer risk among African-American women. *Cancer Causes Control.*1995;6(4):321-31. Ma

244. Schuurman AG, van den Brandt PA, Goldbohm RA. Exogenous hormone use and the risk of postmenopausal cancer: results from the Netherlands Cohort Study.*Cancer Causes and Control.*1995;6:p.420

245. *Ibid.*

246. McPherson K. Third generation oral contraception and venous thrombo-

embolism. *BMJ.* 1996; 312:#7023. http://www.bmj.com/archive/7023e.htm

247. Rosenberg L, Palmer JR, Rao RS, Zauber AG, *et al.,* Case-control study of oral contraceptive use and risk of breast cancer. *Amer J Epidemiol.* 1996;143:25-37

248. *Ibid.*

249. Olsson H, Jernstrom H, Alm P, Kreipe H, Ingvar C, *et al.,* Proliferation of the breast epithelium in relationship to menstrual cycle phase, hormonal use, and reproductive factors. *Breast Cancer Research and Treatment.* 1996;40:p.187

250. *Ibid.,* p.189

251. *Ibid.,* p.190

252. *Ibid.,* p.194

253. Genuis SJ, Genuis SK. Adolescent sexual involvement: time for primary prevention. *Lancet.* 1995;345:240-41.

254. *Ibid.*

255. *Ibid.*

256. *Ibid.*

257. Olsson H, *et al.,* Early oral contraceptive use and breast in Southern Sweden. *Proc Annu Meet Am Soc Clin Oncol.* 1989;8:A367. Ma

258. Ranstam J, Olsson H, *et al.,* Survival in breast cancer and age at start of oral contraceptive usage. *Anticancer Research.* 1991;11:p.2043.

259. Olsson H, Ranstarn J, Baldetorp B, Ewers SB, Ferno M, Killander D, Sigurdsson H. Proliferation and DNA ploidy in malignant tumours in relation to early oral contraception use and early abortions. *Cancer.* 1991;67(5) p.1285

260. "First, as compared with nonusers and late users of oral contraceptives, premenopausal patients with a history of early oral contraceptive use manifested larger tumours, a greater incidence of axilary metasis, lower progesterone and estrogen receptor values, a higher S-phase fraction and frequency of aneuploidy, and poorer survival." Olsson H, Borg A, Ferno M, Ranstam J, Sigurdsson H. Her-2/neu and INT2 Proto-oncogene amplification in malignant breast tumours in relation to reproductive factors and exposure to exogenous Hormones. *J Natl Cancer Inst.* 1991; 83:p.1485

261. Olsson H, Borg A *et al., Cancer Detection and Prevention.* 1991, p.267, Table IV.

262. *Ibid.,* p.269

263   *Ibid.*
264. *Ibid.*
265. Olsson H, Ranstam MA, Baldetrop B, Ewers SB, *op.cit.,* p.1289
266. *Mosby's, op.cit.,* p. 882
267. *Ibid.*
268. Meirik O, Farley TMM, Lund E, Adami HO, Christoffersen T, Bergsjo P. Breast cancer and oral contraceptives: patterns of risk among parous and nulliparous women-further analysis of the Swedish-Norwegian material. *Contraception.* 1989;39(5):471-5.
269. *Ibid.,* p.471
270. *Ibid.,* p.474
271. Rushton L. Jones DR., Oral contraceptive use and breast cancer risk: a meta-analysis of variations with age at diagnosis, parity and total duration of oral contraceptive use. *British Journal Obst Gynae.* 1992; 99(3): 239-46. Ma
272. Colditz GA. Postmenopausal Estrogens and breast cancer. *Society for Gynecologic Investigation.* 1996;3:(2).p.50
273. *Ibid.*
274. *Merck Manual* 16th Ed., *op.cit.,* p.2293-94
275. *Ibid.,* p.2294.
276. Ursin G, Aragaki CC, *et al.,* Oral contraceptives and premenopausal bi-lateral breast cancer: A case-control study. *Epidemiology.* 1992;3(5) p.414.
277. Lund E. Oral contraceptives and breast cancer: A review with some comments on mathematical models. *Acta Oncologia.* 1992 ;31(2): 183-6
278. Weisberg, *Current Therapeutics.* 1994 (Sept) p.51.
279. Chilvers CE, Pike MC, Hermon C, Crossley B. Breast cancer and breast feeding (Meeting abstract) *British Journal of Cancer.* 1992; 66(Suppl xv11):9 Ma
280. *Ibid.*
281. Symons E-K, Pill safety row still unresolved. *The Sunday Telegraph* (Sydney, Aust) 1.10.95; 181
282. NSW Cancer Incidence and Mortality. NSW Central Cancer Registry. Cancer Epidemiology Research Unit 1991. Private correspondence.
283. NSW Central Cancer Registry Cancer Epidemiology Research Unit, NSW Cancer Council. 1994..
284. Sweet, *op.cit.,* 1997
285. Hills Shire Times 13.6.95 (Baulkham Hills NSW Aust)

286. Media Tracking Service. 1995;186:Monday 18th Dec
287. Armstrong D. Breast Cancer - Women's Health Enemy No.1 *Ita.*May 1994. Sydney Aust. , p.27.
288. *Ibid.*
289. Schlesselman, *op.cit.,* p.4
290. *The Sydney Morning Herald* (John Fairfax & Sons, Publishers) 27.6.95 p.9
291. Ferrari J, *The Australian,*(News Ltd, publishers) 27.9.95. p.3.
292. *APPG.* Vol 2. 1996 Trifeme Monograph. p.2341

CHAPTER FOUR.

293. *The Australian Journal of Pharmacy* 1995 ;Vol 76. Feb. p.112
294. Boston Collaborative Drug Surveillance Programme. *Lancet.*1973:1: p.1399
295. *Ibid.,* p.1402.
296. Meade TW, Greenberg G, Thompson SG. Progestogens and cardiovascular reactions associated with oral contraceptives and a comparison of the safety of 50- and 30-ug oestrogen preparations. *Br Med Journ.* 1980:280:p.1157.
297. *Ibid.*
298. Layde P M, Beral V. Further analyses of mortality in oral contraceptive users. *Lancet.* 1981;P.541. Table II.
299. Helmrich SP, Rosenberg L, Kaufman DW, Strom B & Shapiro S. Venous thromboembolism in relation to oral contraceptive use. *Obstet & Gynec.* 1987;69:p.91.
300. The authors did point out that the confidence levels were wide, hence a reduction in DVT risk with reduced oestrogen content cannot be ruled out.
301. Helmich, *loc.cit.*
302. Announcing a new Schering development in oral contraception (gest-odene). Schering Pty.Ltd. Alexandria NSW AUST 2015. Professional marketting material.
303. Stubblefield PG. The effects on hemostasis of oral contraceptives containing desogestrel. *Am J Obstet Gynecol.* 1993;168:p.1047
304. Ehman R. MD. *Problems in Family Planning.* p.14. Heezerweg 345 5643 KG Eindhoven The Netherlands.
305. *Ibid.,* p.15
306. R.H., Was ist da dran?, *Medical Tribune. Internationale Wochenzeitung*

- *Ausgabe fur die Schweiz.* 1989;16,20. Trans. Ania Kurkowski B.Pharm.

307. Women sue over Pill risks. *The Daily Telegraph Mirror,* Thursday, April 13, 1995 p.22

308. *Ibid.*

309. *Mosby's, op.cit.,* p.283.

310. Leroy O, *et al.*, Deep venous thrombosis and antibodies to cyproterone acetate.*Lancet*; 1990; 336:509

311. Beaumont V, Beaumont J-L. Thrombosis and antibodies to cyproterone acetate. *Lancet.* 1991;337; 113

312. Dr.Schueler's *Home Medical Advisor Pro* (CD edition) 1993 Pixel Perfect Inc. 10460 Tropical Trail Merritt, Florida 32952

313. Vandenbroucke J P, *et al.* Increased risk of venous thrombosis in oral contraceptive users who are carriers of factor V Leiden mutation. *Lancet* 1994; 344: p.1454

314. *Ibid.,* pp.1455-1456

315. Rosing J. Tans G, Nicolaes GAF, Thomassen M, van Oerle R, van der Ploeg P et al. Oral contraceptives and venous thrombosis: different sensitivities to activated protein C in women using second- and third-generation oral contraceptives. *Br J Haematology.* 1997;97:p.233

316. "APC resistance is a hereditary disorder that results from a mutation in the gene of blood coagulation factor V and renders the activated form of factor V less susceptible to proteolytic inactivation by APC. Since APC-catalysed factor Va inactivation is a crucial step in the down-regulation of thrombin formation, impaired inactivation of factor Va probably explains the increased risk of venous thrombo-embolism in APC-resistant individuals." *Ibid.*

317. Vandenbroucke, *op.cit.,* p.1455

318. Graham A, Grieve F, Davie, Glasier A. *Lancet.*1995;346:1430 (Letter)

319. Choo V. EU agency asks for more data on oral contraceptives.*Lancet.* 1995;346:1219.(Letter).

320. Lawrence J. Three Pill studies showed increased risk of blood clots. *The Times* (London). 21.10.95

321. Crowe S, Kent S. Pill Panic - Health warning on seven brands. *The Sun-Herald.* Sydney.Aust. 22.10.95

322. *Ibid.*

323. Prudence with the Pill. Health warnings are meant to cause alarm. *The Times.*(London). 21.10.95

324. Crowe, *loc.cit.*

325.   Prudence with the pill., *loc.cit.*

326.   Graham, *loc.cit.*

327.   Cranall D. Controvesry rages over new contraceptive data. *Br Med J.* 1995;311:p.1117-8

328.   Layde, *op.cit.,* p.541-546

329.   *APPG.* 24th Ed 1995, Minulet monograph. p.1540

330.   Watt AH. *Lancet.*1995;346:1430 (Letter)

331.   Persaud R. *Lancet.*1995;346:1431 (Letter)

332.   Ivory Dr K. Pill claims don't make sense. *Medical Observer* 10.11.95, p.5,quoting Dr Edith Weisberg.

333.   Sharp D. Venous thrombosis and the modern pill. *Lancet.*1996;347:181

334.   Prudence with the Pill. *loc.cit.*

335.   McPherson K. Third generation oral contraception and venous thromboembolism. *Br Med J.* 1996;#7023:Vol.312 http://www.bmj.com/archive/7023e.htm

336.   Bloemenkamp KW, Rosendal FR, Helmerhorst FM, Bauller HR, Vandenbrouche JP. Enhancement by factor V Leiden mutation of deep-vein thrombosis associated with oral contraceptives containing third-generation progestagen. *Lancet.* 1995;346:8990:1593-6.

337.   The variation in risk depended upon whether the formulation contained levonorgestrel or norethisterone, and also the amount of ethinyloestradiol. *Ibid.,* p.1594, Table 1.

338.   *Ibid.,* p.1595

339.   (7 multiplied by 120%=7 by 2.2=15.4, 7 multiplied by 280%= 7 by 3.8=26.6)

340.   *Ibid.*

341.   *Ibid.,* p.1596

342.   Spitzer WO, Lewis MA, Heinemann LAJ, Thorogood M, MacRae KD. Third generation oral contraceptives and risk of venous thromboembolic disorders: an international case-control study. *Br Med J.* 1996;312:83-8

343.   *Ibid.,* p.83

344.   *Ibid.*

345.   These results pertained only to England and Germany. Lewis MA, Spitzer WO, LAJ Heinemann, MacRae KD, Bruppacher R, Thorogood M. *Br Med J.* 1996;312:88-90 .

346.   *Ibid.,* p.88

347.   Vandenbroucke JP, Bloemenkamp KWM, Helmerhorst FM, Rosendaal FR. Mortality from venous thromboembolism and myocardial infarction in young women in the Netherlands. *Lancet.*1996;348: #9024.   http://www.thelancet.com/lancet/User/vol348no9024/letters/index.html #Mortalityfrom

348. *Ibid.*
349. *Ibid.*
350. Thomas SHL.. Mortality from venous thromboembolism and myocardial infarction in young adults in England and Wales. *Lancet.*1996;348:#9024. http://www.thelancet.com/lancet/User/vol348no9024/letters/ index.html#Mortalityfrom
351. *Ibid.*
352. *Ibid.*
353. *Ibid.*
354. *Ibid.*
355. *Mosby's Medical Encyclopedia on CD.* Ver.1., 1995.
356. *Ibid.*
357. Rosing, *op.cit.,* p.233
358. *Ibid.*
359. *Ibid.,* p.237
360. *Ibid.*
361. Vandenbroucke JP, Rosendaal FR. End of the line for "third-generation" controvesy? *Lancet.*1997;349:1113-1114
362. *Ibid.,* p.1113
363. *Ibid.,* p.1114
364. Poulter NR, Meirik O. Haemorrhagic stroke, overall stroke risk, and combined oral contraceptives: results of an international, multicentre, case-control study. *Lancet.*1996;348:#9026 http://www.thelancet.com/ lancet/User/vol348no9026/articles/article2.html
365. Poulter NR, Meirik O. Ischaemic stroke and combined oral contraceptives: results of an international, multicentre, case-control study.*Lancet.*1996;348:#9026http://www.thelancet.com/lancet/User/ vol348no9026/articles/article2.html
366. Cooke H. Mother of tragic Pill girls to sue. *Daily Express*(UK) 1996; March 27: p.4.
367. Woodcock J, Hope J. Tragic girl given the Pill at 14. *Daily Mail* (UK). 1996; March 27: p.8.
368. Cooke, *loc.cit.*
369. *Ibid.*
370. Hall C. Girl dies after taking the pill to cure acne. *UK News, Electronic Telegraph,* 5th Feb, 1997, Issue 621. Web Address. *http://www.telegraph. co.uk*
371. Lawson C. Stoke victim doggedly blinks trial testimomy. *The Ottawa Citizen.*April, 1997. <a1a34216@bc.sympatico.ca>

372. Prudence with the Pill. *loc.cit.*
373. Kim MR, Qazi QH, Anderson VM, Valencia GB. A genetic male infant with female phenotype in camptomelic syndrome: A relationship to exposure to oral contraceptives during pregnancy. *Am J Obstet Gynecol.* 1995;172:p.1042
374. Wade ME, McCarthy PM, *et al., Am J Obstet. Gynecol.* (Letter). 1980; March 1:p.698
375. Rahwan, *op.cit.*, p.32
376. *Ibid.,* pp.29-30
377. In *Micromedex* Vol 92. (1) Czeizel A. Increasing trends in congenital malformations of male external genitalia. *Lancet.* 1985;I:462-3. (2) Aarskog D. Clinical and cytogenetic studies in hypospadias. *Acta Paediatr Scand.* 1970: (suppl 203): 1-62. (3) Roberts IF, West RJ. Teratogenesis and maternal progesterone. *Lancet.* 1977; ii, 982. (4) Evans ANW, et al. The ingestion by pregnancy women of substances toxic to the foetus. *Practitioner.* 1980; 224: 315-19. (5) Heinonen OP, et al. Cardiovascular birth defects and antenatal exposure to female sex hormones. *N. Eng. J. Med.* 1977;296:67-70. (6) Mann JR, et al. Transplacental carcinogenesis (adrenocortical carcinoma) associated with hydroxyprogesterone hexanoate. *Lancet.* 1983;ii, 580. (7) Wilkins L. Masculinization of female fetus due to use of orally given progestins. *JAMA.* 1960;172:1028-32 (8) Gal I, et al. Hormonal pregnancy tests and congenital malformation. *Nature.* 1967;216:83. (9) Profumo R, et al. Neonatal choreoathetosis following prenatal exposure to oral contraceptives. *Pediatrics.* 1990;86:648-9
378. *A P P G.* 24th Ed. Microgynon 30 Monograph,1995, p.1508
379. *Micromedex* Vol 89. Oral contraceptives monograph
380. Odeblad, E. Prof. Regolazione Naturale dell Fertilita Femminile. 1988 (Seminar paper)
381. Odeblad, E. Prof. *Families of Australia Foundation International Conference.* Sydney, Australia. p.119-24, July, 1988 (Seminar paper)
382. *Ibid.*

CHAPTER FIVE.

383. Paul C. Depo medroxyprogesterone (Depo-Provera) and risk of breast cancer. *Br. Med. J.* 1989; 299: p.762
384. *Micromedex*, DMPA monograph, Vol. 92, 1997

385. "DMPA causes the endometrium to become atrophic, with small, straight endometrial glands and decidualized stroma.". in Mishell DR. Pharmacokinetics of depot medroxyprogesterone acetate contraception. *J Reprod Med.*1996;41:5 Suppl, 381-90 Ma.

386. Addison AW, *et al.,* The occurrence of adenocarcinoma in endometriosis of the rectovaginal septum during progestational therapy. *Gynecol Oncology* 1979; 8:193., Anon: Depo-Provera debate revs up at FDA. *Science* 1982; 217:424-428., Dabancens A et al: Intraepithelial cervical neoplasia in women using intrauterine devices and long-acting injectable progesterones as contraceptives. *Am J Obstet Gynecol* 1974; 119:1052., *FDA Drug Bulletin:* March-April 1978; 8:2., Powell L & Seymour R: Effects of depo-medroxyprogesterone acetate as a contraceptive agent. *Am J Obstet Gynecol* 1971; 110:36., Richard BW & Lasagna L: Drug regulation in the United States and the United Kingdom: the depo-provera story. *Ann Intern Med* 1987; 106:886-891. In *Micromedex* Vol 86

387. Paul, *op.cit.,* p.760.

388. *Ibid.*

389. Gray RH. Depo medroxyprogesterone and risk of breast cancer. *Br Med J.* 1989;299:1989.

390. "The relevance of experimental studies in rodents [ie rats] to man is often questioned but, in this author's opinion, a case has been established for their inclusion..." King RJB. Biology of female sex hormone action in relation to contraceptive agents and neoplasia. *Contraception.* Imperial Cancer Research Fund. University of Surrey. 1991;43:(6). p.534.

391. *Merck Manual* 16th Ed, pp. 2640-2641

392. King, *op.cit.,* p.530.

393. *Ibid.,* p.533

394 National Alliance if Breast Cancer Organisations (NABCO) Vol 3#4 1989 http://nysernet.org/bcic/

395. Paul, *op.cit.,* p.761

396. Thomas DB, Noonan EA. Breast cancer and depo-medroxyprogesterone acetate: a multinational study. WHO collaborative study of neoplasia and steroid contraceptives. *Lancet.* 1991;338:833-838

397. "What about a biological interpretation of the results? Maximum mitotic activity (cell replication) in glandular mammary epithelium and an increase in the size of terminal ducts and tubules characterise the luteal (post-ovulatory) phase of the normal menstrual cycle, when endogenous progesterone concentrations are highest. Normal mammary epithelium responds similarly, but to a greater extent, to exogenous progestagens.

In addition, progestagens can stimulate human mammary tumour cells in tissue. DMPA could therefore accelerate proliferation of either initiated or fully transformed tumour cells. Stimulation of initiated cells (tumour promotion) would promote development of new tumours that otherwise might not develop. Stimulation of existing tumour cells would accelerate tumour growth and result in breast cancer being diagnosed earlier in users than in non-users, but would not lead to additional tumours. These possibilities are not mutually exclusive...These results are more compatible with stimulation of tumour growth as the predominant mechanism, but the relative risk estimates are not precise enough to distinguish between the two possible modes of action." *Ibid.,* p.857.

398. *A.PPG.* 24th Ed.1995 p.793
399. *Ibid.*
400. Blair JM. Types of Contraception may affect Bone Density in Adolescents. *American Family Physician.* 1995;Sept 15:1181
401. Rowe PM. Investigations into long-term contraceptives. *Lancet.* 1995; 346:693
402. *APPG.* 24th Ed, Premarin Monograph. p.1923
403. Skegg D C , Noonan E, Paul C, Spears GFS, Meirik O, Thomas DB. Depot Medroxyprogesterone Acetate an breast cancer. *Journal of the American Medical Association. (JAMA).* 1995;273:p.804
404. Paul, *op.cit.,* p.761.
405. Thomas, *op.cit.,* p.837
406. Morelli S. Lourdes: Clinic violated teaching. *Binghamton Press & Sun.* 1997 (March 28)

CHAPTER SIX.

407. Epstein KC & Sloat B. Many find side-effects of Norplant intolerable. *The Cleveland Plain Dealer.* (USA) 18.6.95
408. Cooper M. Norplant. *Aust NZ. J Obstet Gynaecol.* 1991;31:p.267
409. Kolata G, Will the Lawyers Kill Off Norplant, *The New York Times.* 28.5.95. page 1&5 Sect 3.
410. Copper, *op.cit.,* p.265
411. I use the term 'pregnant' rather loosely here to mean that the woman does not wish to conceive and implant, and thereby be aware she has an ongoing pregnancy.
412. "The Population Council, which has received patent rights on mifepristone [RU-486] from Roussel Uclaf, will submit an approval for U.S. Food and

Drug Administration approval by the end of 1995". Jackman J. RU-486 wins global praise from women. *The Feminist Majority Report.*Fall 1995 .p.14

413. Davies G C, Newton J R., Subdermal contraceptive implants - a review: with special reference to Norplant. *Br J Fam Planning.* 1991; 17; p.4.

414. Thomas Jr A G, LeMelle S. The Norplant system: where are we in 1995? *The Journal Of Family Practice,*1995; 40: No 2 Feb , p.126

415. Davies, *loc.cit.*

416. Painter K. "As perfect a Method as You Can Have" *USA Today* Dec 6, 1990 (cover story) in "A Hidden Side of Norplant" by Kristine M Severyn, R.Ph., Ph.D. reprinted in *Celebrate Life* July/August 1994

417. Hartmann B, Population and Development Program, Hampshire College, Amherst, MA 01002, USA . 'Population Council report on Norplant in Indonesia'. in *WGNRR Newsletter* 34 Jan - March 1991.p.24

418. Harper V. Agony of women who use Pill implants. *Daily Telegraph* (UK).1996;February 6

419. Davies, *loc.cit.*

420   Thomas, *loc.cit.*

421. Thomas, *op.cit.,* p.125

422. Painter, *op.cit.,* p.16

423. *Ibid.,* pp.16-17.

424. Taylor D. Spare the rod. *The Guardian* (U.K.) March 12, 1996, p11

425. Harper V, *Daily Telegraph* (UK).1996;February 6

426. Taylor, *loc.cit.*

427. Harper, *loc.cit.*

428. America Online:MAXFIELD 28.1.95 Medical legal consultants of Washington: Washington women respond to the dangers of Norplant.

429. Painter K. Norplant gets a shot in the arm. *USA TODAY.* 22.8.95

430. Taylor, *loc.cit.*

431. Harper, *loc.cit.*

432. *Ibid.*

433. *Ibid.*

434. *Ibid.*

435. Taylor, *loc.cit.*

436. Thomas, *op.cit.,* p.127

437. Reynolds R., The 'Modified U' technique: a refined method of Norplant removal. *The Journal of Family Practice,* 1995; 40: No.2 (Feb).p.173.

438. Taylor, *loc.cit.*

439. Steadman MS, Probst JC, Jones WJ, Keisler DL. Norplant prescribing in family practice. *Journal of Family Practice.* 1996;42 (3): p.267

440. Cecil H, Reed D, Holtz J. Norplant removal facilitated by use of ultrasound for localization. *Journal of Family Practice.* 1995;40:(2).p.182

441. Steadman, *loc. cit.*

442. Thomas, *op.cit.,* p.127.

443. Davies, *op.cit.,* p.5

444. Thomas, *op.cit.,* p.126

445. Taylor, *loc.cit.*

446. Thomas, *op.cit.,* p.127

447. Shapiro, *op.cit.,* p.451

448. Thomas, *op.cit.,* p.127.

449. "Recovery of platelet function may occur within 1 day after discontinuation of diclofenac, diflunisal, flurbiprofen, ibuprofen, indomethacin, or sulindac;" United States Pharmacopoeial Dispensing Information (US PDI) *Drug Information for Health Care Professionals.* 12th Ed. 1992. p.463.

450. *Micromedex* Vol 85 Norplant monograph

451. *Merck Manual* 15th Ed. p. 1734.

452. *US PDI.* 12th ED. 1992;IB. p.2344-2345

453. *Merck Manual.* 16th Ed, p. 1483

454. Alder J B , Fraunfelder F.T., Levonorgestrel Implants and Intracranial hypertension. *New Eng J Med.*(Letter) 1995, June 22, p.1720

455. *Ibid.*

456. *Ibid.*

457. *Micromedex,* Vol. 85, Acetazolamide monograph

458. Alder, *loc.cit.*

459. Kolata, *op.cit.,* p.5.

460. *Ibid.*

461. Davies, *op.cit.,* p.6.

462. *Martindale- the Extra Pharmacopoea* 1982-1995 Roy. Pharm. Soc. G.B. in *Micromedex* Vol. 85

463. Spiera H. Scleroderma After Silicone Augmentation Mammoplasty. *JAMA.* 1988;260:236-238

464. Celi BR, Kovnat DM. Acute pneumonitis after subcutaneous injections of silicone. *New Eng J Med.* 1983;309:856-7

465. Hardon A, Norplant: A critical review. *WGNRR Newsletter* 34 Jan-March 1991; p. 17.

466. Cooper, *op.cit.*, p.268
467. Hardon, *op.cit.*, p.17
468. *Ibid.*, p.20
469. Ana Regina Gomes Dos Reis. Norplant in Brazil: Implant strategy in the guise of scientific research. *Issues in Reproductive and Genetic Engineering.* Pergamon Press. 1990; 3, No.2: p.111.
470. *Ibid.*
471. Dos Reis, *op.cit.*, p.112
472. "an 11-year-old Dallas girl, repeatedly raped by her stepfather, was given Norplant, apparently to mask the abuse". Painter K. Norplant gets a shot in the arm. *USA Today.* 1995 Aug 22.
473. Dos Reis, *op.cit.*, p.113
474 *Ibid.*
475. *Ibid.*
476 *Ibid.*
477. *Ibid..*
478. World Health Organisation, Task Force on Methods for the Determination of the Fertile Period, Special Program on Research, Development and Research Training in Human Reproduction, "A prospective Multi-centre Trial of Ovulation Method of Natural Family Planning. 1. The Teaching Phase". *Fertility and Sterility.* 1981;36:152.
479. Dos Reis, *op.cit.*, p.114
480 *Ibid.*
481. *Ibid.*
482. *Ibid.*
483. *Ibid.*, p.115.
484. UBINIG. "The price of Norplant is TK.2000! You cannot remove it." Clients are refused removal in Norplant trial in Bangladesh. *Issues in Reproduction and Gen. Engin.* 1991; 4: (1). 45-46
485. Kolata, *op.cit.*, p.5.
486. *Ibid.*, p.1.
487. *Ibid.*, p.5.

CHAPTER SEVEN.

488. Rowland CW. quoted in 'Expert says condoms unreliable' (letter) *News Weekly* (Melbourme, Australia) 11.9.93.
489. *Merck Manual* 16th Ed., *op. cit.*, p.1773.

490. *USP DI, op.cit.,* p 2504.
491. Llewellyn-Jones, *op.cit.,* p.131.
492. World Health Organisation, *op.cit.,* p.152.
493. *APPG.* 25th Ed. *op. cit.,* Delfen Foam Monograph. p.780.
494. Black C, Houghton VP. A users acceptability study of vaginal spermicides in combination with barrier methods or an IUCD. *Contraception.* 1983;28: 103-110. Lamptey P, Klufio C, Smith SC, *et al.* Ortho vaginal tablets and Emko vaginal tablets in Accura, Ghana. *Contraception.*1985;32:445-454. in *Micromedex* Vol 85. Delfen Foam Monograph.
495. Klebanoff SJ. Effects of spermicidal agent nonoxynol-9 on vaginal micro-flora. *Int Infect Dis.* 1992;165:19-25. in *Micromedex* Vol 85
496. *Merck Manual* 16th Edition., *op.cit.,* p.1786
497. *APPG.* 26th Ed. *op.cit.,* p.782
498. Faich G, Pearson K, Fleming D, *et al.* Toxic shock syndrome and the contraceptive sponge. *JAMA.*1986; 255: 216-218. In *Micromedex* Vol 87 Nonoxynol 9 monograph.
499. *Merck Manual* 15th Ed., *op.cit.,* p.72
500. Jick H, Walker AM, *et al., JAMA.* 1981;245:1329 in Rahwan, *Chemical Contraceptives, Interceptives, and Abortifacients, op.cit.,* p.16.
501. Bird KA. The use of spermicides containing nonoxynol-9 in the prevention of HIV infection. *AIDS;*1991:5. 791-796
502. Hicks D R, Martin LS, *et al.* Inactivation of HTLV-111/LAV- induced cultures of normal human lymphocytes by nonoxynol-9 in vitro (letter). *Lancet.* 1985:2: 1422-1423
503. *Merck Manual* 15th Ed., *op. cit.,* p. 288. There are two key sub-groups of lymphocytes within the immune system - T4 cells, also called helper cells, and T8 cells, also known as suppressor cells.
504. *Merck Manual* 15th Ed., *op. cit.,* p. 288
505. Jeffries DJ. Nonoxynol and HIV infection (letter) *Br Med J.* 1988: 296; 1798
506. Murphy S, Munday PE, *et al.,* Anti-HIV substances for rape victims (letter) *JAMA* 1989; 262:2090-2091 and Murphy S Munday PE, *et al.,* Rape and subsequent seroconversion to HIV (letter) *Br Med J.* 1990;300:118 in *Micromedex* Vol 85 *op.cit.*
507. Rowe PM. Nonoxynol-9 fails to protect against HIV-1. *Lancet.*1997;349:#9058. http://www.thelancet.com/
508. Rowe, *op.cit.*
509. Fihn S.D., Boyko E J, Normand E H, *et al.* Association between use of spermicide-coated condoms and Escherichia coli Urinary Tract Infection

in young women. *Am J Epidem.* 1996;144:512-20

510. *Ibid.*

511. *The Macquarie Dictionary.* Macquarie University, NSW (Aust).
      1982.p.1519

512. *The Concise Oxford Dictionary.* 5Th Ed. Oxford University Press. 1793

513. Food & Drug Administration (FDA) Mailgram. 26/8/87 in *Micromedex*
      Vol 84, 1995

514. Smith R W., 'Safe' sex?. *Bridgetown Evening News.* 25.1.93

515. Smith, *op. cit.*

516. Carey RF, Herman WA, Retta SM, Rinaldi JE, Herman BA, Athey TW.
      Effectiveness of latex condoms as a barrier to human immuno-deficiency
      virus-sized particulars under conditions of simulated use. *Sexually
      Transmitted Diseases.* 1992; 19(4): 230-234

517. Rowland CW., *The Washington Post* (letter), June 25, 1992

518. Further, Rowland says that the voids exist in condoms which are 5 microns
      (5um) in size, being 50 times larger than the AIDS virus. Therefore, the
      AIDS virus is = to 0.1microns (5 divided by 50). Micromedex Vol 84 says
      that the AIDS virus is approximately 125 nM. (Nanometers). One
      nanometer is one billionth of a meter (Mosby's) and a billion, in the
      British measure, is one thousand million, therefore 1 nanometer is one
      thousand millionth of a meter. Thus, 125nM divided by 100 converts
      125nM to 0.125micron or 0.125um which is approximately the measurement
      of 0.1um previously quoted. *Ibid.*

519. Lytle CD, Tondreau SC, Truscott W, Budacz AP, Kuester RK, Venegas L,
      Schmukler RE, Cyr WH. Filtration size of human immunodeficiency virus
      type 1 and surrogate viruses used to test barrier materials. *Applied and
      Enviromental Microbiology.* 1992;58:2:747-749

520. Rowland CW. quoted in 'Expert says condoms unreliable' (letter) *News
      Weekly* (Melbourne, Australia) 11. 9.93. .

521. Conat M, Hardy D, Sernatinger J, Spicer D & Levy J. Condoms prevent
      transmission of AIDS-associated retrovirus (letter) *JAMA.* 1986:255:1706

522. Voeller B, Nelson J, Day C., Viral leakage risk differences in latex condoms.
      AIDS Research and Human Retroviruses. 1994;10; p.708, Mary Ann
      Liebert, Inc., Publishers.

523. *Ibid.,* p.701.

524. Friedman Z, Trivelli L. Condom availability for youth.
      Pediatrics. 1996;97:285 (letter)

525. Collart D. Biochemistry & Molecular Biology. Condom failure for

protection from sexual transmission of the HIV - a review of the medical literature. 5393 Whitney Ct, Stone Mountain. GA 30088

526. Rahwan, 1995, *op.cit.*, p.18.

527. To explain this extrapolation; if the pregnancy rate is used to measure condom failure rates, and if a woman is fertile for only one quarter of her monthly cycle, then she can only become pregnant during a quarter of her cycle. If pregnancy from failed condoms occurs at a rate of 10-30%, it is reasonable to assume that condoms failed outside of the fertile times but are not detected because a pregnancy couldn't occur. The pregnancy rate, as a measure of the condom failure rate, can only give a measure of that failure rate for one quarter of the cycle. Therefore the failure rate must be more than 10-30%. It may indeed be four times that percentage figure.

528. *Micromedex* Vol .84. Drugs Consults. Condom efficacy in preventing HIV transmission.

529. Larriera A. Safe sex drive fails to stop herpes spread. *The Sydney Morning Herald.* (Aust) 8/9/95

530. *Ibid.*

531. Archer WR. Deputy Assistant Secretary for Population Affairs, U.S.Department of Health & Human Services, Washington, D.C. Teens are warned on condom flaws. *The Star-Ledger.* Jan 29 1993

532. *Merck Manual* 15th Ed., *op.cit.,* p. 289

533. Grimes DA. *The Contraception Report.* AIDS Update: The threat to women's health. 1995;6:#2 p.11.

534. *Micromedex* Vol 84, Drug consults topic: barrier method effectiveness against HIV/STD - -1993 CDC report.

535. *Mosby's, op.cit.,* p.953

536 *Ibid.*

537. Beer AE. *JAMA.* 1989;262:3184. quoted in Rahwan, *op.cit.,* p.16.

538. Cohen HS, Savitz DA, Cefalo RC, *et al. JAMA.* 1989;262:3143. quoted in Rahwan, *op.cit.,* p.16.

539. "The disruption of the delicate balance between vasoconstricting, platelet-aggregating prostaglandins (thromboxane A2 and prostaglandin F2a) and vasodilating, platelet-disaggregating prostaglandins (prostacyclin and prostaglandin E) may play an important role in pre-clampsia. Increased thromboxane A2 can cause vasoconstriction (and hypertension) and intravascular coagulation, and decrease prostacyclin can explain endothelial cell injury through impairment to its cytoprotective function." quoted from Rahwan, *op.cit.,* p.16.

CHAPTER EIGHT.

540. Feehery K, Benjamin MD. *National Institute of Health Consensus Development statement on Ovarian Cancer.* University of Pennsylvania. Dept of Oncology. Internet address *OncoLink Home Page, http:// oncolink.upenn.edu*

541. *Merck Manual* 16th Ed., *op. cit.*, p.1772

542. *Ibid.*, p.1827

543. *Ibid.*

544. Lowry S, Russell H, Hickey I, Atkinson R. Incessant ovulation and ovarian cancer.(letter) *Lancet.* 1991; 337:p.1544.

545. *Merck Manual* 15th Ed., *op.cit.,* p.1664

546. *Ibid.*

547. *Ibid.*

548. Greenblatt RB, Roy S, *et al,.* Induction of ovulation. *Am J Obstet Gynec.* 1962;84: 900-909 in *Goodman & Gilman's The Pharmacological Basis of Therapeutics.* 8th Ed., p.1396

549. *The Pharmacological Basis of Therapeutics*, 5th Edition, *op.cit.*, p.1435

550. In part, the formation of ovarian cysts is related to the pharmaco-biological action of clomiphene. In premenopausal women, clomiphene causes a blockage of the oestrogen receptor in the anterior pituitary and the hypothalamus, which disrupts the normal feedback inhibition of GnRH and gonadotropin secretion, resulting in their increased secretion which in some cases leads to the formation of large cystic ovaries. *Goodman & Gilman.* 8th Ed. *op cit.*, p.1396

551. Fathalla M.F. Incessant ovulation - a factor in ovarian neoplasia. *Lancet.* 1971;ii:163

552. *Ibid.*

553. *Ibid.*

554. Obituaries. *The Australian* . Edited by Jennifer McAsey. Jan 16 1996 p 14 (Reprinted from the *Times*)

555. Fathalla, *loc.cit.*

556. Casagrande JT, Pike MC, Ross RK, Louie EW, Roy S, Henderson BE. "Incessant ovulation" and ovarian cancer. *Lancet.*1979;2:p.170.

557. Lowry, *op.cit.*, pp.1544-1545.

558. "The risk [of ovarian cancer] decreased with increasing numbers of live births, with increasing numbers of incomplete pregnancies, and with the use of oral contraceptives. These factors can be amalgamated into a single index of protection - 'protected time' - by considering them all as

periods of anovulation. The complement of protected time — viz., "ovulatory age", the period between menarche and diagnosis of ovarian cancer (or cessation of menses) minus "protected time" — was strongly related to risk of ovarian cancer." Casagrande, *op.cit.,* p.170.

559.   Shu XO, Brinton LA, Gao YT, Yuan JM. Population-based case-control study of ovarian cancer in Shanghai. *Cancer Res* 1989 (Jul 1); 49:13,p.3670

560.   Fishel S, Jackson P. Follicular stimulation for high tech pregnancies: are we playing it safe? *B M J.* 1989;229:p.309

561.   "Most ovarian cancers arise on the epithelial surface of the ovary not the ovary itself. In the normal course of events, the female child has all her oocytes present at birth. These are quiescent for almost 13 years. With the onset of menarche, the oocytes mature. The epithelial surface of the ovary is thereafter ruptured at regular times to release the ovum at ovulation throughout the reproductive years. Following each rupture these epithelial tears repair by cell division. When repair is complete, growth ceases. It is proposed that this repetitive proliferation allows the promotion of cells bearing allele loss and, by inference, those carrying inactivated tumour-suppressor genes. This may lead to uncontrolled cell division and malignant transformation." Lowry, *op.cit.,* p.1544-45.

562.   Fathalla, *loc.cit.*

563.   Fishel, *op.cit.,* p.310.

564.   Lowry, *op.cit.,* p.1544-1545.

565.   Dietl L. K. Ovulation and ovarian cancer. *Lancet.*1991;338:445.

566.   "...and the omentum (fat-skin) majus (FIGO stage IIIb) was detected." *Ibid.*

567.   with intervening treatment for endometriosis genitalis externa. *Ibid.*

568.   Whittelmore AS, Harris R, Itnyre J, and the Collaborative Ovarian Cancer Group (COCG). *Amer J Epidem.* 1992: 136:1184-1203. The Johns Hopkins University School of Hygiene and Public Health. (OR 2.8, CI 95% 1.3-6.1, c =1.4,p=0.50).

569.   *Ibid.,* p.1189, Table 3.

570.   *Ibid.,* p.1188.

571.   "Each month of breast feeding was associated with an overall risk reduction of 0.99..." in *Ibid.,* p.1192.

572.   *Ibid.,* p.1189.

573.   Spirtas R, Kaufman SC, Alexander N., Fertility dugs and ovarian cancer: red alert or red herring ? *Fertility & Sterility.* 1993; 59: p.291.

574.   *Ibid.*

575. "One problem ... is choosing women lacking a history of infertility as the reference group for the odds-ratio calculations... Although ideal conditions are, of course, impossible to achieve, ... More importantly, the study's small numbers result in very wide confidence intervals, with lower limits as low as 1.3... Other weakness include lack of information on the diagnostic efforts made to determine the cause of each woman's infertility, infertility type, specific fertility drug combination used, treatment dosage and duration, and histological type of ovarian cancer. The COCG has been appropriately cautious in interpreting their results." *Ibid.*, p.292.

576. *Ibid.*

577. *Micromedex*. Drug Monograph on Gonaderilin Vol. 85

578. Rossing M.A. Ph.D. Daling J.R. et al Ovarian tumors in a cohort of infertile women *N Eng J Med.* 1994: 331: p.772.

579. *Ibid.*, p.773. (Age-standardized incidence ratio associated with clomiphene use, 3.1, CI 1.4-5.9).

580. *Ibid.*, p.774.

581. HMG = human menopausal gonadotropin, FSH= follicle stimulating hormone.

582. Buhle EL PhD,. Infertility Drugs and Ovarian Cancer, University of Pennsylvania. *OncoLink Home Page, Internet address is http://oncolink.upenn.edu*

583. Whittlemore AS. The risk of ovarian cancer after treatment for infertility. *NEJM.* 1994;331;12;805-6.

584. Priore GD, Robischon K, Phipps W. (Letter),*NEJM.* 1995; 332: 1300-1302

585. Kurman R, Wallach EE, Zacur HA. (Letter)*NEJM.*1995;332:1300-1302

586. Shapiro S. (Letter). *NEJM.* 1995;332:1300-1302

587. Rossing MA, Daling JR, Weiss NS. Letter.*NEJM.*1995;332:1300-1302

588. Shushan A, Paltiel O, Iscovich J, Elchalal U, Peretz T, Schenker JG. Human menopausal gonadotropin and the risk of epithelial ovarian cancer. *Fertility and Sterility.*1996;65:p.16

589. *Micromedex* Vol 92. Menotrophins drug evaluation monographs.

590. Shushan, *op.cit.,* p.17

591. *Ibid.*

592. Hull ME, Kriner M, Schneider E, Maiman M. Ovarian cancer after successful ovulation induction: a case report.*J Reprod Med.*1996 (Jan); 41:1,52-4

593. Shushan, *op.cit.,* p.17

594. *Ibid.*

595. Coney S, Long-term effects of assisted conception.*Lancet.* 1995:345:976

596. *Ibid.*
597. *Ibid.*
598. Shanner L, Informed consent and inadequate medical information. *Lancet.*1995;346:251
599. *Ibid.*
600. *Ibid.*
601. *Ibid.*
602. *Ibid.*
603. Stanford JL. Oral contraceptives and neoplasia of the ovary. *Contraception.* 1991;43:(6). p.543

CHAPTER NINE.

604. Klein R, Raymond J, and Dumble L. *"RU-486; Misconceptions, Myths and Morals."* Spinifex Press 1991. p52
605. Olsen D, Pill policy will help victims of rape: hospital. *The Peoria Journal Star.* Monday, November 13, 1995. (USA)
606. Kessler DA. Prescription drug products; certain combined oral contraceptives for use as postcoital emergency contraception;Notice. *Federal Register.*1997;62:37. http://www.fda.gov
607. Grou F, Rodrigues I. The morning - after pill; How long after? *Am J Obstet Gynecol*1994;171: 1529-34
608. Harper, *op.cit.,* p.149.
609. Rabone D. Postcoital contraception - coping with the Morning After. *Current Therapeutics.*1990; p.46
610. *Martindale-The Extra Pharmacopoeia.* In *Micromedex* Vol. 92 (Hormonal Contraceptives Monograph)
611. Rahwan, *op.cit.,* p.7
612. Rabone, *op.cit.,* p.45
613. Dixon GW.*JAMA.* 1980; 244:1336 in *Micromedex* Vol 85
614. Mogia *et al.*, 1974; Larranaga *et al.,* 1975 in *Micromedex* Vol 85
615. Ellertson, *op.cit.,* p.252
616. Rabone, *op.cit.,* p.47
617. *USP DI.* 12th Ed., 1992, *op.cit.,* p.1355
618. Rabone, *op.cit.,* p.45
619. Olsen D. Pill policy will help victims of rape:hospital. *The Peoria Journal Star* (Illonois, USA) Monday , November 13, 1995.
620. *Merck Manual* 16th Ed *op.cit.,* p.1762-63
621. *Ibid.*

622. *Mosby's, op.cit.* p. 471. "Fertile period - the time in the menstrual cycle during which fertilization may occur. Spermatozoa can survive for 48-72 hours; the ovum lives for 24 hours. Thus, the fertile period begins 2 to 3 days before ovulation and lasts 2 to 3 days afterwards."

623. Klein, *op.cit.,* p.13.

624. Jackman J. *The Feminist Majority Report.* Fall 1995 p.5.

625. Bachorik L. FDA issued approvable letter for mifepristone. Sept.18, 1996. http://www.fda.gov

626. *Reuters* - Hoechst gives away patent to RU-486 in Europe. Apr.4 1997 http://www.reutershealth.com

627. *Ibid.*

628. *Ibid.*

629. *Ibid.*

630. RU 486 also has a strong anti-glucocorticoid and weak anti-androgen action. Klein, *op.cit.,* p.67.

631. "With the *exception of progesterone*, progestins have no proven value in the treatment of threatened abortion and are no longer recommended for its use" *USP DI.* 12th Ed., 1992, *op.cit.,* p.2344

632. *Martindale - The Extra Pharmacopoeia* 29th Ed p.1590

633. Duffy A, Santamaria Dr J. The How and the why of RU 486. *Thomas More Centre Bulletin.* 1990;2:(3):p.2.

634. Klein, *op.cit.,* p.11

635. Herranz G. RU-486: The Abortion Pill. *Catholic International.* 1991;2. #14:p.673

636. Delaney A. ABC Radio National: *The Health Report* 22.4.91 (Transcript)

637. *Mosby's, op.cit.,* p.973

638. Nalador, from Schering Germany is not indicated for use with RU-486. in Klein, *op.cit.,* p.86

639. Cytotec, manufactured by Searle, is NOT endorsed by the company as part of the RU-486 abortion procedure. *APPG.* 1991 p.584 says " Cytotec is contra-indicated in pregnancy"

640. The indications for its use are " for softening and dilation of the cervix uteri prior to transcervical, intrauterine operative procedures in the first trimester of pregnancy". Cervagem Pessaries , from May & Baker, as listed in the *APPG.* 1991 p.478.

641. *Ibid.*

642. Klein, *op.cit.,* p.27

643. Ince S. The trouble with RU-486. *Vogue (American Edition)* July 1991. p. 88

644. Klein, *op.cit.,* p.28
645. Ince, *loc.cit.*
646. Klein, *op.cit.,* p.35
647. Duffy, *op.cit.,* p.3
648. Coppess M H, "Who's Pushing the Abortion Pill" *Focus on the Family Citizen* 21.1.91 p.13
649. Klein, *op.cit.,* pp.27-28, 51
650. Interview, *Le Monde* Aug 1 1990, reprinted in *"Guardian Weekly"* UK August 19 1990.
651. French report on death in abortion pill treatment. *Dayton Daily News.* Dayton. OHIA, USA. 9th April, 1991
652. Klein, *op.cit.,* p.23
653. Lefevre T. To verify, phone +33 1 47 901998, fax +33 1 47 338187 or e-mail tdd1001@ibm.net
654. *Micromedex* Vol 87. Nalador Drug Monograph.
655. Klein, *op.cit* p.23
656. *Le Monde* 10.4.91, *Le Figaro* 9.4.91
657. Delaney, *loc.cit..*
658. El-Refaey H, *et al.* Induction of abortion with mifepristone (RU486) and oral or vaginal misoprostol. *N Eng J Med.* 1995;332:p.983.
659. "Le Quotidien de Medecin Paris" 30.4.90.
660. Herranz, *op.cit.,* p.674.
661. Ince, *op.cit.,* p.88
662. Coppess, *op.cit.,* p.13
663. Klein, *op. cit.,* p.32-33
664. Ince, *op. cit.,* p.89
665. El-Refaey, *op.cit.,* p.986
666. Weiner JJ & Evans WS. Uterine rupture in mid-trimester abortion: a complication of gemeprost vaginal pessaries and oxytocin-a case report. *Br J Obstet Gynaecol.* 1990;97:1061-62 in *Micromedex* Vol 87
667. Coppess, *op.cit.,* p.13
668. Darton N, Surprising journey for abortion drug. *New York Times.* 23rd March 1995 p. C12
669. *Ibid.*
670. "Abortion Drug Further Discredited" *News Weekly.* (Melbourne, Australia) June 22nd 1991 p.10.
671. *Micromedex* Vol 87
672. Klein, *op. cit.,* pp.44-45
673. *The Australian,* 13-14th April 1991

674. Klein, *op.cit.*, p.34
675. Delaney, *loc.cit.*
676. Ince, *op. cit.*, p.89
677 Klein, *op.cit.*, p.52
678. *Ibid.*, p 47-48
679. Francis B, *The Age* (Melbourne, Australia) Letters. 23.7.90
680. Ince, *op.cit.*, p.88
681. *Ibid.*
682. Ministry of Health, 1 Place de Fontenoy Paris 12th April 1990. in *Human Life International Reports.* Oct. 1990
683. El-Refaey, *op.cit.*, p.983.
684. Ince, *op.cit.*, p.90
685. Ince, *op.cit.*, p.89.
686. Delaney, *loc.cit.*
687. Herrantz, *op.cit.*, p.674
688. Coppess, *op.cit.*, p.13
689. "This is why French women must sign a form that says they will agree to a conventional termination if RU486/PG fails." Klein, *op.cit.*, p.79
690. A. Jost. C.R. *Acad Sc Paris Ser.* 111. 303. 1986, pp.281-284. in International Inquiry Commission on RU 486, BP 167 - 92805 Puteaux - France.
691. Schonhofer PS, *et al.*, Brazil: misuse of misoprostol as an abortifacient may induce malformations. *Lancet.* 1991;337:1537-5
692. Fonseca W, *et al.*, Congenital malformations of the scalp and cranium after failed first trimester abortion attempt with misoprostol. *Cli Dysmorph* 1993;2:76-80
693. Gonzalez CH, *et al.*, Limb deficiency with or without Mobius sequence in seven Brazilian children associated with misoprostol use in the first trimester of pregnancy. *Am J Med Genet.* 1993;47:59-64
694. Costa SH, Vessey MP. Misoprostol and illegal abortions in Rio de Janeiro, Brazil. *Lancet.* 1993;341:1258-61
695. Barbosa RM, *et al.*, The Brazilian experience with Cytotec (misoprostol) *Stud Fam Planning.* 1993;24:236-240
696. Collins FS, Mahoney MJ. Hydrocephalus and abnormal digits after failed first-trimester prostaglandin abortion attempt. *Journ Ped.* 1983; 102 (4):p.620
697. Burnell, P. *The Universe* (U.K.). Sunday July 28,1991
698. Right To Life Of Greater Cincinnati, *Newsletter* April 1991.
699. *Sixty Minutes,* U.S.A., C.B.S. TV April 9 1989. (Transcript)
700. Duffy, *op.cit.*, p.4.

701. Fife-Yeomans J. On trial: oral contraceptive safety and corporate honesty. *The Australian*. 20.1.96

702. *Alliance for Life* Newsletter, 1990 (Winnipeg-Canada)

703. Tonti-Filippini N. RU-486: Dispelling Some Myths. *St. Vincents Bioethics Newsletter* 1990.Vol.8, No.2,

704. *Ibid.,* p.3

705. Cekan S, Aedo AR, SegerstAEeen E, Van Look P, *et. al.*, Levels of the antiprogestin RU486 and its metabolites in human blood and follicular fluid following oral administration of a single dose. *Hum Reprod.* 1989 Feb;4(2):131-5.

706. Klein, *op.cit.,* p.76.

707. *Ibid.,* p.88

708. *Le Monde* 10.4.91, *Le Figaro* 9.4.91

709. *Lancet.* 1991; 337: 969-70

710. Delaney, *loc.cit.*

711. Klein, *op.cit.,* p.82

712. Robinson Assoc. Prof M, Benrimoj Prof. C, Kot T, Dight D, Parker J. *CNS Medicines - Drug Information for Health Care Pharmacists.* University of Queensland. (Aust).1992

713. *APPG.* 1996, 25th Ed., *op.cit.,* p.606.

714. Klein, *op.cit.,* p.82

715. *Ibid.* p.82

716. *Ibid.* p.84

717. *Ibid.* p.78

718. Regelson W. Beyond Abortion: RU-486 and the Needs of the Crisis Constituency. *JAMA.* 1990; 264, #8:1027 p.1027

719. Glasow R D, "National Right to Life Newsletter" Jan.8.91 (U.S.A.) from *Nature.* 29.11.1990

720. Van Voorhis BJ, Anderson DJ, Hill JA. The Effects of RU-486 on Immune Function and Steroid-Induced Immunosuppression In Vitro. *Journ Clinical Endoc Metab.*1989; 69, #6,p.1195

721. Regelson, *op.cit.,* p.1026

722. Klein, *op.cit.,* p.70

723. Glasow, *loc.cit.*

724. Bowden T, Hissom JR, Moore MR. Growth Stimulation of T47D human Breast Cancer Cells by the Anti-Progestin RU-486. *Endocrinology* 1989; 124 No.5. p. 2642

725. Glasow, *loc.cit.*

726. Powles TJ, Hardy JR, *et al.*, A pilot trial to evaluate the acute toxicity and feasibility of tamoxifen for prevention of breast cancer. *Br J Cancer* 1989; 60: p.126

727. Perrault D, Eisenhauer EA, Pritchard KI, *et al.*, Phase II study of the progesterone antagonist mifepristone in patients with untreated metatastic breast carcinoma: A National Cancer Institute of Canada Clinical Trials Group Study. *Journal of Clinical Oncology.* 1996 (Oct);14: p.2711 [The authors also noted that the combined use of an anti-progesterone (RU-486) plus an anti-estrogenic (tamoxifen) may offer an additive, if not synergistic benefit in breast cancer treatment. Further research was suggested.]

728. *Davidson's Principles and Practice of Medicine.* 11th Ed. Churchill Livingstone. 1975. p.658

729. Nieman LK, Chrousos GP, Kellner C, *et al.* Successful Treatment of Cushings Syndrome with the Glucocorticoid Antagonist RU-486. *Journ Clin Endocrin Metabol.* 1985;161: 536-540

730. As indicated, Cushing's Disease is due to a pituitary gland tumour whereas the syndrome is associated with a tumour on the adrenal gland or a small cell carcinoma of the lung (ectopic ACTH syndrome). The pituitary gland is located in the brain, the adrenal gland is found on the kidney's. See *Merck Manual* 16th Edition, p.1093 and Dr Schuelers's *Home Medical Advisor Pro* CD.

731. Nieman, *op.cit.,* p.539

732. Rowe PM, IOM (Institute of Medicine -USA) report calls for research into new contraceptives. *Lancet.* 1996;347:1611

733. Spinnato JA. Mechanism of action of intrauterine contraceptive devices and its relation to informed consent. *Am J Obstet Gynecol.* 1997;176.p.503

734. *Ibid.*

735. *Merck Manual* 15th Ed., p.1223

736. *Ibid.,* p.1245

737. *Ibid.,* 15th Ed. pp.1222-1223

738. Stryer L. *Biochemistry.* 2nd Ed., p.511

739. *Merck Manual* 16th Ed., p.1858

740. 'Blastocyst' - the name given to the fertilized ovum prior to implantation, whence it will be referred to as an embryo until the end of week eight, then fetus until birth. *Mosby's, op.cit.,* pp.,152, 415,473

741. Floridon C, Mielsen O, Byrjalsen C, *et al.*, Ectopic pregnancy: histopathology and assessment of cell proliferation with and without methotrexate treatment. *Fert Ster.* 1996;65(4).p730

742. Hausknecht R. Methotrexate and misoprostol to terminate early pregnancy. *New Eng J Med.* 1995;333:537-540 p. 537
743. *Ibid.,* p.538
744. *Mosby's, op. cit.,* p.1119
745. *APPG.* 24th Ed., *op.cit.,* p.1484.
746. *Micromedex* Vol 85. Methotrexate Monograph
747. "Carcinogenicity studies with methotrexate in animals have been inconclusive. However, there is evidence that methotrexate causes chromosomal damage in animal somatic cells and human bone marrow cells". *USP DI* 12th Ed. 1992 Vol 1B. p.1865.
748. *APPG., op. cit.,* p.1483
749. Hausknecht, *op. cit.,* p.539
750. *APPG. op.cit.,* p.1485.

CHAPTER TEN.

751. *Media Tracking Service.* Monday, August 21, 1995 No.177
752. *Merck Manual,* 15th Ed., *op.cit.,* p.1713
753. *Mosby's, op.cit.,* p.740
754. *Merck Manual, op.cit.,* p.1713
755. *Mosby's, op.cit.,* p.740
756. *Goodman and Gilman's,* 5th Ed., *op.cit.,* p.1432.
757. *Goodman and Gilman's,* 8th Ed., *op.cit.,* p.1389.
758. Lafferty FW, Spencer G E, Pearson O H. Effects of androgens, estrogens, and high calcium intakes on bone formation and resorption in osteoporosis. *Am J Med.,* 1964, 36, 514-528 in *Goodman & Gilman's,* 5th Ed. *op. cit.,* p.1434.
759. *Goodman & Gilman's,* 5th Ed., *op.cit.,* p.1432
760. In Hunt K, Vessey M, McPherson K, Voleman M. Long-term surveillance of mortality and cancer incidence in women receiving hormone replacement therapy. *Br J Obstet Gyn.* 1987;94:pp. 620-621.
761. In Brinton L A, Hoover R, Fraumeni JF. Menopausal oestrogens and breast cancer risk: an expanded case-control study. *Br J Cancer.* 1986; 54; p. 825.
762. *Ibid.*
763. *Ibid.,* pp.826-827.
764. *Ibid.,* p. 831
765. *Goodman & Gilman's, op. cit.,* p.1425

766. King, *op.cit.,* p.532
767. Key TJA, Pike MC., The role of oestrogens and progestagens in the Epidemiology and prevention of Breast Cancer. *Eur J Cancer Clin Oncol.* 1988;24:1:p.30.
768. Two alternate theories pertaining to breast cancer are known as the 'oestrogen (E2) plus progestagen (Pg) hypothesis', and the 'oestrogen (E2) alone hypothesis'. The former states that "increased exposure to oestrogen alone causes some increase in breast cancer risk, but that risk will be increased much more by exposure to both oestrogen and progesterone". The latter theory states that "oestrogen alone increases risk and that progestagens are irrelevant". Key & Pike, *op.cit.,* p.32 The basis for these alternate views are thus: "Two interpretations of the evidence relating to the hormonal control of breast cell division have to be seriously considered. A simple explanation of the biopsy and autopsy studies [done on breast cell cultures exposed to varying levels of E2 and Pg] is that E2 alone (in the follicular -pre ovulatory - phase) induces some cell division, but that E2 and Pg together (in the luteal -post ovulatory - phase induce more cell division. The failure of the laboratory studies to show a significant mitotic - cell division - effect of Pg suggests an alternate explanation: breast cell division is induced only by oestrogens with Pg having little or no effect." *Ibid.* The third theory , known as the 'unopposed oestrogen hypothesis', a theory proven to be relevant in endometrial cancer, is rejected in the case of breast cancer because "current evidence provides little support for (it) ...". *Ibid.,* p.38
769. King, *op.cit.,* p.534
770. Llewellyn-Jones, *op.cit.,* p.38-43
771. Key & Pike, *op.cit.,* p.30.
772. *Ibid.,* p.32
773. The follicular phase (reasonably coinciding with what is also called the proliferative phase) is the first part of the menstrual cycle, when ovarian follicles grow to prepare for ovulation. The luteal phase (also known as the secretory phase) is the phase of the menstrual cycle after the release of an ovum from a mature ovarian follicle. *Mosby's, op.cit.,* p. 488
774. Progesterone; a *natural* female hormone produced by both the corpus luteum (the structure formed by the follicle after it has released an ovum), and by the adrenal cortex (structures located on the kidneys). The term progestogen refers to "any synthetic or natural progestational hormone. Also spelt *progestagen.* Also called *progestin."* Progestin; " any of a group of hormones, natural or synthetic, secreted by the corpus luteum,

placenta or adrenal cortex that have a progesterone-like effect on the uterus". *Mosby's, op. cit.,*p.969

775.   "Estrogens increase endometrial proliferation and progestins counteract that response. These effects are relevant to the genesis of endometrial carcinoma but additional events are also important." King ,*op.cit.,* p.532.

776.   Bergkvist L, Adami Hans-Olov, *et al.,* The risk of breast cancer after estrogen and estrogen-progestin replacement. *New Eng J Med.* 1989; 321: p.293.

777.   "Pg (progesterone) opposes the stimulatory effect of E2 (oestradiol) on the endometrium mainly by reducing the concentration of E2 receptors, but also by increasing the metabolism of E2 to the less active oestrone." Key & Pike, *op.cit.,* p.30

778.   Mosby's, *op. cit.*, p. 89

779.   See previous lengthy footnote apropos breast cancer. Key & Pike, *op.cit.,* pp.37-38.

780.   Hunt K, Vessey M, McPherson K, Coleman M. Long term surveillance of mortality and cancer incidence in women receiving hormone replacement therapy. *Br J Obstet Gynace* 1987;94:p.633

781.   National Alliance of Breast Cancer Organisations. (NABCO) Vol 3 #4, 1989 *Internet address http://nysernet.org/bcic/*

782.   Hunt, *op.cit.,* p.633.

783.   *Goodman & Gilman's,.* 8th Ed. *op.cit.,* p.1393

784.   NABCO, *op.cit.,* 1989

785.   Bergkvist, *op.cit.,* pp.293-297

786.   NABCO, *Ibid.*

787.   *Ibid.*

788.   *Ibid.*

789.   *Ibid.*

790.   Colditz GA, Hankinson SE, *et al* . The use of estrogens and progestins and the risk of breast cancer in post-menopausal women. *New Eng. J. Med.* 1995;332:p.1591 & p.1592.

791.   *Ibid.,* p.1591.

792.   *Ibid.,* p.1590

793.   *Ibid.,* p.1592

794.   *Ibid.,* p.1592

795.   Patel S. Current and potential future drug treatments for osteoporosis. *Ann Rheum Dis.*1996;55:10,700-14. Ma

796.   Daly E, Vessey MP, Hawkins MM, Carsons JL, Gough P, Marsh S. Risk of venous thromboembolism in users of hormone replacement therapy.

*Lancet.*1996;348:#9033. (http://www.thelancet.com/lancet/Users/ vol348no9033/articles/article1.html)

797.   Colditz GA, Willett WC, Speizer FE. (Letter).*NEJM.*1995; 333:1355-1358. http://www.nejm.org/publicM/1995/0333/0020/1355/1.htm

798.   Colditz,*NEJM,* 1995.*op.cit.,* p.1592

799.   Colditz,*J Soc Gynecol Invest.,* 1996,*op.cit.,* p.55

800.   *Ibid.*

801.   *Goodman & Gilman's, op.cit.,* p.1395

802.   Abbott TA 3d, Lawrence BJ, Wallach S. Osteoporosis: the need for comprehensive treatment guidelines.*Clin Ther.*1996;Jan-Feb,18:1: pp.127-49 Ma

803.   Isenbarge DW, Chapin BL. Osteoporosis. Current pharmacologic options for prevention and treatment.*Postgrad Med.* 1997 Jan, 101:1,129-32,136-7, 141-2. Ma

804.   Colditz, p.1591, Table 2

805.   Isenbarge DW, Chapin BL. *op.cit.,* Ma.

806.   "The most common type of PE is a thrombus that usually has formed in a leg or pelvic vein.". *Merck Manual*, 15th Ed, *op.cit.,* p.649

807.   Vandebroucke JP, Helmerhorst FM. Risk of venous thrombosis with hormone-replacement therapy. *Lancet.*1996;348:#9033. (commentary). http://www.thelancet.com/lancet/Users/vol348no9033/editorial/ commentary.html

808.   Jick H, Derby L, Myers MW, Vasilakis C, Newton KM. Risk of hospital admission for idiopathic venous thromboembolism among users of postmenopausal oestrogens. *Lancet.*1996;348#9033. http://www. thelancet.com/lancet/Users/vol348no9033articles/article2.html

809.   *Ibid.*

810.   Daly E,*op.cit.*

811.   Grodstein F, Stampfer MJ, Goldhaber SZ, Manson JE, Colditz GA, Speizer FE, Willett WC, Hennekens CH. Prospective study of exogenous hormones and risk of pulmonary embolism in women. *Lancet.*1996; 348:#9033. http://www.thelancet.com/lancet/Users/vol348no9033/articles/ article3.html.

812.   Vandenbroucke JP, Helmerhorst FM,*Ibid.*

813.   *loc.cit.*

814.   Gutthann, SP, Rodriguez LA, Castellsague J, Oliart AD. Hormone replacement therapy and risk of venous thromboembolism: population based case-control study. *BMJ.*1997;314#7083. http://www.bmj.com.

815.   Hemminki E, McPherson K. Impact of postmenopausal hormone therapy

on cardiovascular events and cancer: pooled data from clinical trials. *BMJ*.1997;315:#7101

816.	Grady D, Furberg C. Venous thromboembolic events associated with hormone replacement therapy (Letter). *JAMA*.1997;278:477

817.	Lowe G, Rumley A, Woodward M, Reid E. (Letter).*Lancet*.1997;349:1623

818.	A review of the approved drug information reports that side-effects are limited to the gastro-intestinal tract (nausea, stomach pain, diarrhoea, wind and reflux), plus muscle cramps, headaches, dizziness and altered taste. Further, since alendronate is tissue specific for bone, it is difficult to see how it would interact with the cellular structure of breast or cervical tissue.*MIMS on CD. V2* 1 Feb- 20 April 1997. MIMS Australia. 2 Chandos St, St. Leonards. N.S.W. Aust.

819.	Alendronate Drug Evaluation Monograph.*Micromedex* Vol 92. 1997

820.	McClung MR. Current bone mineral density data on bisphosphates in postmenopausal osteoporosis.*Bone*.1996;19:5 (suppl)195S-198S.

821.	*Merck Manual* 16th Ed., *op.cit.,*p.1357

822.	McClung, *loc.cit.*

823.	Alendronate Drug Evaluation Monograph.*Micromedex* Vol 92. 1997

824.	Liberman UA, Weiss SR, Broll J, Minnie HW, *et al.*, Effects of oral alendronate on bone mineral density and the incidence of fractures in postmenopausal osteoporosis.*N.E.J.M.*1995;333:1437-1443.

825.	Adami S, Passeri M, Ortolani S, Broggini M, *et. al.,* Effects of oral alendronate and intranasal salmon calcitonin on bone mass and biochemical markers of bone turnover in postmenopausal women with osteoporosis.*Bone.*1995 Oct, 17:4; 383-90 Ma

826.	Sambrook PN. The treatment of postmenopausal osteoporosis. *N.E.J.M.*1995;333:1495-1496

827.	Karpf DB, Shapiro DR, Seeman E, Ensrud KE, *et. al.,* Prevention of nonvertebral fractures by alendronate. (A meta-analysis). *JAMA.*1997;227:1159-1164 Ma

828.	The writing group for the PEPI trials. Effects of hormone therapy on bone mineral density. Results from the postmenopausal estrogen/progestin interventions (PEPI) trial.*J.A.M.A.* 1996;276:1389-1396

829.	Eiken P, Kolthoff N, Nielsen SP. Effects of 10 years' hormone replacement therapy on bone mineral content in postmenopausal women. *Bone.*1996 Nov, 19:5 Suppl, 191S-193S Ma

830.	"The efficacy and safety of alendronate were compared with those of estrogen/progestin in a 6- yr, double-blind, placebo-controlled study (i.e., the EPIC study) of 1609 healthy postmenopausal women (age 45-59 yr). The study was divided into 2 strata:435 women in stratum 1 were randomised to either blinded or open-label treatment with estrogen/progestin (E/P; n=110) while 117 in statum 2 were randomised to receive alendronate 2.5mg or 5mg/day or placebo. In the U.S., the women in stratum 1 were given conjugated equine oestrogens 0.625 mg/day and medroxyprogesterone acetate 5mg/day (CEE/MPA); in Europe, the women were given monthly cycles of 17-b-estradiol 1-2 mg/day and norethisterone acetate 0.1 mg/day (E2/NEA). BMD changes from baseline in the spine, hip, and total body were measured after 2 yr. Placebo reduced BMD whereas alendronate and estrogen/progestin prevented loss. For example, placebo, alendronate 2.5mg, alendronate 5mg, CECE/MPA, and E2/NEA changed BMD by -1.78%, 2.28%, 3.46%, 4.04% and 5.14% respectively. Serum osteocalcin was reduced about 45% with alendronate 5mg and by 50-56% with E/P. ..." Hosking DJ, McClung MR, Ravn P, Wasnich RD, Thompson RD, Daley MS, Yates AJ. Alendronate in the prevention of osteoporosis:Epic study two-year results. *J.Bone. Miner.Res.*11 (Suppl. 1):S133-S133, Aug.1996 (in Soc. Proc.)

831. *Ibid.*
832. Science News Update April 9, 1997. http://www.ama-assn.org/sci-pubs/sci-news/1997/snr0409.htm#oc7194
833. Hodsman A, Adachi J, Olsznski W. Prevention and management of osteoporosis: consensus statement from the Scientific Advisory Board of the Osteoporosis Society of Canada. 6. Use of bisphophonates in the treatment of osteoporosis. *Can Med Assoc J.* 1996 Oct 1, 155:7,945-8 Ma
834. Colditz GA, Willett WC, Speizer FE. *NEJM.* (Letter) 1995;333:1355-1358
835. Taylor S, Armour C. The debate is on: should men receive equal osteoporosis treatment? *Retail Pharmacy.* May 1997 p.18
836. Abbott TA, Lawrence BJ, Wallach S. Osteporosis: the need for comprehensive treatment guidelines. *Clin Ther.*1996;Jan-Feb,18:1: pp127-49 Ma
837. Sambrook,*op.cit.,* p.1495
838. Clarke C, Foundation chief executive, Menopause Foundation. *The Australian Journal of Pharmacy.* 1996;77:117
839. Key & Pike. *op.cit.,* p.30
840. *Ibid.*
841. Pike MC, Spicer DV, Dahmoush L, Press MF. Estrogens, progestogens, normal breast cell proliferation, and breast cancer risk. *Epidemiologic Reviews.*1993;Vol 15, 1, p.18

842. *Ibid.*

843. *Ibid.*

845. *Ibid.*

845. *Ibid,* p.19

846. Rosner B, Colditz GA, Willett WC. Reproductive risk factors in a prospective study of breast cancer: the Nurses' Health Study. *AmJ Epidem.*1994;139: p.834

847. Colditz, Hankinson, *et al., NEJM.* 1995, *op.cit.,* p.1549

848. Key TJ, Hormones and cancer in humans. *Mutat. Res.* 1995;333(1-2):97-9

849. Colditz, *J Soc Gynecol Invest.* 1996, *op.cit.,* p.51

850. *Ibid.,* p.53 (95% CI 1.00-1.06).

851. *Ibid.,* pp.52-53

852. Ewertz M. Epidemiology of breast cancer: the Nordic contributions. *Eur J Surg.*1996;162(2):97-9 Ma

CHAPTER ELEVEN.

853. *APPG.* 25th Ed., o*p.cit.,* p.4

854. Reynolds C. School of Law, Flinders University of South Australia, Adelaide. Common law duties of prescribers. *Aust. Prescriber.* 1996; 19(1):18-20

855. *Ibid.,* p.19

856. *APPG.* 25th Ed., o*p.cit.,* p.4

857. *APPG.* Vol. 2 1996. Relevant drug monograph.

858. *MIMS* on CD. Ver. 2 1997

859. *APPG.* Vol. 2 1996 . Relevant drug monograph.

860. *MIMS* on CD. Ver. 2 1997

861. How to use your 28 day pack . Nordette, Nordiol , Triphasil, Biphasil. Wyeth Pharmaceuticals, Gregory Place, Parramatta, NSW 2150 Aust. Product Information

862. Patient information leaflet- Microgynon 30 ED, Levlen ED, Logynon ED. Schering AG. Product Information.

863. "several studies of oral contraceptives and breast cancer have also reported that current or recent use of oral contraceptives is associated with higher risk of breast cancer than more distant use". Gray R. Depot medroxyprogesterone and risk of breast cancer. *Br Med J.* 1989; 1099

864. Patient information leaflet- Microgynon 30 ED, Levlen ED, Logynon ED. Schering AG. Product Information .

865. (see Chapter 5, Upjohn's rejection of FDA criticism of animal study results)

866. *APPG.* 25th Ed., 1996. Approved Product Information. pp.1030,1556,2345, 2348.

867. "Although gestrinone (used to treat endometriosis) inhibits ovulation, patients need to use barrier contraception while taking the drug. This is because the drug is *embryotoxic* in some animals and can cause masculinization of a female fetus." *Australian Prescriber.* An independent review. 1996;19;1; p.26

868. King, *op cit.,* p.534 (For further detailed information on this topic I refer the reader to the following: Russo J, Gusterson BA, Rogers AE, Russo IH, Wellings SR, van Zwieten MJ. Biology of Disease: comparative study of human and rat mammary tumourogenesis. *Lab Invest.* 1990;62:244-78.)

869. "Additional evidence from animal studies support this [Fathalla] hypothesis." Casagrande, *op.cit.,* p.172.

870. "Overall, these five studies indicate that ovulation did not appear to be prevented in rabbits;" Grou F, Rodrigues I. The morning-after pill; How long after? *Am J Obstet Gynecol.* 1994;171:6:1529-1534

871. "Hormonal steroids are capable of promoting the development of cervical cancer in animals." Brinton, *Contraception.* 1991, *op.cit.,* p.589.

872. "Experimental evidence indicates that oestrogens are involved in carcinogenic promotion of mouse mammary tumours." Powles, *Br. J. Cancer.* 1989 *op.cit.,* p.126

873. Cooper, *op.cit.,* p.266 It was precisely *because* beagle dogs reportedly developed breast nodules that certain progestagens under active consideration as 'candidates' for use in Norplant were rejected.

874. "The closer births are spaced after the first birth, the lower the risk of breast cancer. This is consistent with data from animal experiments ...". Colditz G, *J. Soc. Gynecol. Invest.* 1996. *op.cit.,* p.51

875. *'Clomid - A Guide for Women'* (Marion Merrell Dow, Pub. 1993). Patient Booklet

876. *Micromedex* Vol 87. Clomiphene monograph.

877. *'Clomid - A Guide for Women'. op.cit.,* p.6

878. The primary cause of death was a stroke but this was in turn caused by OHSS as a consequence of IVF treatment. Shanner L, Informed consent and inadequate medical information. *Lancet.* 1995;346:251

879. *APPG.* 24th Edition, p.1954

880. *Ibid.,* p.1195

881. *Ibid.,* p.1494

882. *Ibid.,* p.373

883. 70% of women given Clomid will ovulate, of these, "about 30% will become

pregnant." Therefore, 30% of 70% is 21%. Clomid approved product information. *APPG.* 1995, p.664.

884.   Trisequens/Trisequens Forte Consumer product Information. Novo Nordisk Pharmaceuticals Pty Ltd. 22 Loyalty Rd, North Rocks NSW 2151.

885.   *Ibid.*

886.   Estraderm and how to use it. A change for the better. Ciba-Geigy Aust. Ltd. Patient Booklet

887.   *A small book of questions and answers about the 'pill'*. 5th Ed. Presented by Wyrth Pharmaceuticals and the Family Planning Association of NSW. "The views expressed in this booklet are not necessarily those of Wyeth Pharmaceuticals." Dated 10/92. NB The edition dated 12/94 has the same question and answer.

888.   *Ibid.*

889.   *Mosby's, op.cit.,* p.573

890.   Evans R. Letters to the Editor. *Pharmacy Connection* (Canada) May/ June 1995

891.   Berg M op ten, Desogestrel: using a selective progestogen in a combined oral contraceptive. *Advances in Contraception.* 1991;17 No. 2/3 :241-250.

892.   Cullberg G, *et al.,* Central and peripheral effects of desogestrel 15-60ug daily for 21 days in healthy female volunteers. *Acta Obstet Gynecol Scand.* 1982;111:21-28

893.   Modern Oral Contraceptives. Your questions answered. Schering Pty. Ltd 27-31 Doody St. Alexandria NSW. Patient Booklet.

894.   Rodriguez C, Tatham LM. Thun MJ, Calle EE, Heath CW Jrn. Smoking and fatal prostate cancer in a large cohort of adult men. *AJE.* 1997;145: No.5. p.473

895.   Law MR, Hackshaw AK. Environmental tobacco smoke. *Br Med Bull.* 1996;52:1,22-34

896.   Higginson J, Muir CS, Munoz N. Human cancer:epidemiology and enviromental causes. Cambridge University Press. Tables 34.2 & 34.3. pp.338-339

897.   Moore P. Smoking in pregnancy may cause limb defects. *Lancet.*1997; 349: #9051

898.   Bennicke K, Conrad C, Sabroe S, Sorensen T. Cigarette smoking and breast cancer. *BMJ.*1995;310:#6992

899.   Olsson H & ML, Moller TR, Ranstam J, Holm P. *Lancet.*(Letter) 1985. *op.cit* p.748-49.

900.   Olsson H, *et al., J Nat Can Inst.* 1989; *op.cit.*

901.   Thomas DB, Ray RM . Oral contraceptives and invasive adenocarcinomas

and adenosquamous carcinomas of the uterine cervix. *Am J Epid.* 1996; 144:p284. Table 2

902. Vandebroucke JP, Rosendaal FR. End of the line for "third-generation-pill" controversy? *Lancet.*1997;349:1113-1114.

903. Rahwan, *op.cit.,* pp. 29-30

904. Kennedy F. Death prompts tampon inquiry. *The Australian.* Feb.1. 1995. p.3

905. Schlesselman, *op.cit.,* p. 9

906. McPherson K, Vessey MP, Neil A, *et al. Br J Cancer.* 1987. p.658

907. *Ibid.,* p.659

908. *Ibid.*

909. Paul, *BMJ.* 1989, *op.cit.,* p.759

910. Skegg, *JAMA. op.cit.,* pp.799-804

911. *Ibid.,* p.803.

912. Collaborative Group on Hormonal Factors in Breast Cancer. Breast cancer and hormonal contraception: collaborative reanalysis of individual data on 43297 women with breast cancer and 100,239 women without breast cancer from 54 epidemiological studies. *Lancet.*1996;347:1713-27

913. Meirik O, Adami H-O, Christoffersen T, Lund E, Bergstrom R, Bergsjo P. Oral Contraceptive use and Breast Cancer in Young Women.*Lancet.* 1986; 2; p.653

914. Rookus M A, E van Leeuwen. Oral contraceptives and risk of breast cancer in women aged 20-54 years. *Lancet* 1994; 334; p.844

915. Olsson H, *et al.* Early oral contraceptive use and breast cancer among premenopausal women: Final report from a study in Southern Sweden. *Journal of the National Cancer Institute.* 1989; 81(12):1000-4, Ma

916. Two examples are: McPherson K, Vessey M.P, Neil A, Doll R, Jones L & Roberts M. Early oral contraceptive use and breast cancer: Results of another case-control study. *Br J Cancer.* 1987;56:653-660 [a 160% increased risk for 4+ years of use before FFTP] and Chilvers C, *et al.* Oral contraceptive use and breast cancer risk in young women. *Lancet.* 1989 6th May 973-982. UK National Case-Control Group, *op.cit.,*p.973 [Chilvers and co-worker's reported that "there was a highly significant trend in risk of breast cancer with total duration of OC use with relative risks of 1.43 [a 43% risk increase] for 49-96 months use, and 1.74 [a 74% risk increase] for 97 months or more.".

917. Crowe S, Kent S. Pill Panic. *The Sun-Herald* (Sydney) 22.10.95

918. Watt AH. Oral contraceptives and venous thromboembolism. *Lancet.* 1995;346:1430

919.   The rationale behind advocating the pill as a means of avoiding pregnancy is predicated upon the oft touted justification that pregnancy is dangerous and should be avoided. Yet recent figures released in a draft report by an expert panel advising the National Health & Medical Research Council (Aust) shows that the maternal mortality rate for 1977-1981 was 7.9/100,00 women. As a comparison, the maternal mortality rate for surgical abortion *at 16-20 weeks* is 7.1/100,000 women. Given that the mortality rate from surgical abortion " rises progressively with each advancing gestational week", it would seem that abortion may have a higher risk after 20 weeks than a full-term delivery. Given that abortion is perceived to be a safe procedure, a full-term delivery must be *safer.Services for the Termination of Pregnancy in Australian: A Review. Draft Consultation Document* Sept 1995. National Health & Medical Research Counsel. (NH & MRC)

920.   Armstrong D. Breast Cancer- Women's Health Enemy No.1. *Ita*, May, 1994.Sydney. p.27

921.   Toynbee P. The pill is still a girl's best friend. *The Independent*. 20.10.95. (U.K.)

922.   Sieghart M A. What is their Pill doing to my body? *The Times*. 21.10.95. (U.K.)

923.   Symons E-K. Pill safety row still unresolved. *The Sunday Telegraph*. (Sydney, Aust.) October 1, 1995 p. 181

924.   Armstrong, *loc.cit.*

925.   *Ibid.*

926.   *Ibid.*

927.   Mackenzie Dr.F. "Healthwise", *Australian Women's Weekly* May 1991

928.   This event was reported by *AAP* (25.3.91), the *Australian* (13-14th April 1991), *Daytona Daily News* (9th April 1991) and confirmed on 8 April 1991 by the French Ministry of Health in an official *Communique*.

929.   Klein, *op.cit.,* p.5

930.   *Ibid.,* p.9

931.   Wiles J. Contraception: what's new, what works. *Australian Women's Weekly.* 1997 (Feb) p.33

932.   Bloemenkamp, 1995 *op.cit.*, p.1596

933.   Spitzer WO, Lewis MA, Heinemann LAJ, Thorogood M, MacRae KD. Third generation oral contraceptives and risk of venous thromboembolic disorders: an international case-control study. *BMJ*. 1996;312:83-8

934.   Delaney A, *loc.cit.*

935.   Kerekovic S, Women's Health Conference. *Australian Journal of*

Pharmacy. 1996;77:117.

936.   Camelotti W. Editor. *The essentials*. Autumn 1996 p.3.

937.   Cranston L. The Pill - debunking the myths. *The essentials*. Autumn 1996. p.16.

APPENDICES.

938.   *APPG*. 24th Ed. 1995 Vol 2 p 1511

939.   Schedule of Pharmaceutical Benefits. Australian Commonwealth Department of Human Services and Health. 1995

940.   Garland S, Faulkner-Jones B, Fortune D *et al*., Cervical cancer-what role for human papillomavirus ? *Med J Aust*. 1992;156; 204-212

941.   *Merck Manual* 16th Ed., *op.cit*., p.1824-25

942.   Brinton, *Contraception, op.cit.,* p.588

943.   *Mosby's, op.cit.,* p.197.

944.   Bartagol R (ed) : *Drugs In Pregnancy*. The Royal Women's Hospital, CSL Limited, Victoria, Australia 1993

GLOSSARY.

945.   *Mosby's Medical, Nursing and Allied Health Dictionary* 3rd Edition 1990 N. Darlene Como (Ed)

946.   Garland, *op.cit.,* p.204-212

15. BIBLIOGRAPHY.

1. Aarskog D. Clinical and cytogenetic studies in hypospadias. *Acta Paediatr Scand*. 1970: (suppl 203): 1-62.

2. Abbott TA 3rd, Lawrence BJ, Wallach S. Osteoporosis: the need for comprehensive treatment guidelines. *Clin Ther*.1996;Jan-Feb,18:1: pp.127-49 Ma

3. Adami S, Passeri M, Ortolani S, Broggini M, *et al.,* Effects of oral alendronate and intranasal salmon calcitonin on bone mass and biochemical markers of bone turnover in postmenopausal women with osteoporosis. *Bone*.1995 Oct, 17:4; 383-90 Ma

4. Addison AW, *et al.,* The occurrence of adenocarcinoma in endometriosis of the rectovaginal septum during progestational therapy. *Gynecol Oncology* 1979; 8:193.

5. Alder JB, Fraunfelder FT. Levonorgestrel Implants and Intracranial hypertension. *The New England Journal of Medicine*. 1995; June 22: 1720 (Letter).

6. Alliance for Life Newsletter, 1990 (Winnipeg-Canada).

7. America Online:MAXFIELD 28.1.95 Medical legal consultants of Washington: Washington women respond to the dangers of Norplant.

8. Ana Regina Gomes Dos Reis. Norplant in Brazil: Implant strategy in the guise of scientific research. *Issues in Reproductive and Genetic Engineering*. 1990; 3: (2) 111-118

9. Anon: Depo-Provera debate revs up at FDA. *Science* 1982; 217:424-428.

10. Anon. Oral contraceptive use and breast cancer risk in young . UK National Case-control study group. *Lancet*. 1989;1(8645):973-82. Ma

11. Approved Product Information. Femoden ED and Trioden ED 24 June 1994

12.   Archer WR. Deputy Assistant Secretry for Population Affairs,
       U.S.Department of Health & Human Services, Washington, D.C. Teens
       are warned on condom flaws. *The Star-Ledger.*Jan 29 19.93

13.   Armstrong B. Human papillomavirus and cervical cancer.
       *Lancet.*1988:April 2;756-57

14.   Armstrong D. Breast Cancer - Women's Health Enemy No.1 *Ita.* May
       1994. Sydney, Aust.

15.   *Australian Prescription Products Guide (APPG)* 1991 (20th Ed), 1995
       (24th Ed.) & 1996 (25th Ed) Australian Pharmaceutical Publishing Co.
       40 Burwood Rd, Victoria 3122 .

16.   Bachorik L. FDA issued approvable letter for mifepristone. Sept.18,
       1996. Http://www.fda.gov

17.   Baciewicz AM. Oral Contraceptive Drug Interactions (Review).
       Therapeutic Drug Monitoring. 1985;7:26-35. Raven Press. New York

18.   Barbosa RM, *et al.,* The Brazilian experience with Cytotec
       (misoprostol) *Stud Fam Planning.* 1993;24:236-240

19.   Barnard M. Pill to hard to swallow. *The Melbourne Age.* 7.6.91

20.   Bartagol R (ed) : *Drugs In Pregnancy.* The Royal Women's Hospital,
       CSL Limited, Victoria, Australia 1993

21.   Beaumont V, Beaumont J-L. Thrombosis and antibodies to cyproterone
       acetate. *Lancet.* 1991;337; 113

22.   Beer AE.*JAMA.* 1989;262:3184

23.   Bennicke K, Conrad C, Sabroe S, Sorensen T. Cigarette smoking and
       breast cancer.*BMJ.*1995;310:#6992   http://www.bmj.com

24.   Beral V, Hannaford P, Kay C. Oral contraceptive use malignancies of
       the Genital Tract. *Lancet.* 1988; Dec 10:1331-1335

25.   Beral V, Colwell L. Randomised trial of high doses of stilboestrol and ethisterone in pregnancy: long-term follow-up of mothers. *BMJ.* 1980; 281:1098-1101

26.   Berg M op ten . Desogestrel: using a selective progestogen in a combined oral contraceptive. *Advances in Contraception.* 1991;Vol7 No. 2/3 :241-250.

27.   Bergkvist L, Adami Hans-Olov, Persson I, Hoover R, Schairer MS. The risk of breast cancer after estrogen and estrogen-progestin replacement. *N Eng J Med.* 1989; 321: 293-297.

28.   Bird KA. The use of spermicide containing containing nonoxynol-9 in the prevention of HIV infection. *AIDS.* 1991;5: 791-796

29.   Black C, Houghton VP. A users acceptability study of vaginal spermicides in combination with barrier methods or an IUCD. *Contraception.* 1983;28:103-110.

30.   Blair JM. Types of Contraception may affect Bone Density in Adolescents. *American Family Physician.* 1995;Sept 15:1181

31.   Blankenstein MA,Van't Verlaat JW, Croughs RJM. Hormone dependency of meningiomas. *Lancet* 1989;i :1381-1382

32.   Bloemenkamp KW, Rosendal FR, Helmerhorst FM, Bauller HR, Vandenbrouche JP. Enhancement by factor V Leiden mutation of deep-vein thrombosis associated with oral contraceptives containing third-generation progestagen. *Lancet.* 1995;346:8990:1593-6.

33.   Bosch FX, Manos MM, MuAnoz N, Sherman M, Jansen AM, Peto J, Schiffman MH, Moreno V, Kurman R, Shah KV. Prevalence of human papillomavirus in cervical cancer: a worldwide perspective. International biological study on cervical cancer (IBSCC) Study Group. *J Natl Cancer Inst.*1995 (June7);87:,796-802 Ma

34.   Boston Collaborative Drug Surveillance Programme. *Lancet*;1973: 1:1399-1404

35. Bowden T, Hissom JR, Moore MR. Growth Stimulation of T47D human Breast Cancer Cells by thr Anti-Progestin RU-486 *Endocrinology* 1989; 124(5) 2642-2644

36. Boyce JG, Lu T, Nelson JH, Fruchter RG. Oral contraceptives and cervical carcinoma. *Am J Obstet Gynec* 1977; 128: 761-66

37. Brinton LA, Hoover R, Fraumeni JF. Menopausal oestrogens and breast cancer risk: an expanded case-control study. *Br J Cancer*. 1986; 54; 825-832

38. Brinton LA, Reeves WC, Brenes MM, Herrero R, de Britton RC, Gaitan E, Tenorio F, Garcia M, Rawls WE. Oral contraceptive use and risk of invasive cervical cancer. *International Journal of Epidemiology*. 1990;19(1): 4-11, Ma

39. Brinton LA. Oral contraceptives and cervical neoplasia. *Contraception*. 1991;43(6): 581-95,

40. Brisson J, Morin C, Fortier M, Roy M, Bouchard C, Leclerc J, Christen A, Guimont C, Penault F and Meisels A. Risk Factors for Cervical Intraepithelial Neoplasia: Differences between Low-and High-Grade Lesions. *American Journal of Epidemiology*, 1994;140:(8)700-710.

41. Brock KE, Berry G, Brinton LA, *et al.* Sexual, reproductive and contraceptive risk factors for carcinoma-in-situ of the uterine cervix in Sydney. *Medical Journal of Australia.* 1989;15: 125-130

42. Buhle EL. Infertility Drugs and Ovarian Cancer, University of Pennsylvania. OncoLink Home Page. *http://oncolink.upenn.edu*

43. Burnell P. *The Universe.(U.K.)* Sunday July 28,1991

44. *Butterworth's Medical Dictionary* 2nd Ed 1978 MacDonald Critchley (ed).

45. Camelotti W. Editor. The pill- debunking the myths. Easy, safe and effective birth control. *The essentials*. Autumn 1996

46.   CancerNet News - Oral Contraceptives and Risk for Breast Cancer in Young Women- *National Cancer Institute.* August 1995. *Internet address* - *http://oncolink.upenn.edu/cancer_new/*

47.   Carey RF, Herman WA, Retta SM, Rinaldi JE, Herman BA, Athey TW. Effectiveness of latex condoms as a barrier to human immuno-deficiency virus-sized particulars under conditions of simulated use. *Sexually Transmitted Diseases.* 1992;19:(4): 230-234

48.   Cranall D. Controversy rages over new contraceptive data. *BMJ.*1995;311:1117-8. *http://www.tecc.co.uk/bmj/archive/7031n.htm*

49.   Casagrande JT, Pike MC, Ross RK, Louie EW, Roy S, Henderson BE. "Incessant ovulation" and ovarian cancer. *Lancet.*1979;2:170-173

50.   Cecil H, Reed D, Holyz J. Norplant removal facilitated by use of ultrasound for localization. *Journal of Family Practice.* 1995; 40:(2). 182-186.

51.   Celi BR, Kovnat DM. Acute pneumonitis after subcutaneous injections of silicone. *N Eng J Med.* 1983;309:856-7

52.   Cekan S, Aedo AR, SegerstAEeen E, Van Look P, Messinis I, Templeton A. Levels of the antiprogestin RU486 and its metabolities in human blood and follicular fluid following oral administration of a single dose. *Hum Reprod.* 1989; 4(2):131-5.

53.   Chang AR. Hormonal contraceptives, human papillomavirus and cervical cancer; some observation from a colposcopy clinic. *Aust NZ. Obstet Gynec.*1989;29:329-331 in Dunn, H.P. *The Doctor and the Christian Marriage.* Alba House, New York. 1992 p.68

54.   Chen Y-H, Huang L-H, Chen T-M. Differential effects of progestins and estrogens on long control regions of human papillomavirus types 16 and 18. *Biochemical and Biophysical Research Communications.* 1996;224:651-659 (Article No. 1080)

55.   Chilvers C, McPherson K, Peto J, Pike MC, Vessey MP. Oral contraceptive use and breast cancer risk in young women. *Lancet.* 1989;6th May: 973-982. UK National Case-Control Group.

56.   Chilvers C. Breast cancer and depo-medroxyprogesterone acetate. A
        review. *Contraception.* 1994;49:211-222

57.   Chilvers CE, Pike MC, *et al.* Breast cancer and breast feeding (Meeting
        abstract) *British Journal of Cancer.* 1992;66 (Suppl xv11):9, Ma

58.   Choo V. EU agency asks for more data on oral contraceptives *Lancet.*
        1995;346:1219.

59.   *'Clomid - A Guide for Women'* (Marion Merrell Dow).1993.Sydney.

60.   Clarke C, Foundation chief executive, Menopause Foundation.
        Australian Journal of Pharmacy. 1996;77:117

61.   Cohen HS, Savitz DA, Cefalo RC, *et. al. JAMA.* 1989; 262:3143

62.   Colditz GA, Hankinson SE, *et. al.* The use of estrogens and progestins
        and the risk of breast cancer in post-menopausal women. *N Eng. J.
        Med.* 1995;332:1589-1593

63.   Colditz GA, Willett WC, Speizer FE. (Letter). *NEJM.*1995;333:1355-1358.
        http://www.nejm.org/publicM/1995/0333/0020/1355/1.htm

64.   Colditz GA. Postmenopausal estrogens and breast cancer. *Society for
        Gynecologic Investigation.* Elsevier Science Inc. (Pub) 1996;3:(2):50-56

65.   Collabarative Group on Hormonal Factors in Breast Cancer. Breast
        cancer and hormonal contraceptives: collaborative reanalysis of
        individual data on 53,297 women with breast cancer and 100,239
        women without breast cancer from 54 epidemiological studies. *Lancet.*
        1996;347:1713-27

66.   Collart D. Condom failure for protection from sexual transmission of
        the HIV - a review of the medical literature.*Biochemistry & Molecular
        Biology.* 5393 Whitney Ct, Stone Mountain. GA 30088

67.   Collins FS, Mahoney MJ. Hydrocephalus and abnormal digits after
        failed first-trimester prostaglandin abortion attempt. *Journ Ped.* 1983;
        102 (4):620-621

316   A Consumer's Guide to the Pill and other Drugs.

68.   Conat M, Hardy D, *et. al.* Condoms prevent transmission of AIDS-associated retrovirus (letter) *JAMA.* 1986;255:1706

69.   *Concise Oxford Dictionary.* 5Th Ed.OUP. 1793

70.   Coney S. Long-term effects of assisted conception. *Lancet.* 1995; 345: 976

71.   Cooke H. Mother of tragic Pill girls to sue. *Daily Express*(UK) 1996; March 27

72.   Cooper M. Norplant. *Aust NZ J Obstet Gynaecol* 1991;31:3.265-272.

73.   Coppess M H. Who's Pushing the Abortion Pill. *Focus on the Family Citizen.* 21.1.91

74.   Corson S. Contraceptive efficacy of a monophasic oral contraceptive containing desogestrel. *Am J Obstet Gynecol.* 1993;168:1017-20

75.   Costa SH, Vessey MP. Misoprostol and illegal abortions in Rio de Janeiro, Brazil. *Lancet.* 1993;341:1258-61

76.   Cox JT. Epidemiology of cervical intraepithelial neoplasia: the role of human papillomavirus. *Baillieres Clin Obstet Gynaecol.* 1995;9:1,1-37 Ma

77.   Crowe S, Kent S. Pill Panic - Health warning on seven brands. *The Sun-Herald* . Sydney, Aust. 22.10.95

78.   Cullberg G, Lindstedt G, Lundberg PA, Steffensen K. Central and peripheral effects of desogestrel 15-60ug daily for 21 days in healthy female volunteers. *Acta Obstet Gynecol Scand.* 1982;111:21-28

79.   Czeizel A. Increasing trends in congenital malformations of male external genitalia. *Lancet.* 1985;I:462-3

80.   Dabancens A, Prado R, Larraguibel R, *et al.* Intraepithelial cervical neoplasia in women using intrauterine devices and long-acting

injectable progesterones as contraceptives. *Am J Obstet Gynecol.* 1974; 119:1052.

81.   Daly E, Vessey MP, Hawkins MM, Carsons JL, Gough P, Marsh S. Risk of venous thromboembolism in users of hormone replacement therapy. *Lancet.*1996;348:#9033. *http://www.thelancet.com/lancet/Users/vol348no9033/articles/article1.html*

82.   Darton N. Surprising journey for abortion drug. *New York Times.* 23rd March 1995 p. C12

83.   *Davidson's Principles and Practice of Medicine.* 11th Ed. Churchill Livingstone. 1975.

84.   Davies G C, Newton J R. Subdermal contraceptive implants - a review: with special reference to Norplant. *Br J Fam Planning.* 1991; 17; 4-8

85.   Delaney A. ABC Radio National: *The Health Report* 22.4.91 (Transcript)

86.   Delgado-Rodriguez M, *et al.* Oral contraceptives and cancer of the cervix uteri. A Meta-analysis. *Acta Obstetricia et Gynecologia Scandinavica.* 1992;71:(5):368-76, Ma

87.   Dietl L. K. Ovulation and ovarian cancer. *Lancet.* 1991;338:445.

88.   Dr Schueler's *Home Medical Advisor Pro* (CD edition) 1993 Pixel Perfect Inc. 10460 Tropical Trail Trail Merritt, Florida 32952

89.   Duffy A, Santamaria Dr J. The How and the why of RU 486. *Thomas More Centre Bulletin.* 1990;2:(9).1-5

90.   Editorial: After the morning after and the morning after that. *Lancet.* 1995;345:1381-1382

91.   Ehman R. MD. *Problems in Family Planning.* p.14. Heezerweg 345 5643 KG Eindhoven The Netherlands.

92.   Eiken P, Kolthoff N, Nielsen SP. Effects of 10 years' hormone replace-
       ment therapy on bone mineral content in postmenopausal women.
       *Bone.*1996; Nov, 19:5 Suppl, 191S-193S Ma

93.   Ellertson C, Winikoff B, Armstrong E, Camp S, Senanayake P.
       Expanding Access to Emergency Contraception in Developing
       Countries. *Studies in Family Planning.* 1995;26,5:251-263

94.   El-Refaey H, Rajasekar D, Abdalla M. Calder L, Templeton A.
       Induction of abortion with mifepristone (RU486) and oral or vaginal
       misoprostol. *N Eng J Med.* 1995;332:983-987

95.   Epstein KC, Sloat B. Many find side-effects of Norplant intolerable.
       The Cleveland Plain Dealer. 18.6.95

96.   Estraderm and how to use it. A change for the better. Ciba-Geigy Aust.
       Ltd

97.   Evans ANW, *et al.* The ingestion by pregnant women of substances
       toxic to the foetus. *Practitioner.* 1980; 224: 315-19

98.   Evans R. Letters to the Editor. *Pharmacy Connection Canada* May/
       June 1995

99.   Ewertz M. Epidemiology of breast cancer: the Nordic contributions.
       *Eur J Surg.*1996;162(2):97-9 Ma

100.   Faich G, Pearson K, Fleming D, *et al.* Toxic shock syndrome and the
       contraceptive sponge.*JAMA.*1986; 255: 216-218

101.   Family Planning Association (FPA) of NSW. Presented by Wyeth P/L.
       A small book of questions and answers about the 'pill'. Prepared by
       the F.P.A.

102.   Fathalla M.F. Incessant ovulation - a factor in ovarian neoplasia.
       Lancet. 1971;ii:163

103.   FDA Mailgram 26/8/87 in *Micromedex* Vol. 84, 1995

104.   Ferrari J. *The Australian*,(News Ltd, publishers) 27.9.95.

105.   Fife-Yeomans J. On trial: oral contraceptive safety and corporate honesty. *The Australian*. 20.1.96

106.   Fishel S, Jackson P. Follicular stimulation for high tech pregnancies: are we playing it safe? *BMJ*.1989;229:309-311

107.   Floridon C, Mielsen O, Byrjalsen C, Holund B, Kerndrup G, Thomsen S, Anderson J. Ectopic pregnancy: histopathology and assessment of cell proliferation with and without methotrexate treatment. *Fert Ster*. 1996;65(4).730-738

108.   Fonseca W, *et al*. Congential malformations of the scalp and cranium after failed first trimester abortion attempt with misoprostol. *Clin Dysmorph* 1993;2:76-80

109.   Francis B. "Letters" *The Melbourne Age* 23.7.90

110.   French Ministry of Health, 1 Place de Fontenoy Paris 12th April 1990.in *Human Life International Reports* Oct 1990.

111.   French report on death in abortion pill treatment. *Dayton Daily News*. Dayton. OHIA, USA. 9th April, 1991

112.   Friedman Z, Trivelli L. Condom availability for youth. *Pediatrics*. 1996; 97:285 (letter)

113.   Gal I, *et al*. Hormonal pregnancy tests and congenital malformation. *Nature*. 1967;216:83.

114.   Garland M S, Faulkner-Jones B, Fortune D, *et al*. Cervical cancer - what role for human papillomavirus. *Med Journ Aust*. 1992;156: 204-212

115.   Genuis SJ, Genuis SK. Adolescent sexual involvement: time for primary prevention. *Lancet*. 1995;345:240-41.

116.   Gitsch G, Kainz C, Studnicka M, *et al*. Oral contraceptives and human

papillomavirus infection in cervical intraepithelial neoplasia. *Arch Gynae. Obstet.* 1992:252(1):25-30

117. Gitsch G, *et al.* Oral contraceptives and human papilloma virus infection in cervical lesions. *Nineteenth Eurpoean Congress of Cytology.* June 17-20, 1991, Turku,Finland,

118. Glasow R D. *National Right to Life Newsletter* Jan.8.91 (U.S.A.) from *Nature.* 29.11.1990

119. Gonzalez CH, *et al.* Limb deficiency with or without Mobius sequence in seven Brazilian children associated with misoprostol use in the first trimester of pregnancy. *Am J Med Genet.* 1993;47:59-64

120. *Goodman & Gilman's The Pharmacological Basis of Therapeutics.* 5th Ed. Macmillan Pub. Co. N.Y.1975

121. *Goodman & Gilman's The Pharmacological Basis of Therapeutics.* 8th Ed. Pergamom Press 1990

122. *Gould Medical Dictionary.* 4th Ed.1979. McGraw-Hill Book Co.

123. Graham A, Grieve F, Davie, Glasier A. (Letter) *Lancet.*1995;346:1430

124. Gram IT, *et. al.* Oral contraceptive use and the incidence of cervical intraepithelial neoplasia. *American Journal of Obstetrics and Gynecology.* 1992; 167(1):40-4,

125. Gray RH. Depo-medroxyprogesterone and risk of breast cancer. *Br Med J.* 1989;299:1989

126. Greenblatt RB, Roy S, *et. al.* Induction of ovulation. *Am J Obstet Gynec.* 1962;84: 900-909

127. Grimes DA, Godwin AJ, Rubin A, Smith J, Lacarra M. Ovulation and follicular development associated with the low-dose oral contraceptives:a randomised controlled trial. *Ob. & Gynae.* The American College of Obstetricans & Gynaecologists. 1994;83:(1).29-34

128.   Grimes DA. AIDS Update: The threat to women's health. *The Contraception Report.* 1995;6:#2 p11.

129.   Grou F, Rodrigues I. The morning - after pill; How long after? *Am J Obstet Gynecol.* 1994;171:1529-34

130.   Gutthann, SP, Rodriguez LA, Castellsague J, Oliart AD. Hormone replacement therapy and risk of venous thromboembolism: population based case-control study. *BMJ.* 1997;314#7083. *http://www.bmj.com.*

131.   Hall C (Med.Ed.), Girl dies after taking the pill to cure acne. *UK News, Electronic Telegraph* Feb.2.97 Issue 621. *http://www.telegraph.co.uk*

132.   Hardon Anita, Norplant: A critical review. *WGNRR Newsletter* 34 Jan-March 1991

133.   Harper C, Ellerton C. Knowledge and perceptions of emergency contraceptive pills among a college-age population: A qualitative Approach. *Fam Plan Perspectivies.* 1995;27:149-154

134.   *Harrup's Dictionary of Medicine and Health* Ist Ed. 1988. London

135.   Hartmann B, Population and Development Program, Hampshire College, Amherst, USA. Population Council report on Norplant in Indonesia. in *WGNRR Newsletter* 34 Jan - March 1991

136.   Hausknecht R. Methotrexate and misoprostol to terminate early pregnancy. *New Eng. J. Med.* 1995;333:537-540

137.   Heinonen OP, *et al.* Cardiovascular birth defects and antenatal exposure to female sex hormones. *N Eng J Med.* 1977;296:67-70

138.   Helmrich SP, Rosenberg L, Kaufman DW, Strom B, Shapiro S. Venous thromboembolism in relation to oral contraceptive use. *Obstet Gynec.* 1987;69:91-95

139.   Hemminki E, McPherson K. Impact of postmenopausal hormone therapy on cardiovascular events and cancer: pooled data from clinical trials. *BMJ.* 1997;315:#7101

140.   Herranz Prof.G., RU-486: The 'Abortion Pill'. *Catholic International*
       1991;2:#14 673-677.

141.   Hicks D R, Martin LS, *et al.* Inactivation of HTLV-111/LAV- induced
       cultures of normal human lymphocytes by nonoxynol-9 in vitro (letter).
       Lancet. 1985:2: 1422-1423

142.   Hildesheim A, Reeves WC, *et al.* Association of oral contraceptive
       use and human papillomaviruses in invasive cervical cancers.
       International Journal of Cancer. 1990;45(5):860-4, Ma

143.   *Hills Shire Times* 13.6.95 (Baulkham Hills, NSW, AUST)

144.   Ho GY, Burk RD, Klein S, Kadish AS, Chang CJ, Palan P, Basu J,
       Tachezy R, Lewis R, Romney S. Resistent genital human
       papillomavirus infection as a risk factor for persistent cervical
       dysplasia. *J.Natl. Cancer. Inst.* 1995; 87:18,1365-71

145.   Hodsman A, Adachi J, Olsznski W. Prevention and management of
       osteoporosis: consensus statement from the Scientific Advisory Board
       of the Osteoporosis Society of Canada. 6. Use of bisphophonates in
       the treatment of osteoporosis. *Can Med Assoc J.* 1996 Oct 1, 155:7,945-
       8 Ma

146.   Hosking DJ, McClung MR, Ravn P, Wasnich RD, Thompson RD,
       Daley MS, Yates AJ. Alendronate in the prevention of osteo-
       porosis:Epic study two-year results. *J Bone Miner Res.* 11 (Suppl.
       1):S133-S133, Aug.1996 (in Soc. Proc.)

147.   How to use your 28 day pack. Wyeth Pharmaceuticals, Gregory Place,
       Parramatta, NSW 2150 Aust.

148.   Hull ME, Kriner M, Schneider E, Maiman M. Ovarian cancer after
       successful ovulation induction: a case report. *J Reprod Med.* 1996
       (Jan);41:1,52-4 Ma

149.   Hume K., The Pill and other potions in perspective. *Health care Bio-*
       ethics perspectives. 27.7.1991

150. Hunt K, Vessey M, McPherson K, Coleman M. Long-term surveillance of mortality and cancer incidence in women receiving hormone replacement therapy. *Br J Obstet Gyn.* 1987;94: 620-635

151. Ince S. The trouble with RU-486. *Vogue* (American Edition). July, 1991: 88-90

152. Interview, *Le Monde* Aug 1 1990, reprinted in *Guardian Weekly.* UK August 19 1990.

153. Isenbarge DW, Chapin BL. Osteoporosis. Current pharmacologic options for prevention and treatment. *Postgrad Med.* 1997 Jan, 101:1,129-32,136-7, 141-2. Ma

154. Isselbacher *et al. Harrison's Principles of Internal Medicine.* 13th Ed.1994. Ch. 150.

155. Ivory Dr K. Pill claims don't make sense. *Medical Observer* (Aust) 10.11.95

156. Jackman J. RU-486 wins global praise from women. *The Feminist Majority Report.* Fall 1995, pp.5 &14.

157. Jeffries DJ. Nonoxynol and HIV infection (letter).*BMJ.* 1988: 296;1798

158. Jick H, Walker AM, *et al. JAMA.* 1981;245:1329

159. Jick H, Derby L, Myers MW, Vasilakis C, Newton KM. Risk of hospital admission for idiopathic venous thromboembolism among users of postmenopausal oestrogens. *Lancet.*1996;348#9033. *http://www. thelancet.com/lancet/Users/vol348no9033articles/article2.html*

160. Johnson JH., Weighing the evidence on the pill and breast cancer. *Family Planning Perspectives.* 1989; 21(2):89-92, Ma

161. Jost. C.R.*Acad. Sc. Paris. Ser.* 111. 303. 1986; p.281-284.

162.   Karpf DB, Shapiro DR, Seeman E, Ensrud KE, *et al.* Prevention of nonvertebral fractures by alendronate. (A meta-analysis). *JAMA.*1997; 227:1159-1164 Ma

163.   Kennedy F. Death prompts tampon inquiry. *The Australian.* Feb.1. 1995. p.3

164.   Kenney JW. Risk factors associated with genital HPV infection. *Cancer Nurse.* 1996 (Oct);19:5, 353-9

165.   Kessler DA. Prescription drug products; certain combined oral contraceptives for use as postcoital emergency contraception;Notice. *Federal Register.*1997;62:37. *http://www.fda.gov*

166.   Kerekovic S. Women's Health Conference. *Australian Journal of Pharmacy.* 1996;77:116-117.

167.   Key TJA, Pike MC. The role of oestrogens and progestagens in the epidemiology and prevention of breast cancer. *Eur J Cancer Clin Oncol.* 1988;24:29-43 Pergamon Journals Ltd.

168.   Key TJ. Hormones and cancer in humans.*Mutat Res.*1995;333(1-2) :97-9

169.   Khoo SK. Contraceptive efficacy of the Pill. *Med J Aust* 1989;150: 548-549

170.   King RJB. Biology of female sex hormone action in relation to contraceptive agents and neoplasia. *Contraception.* Imperial Cancer Research Fund. University of Surrey. 1991;43:(6)527- 542

171.   Kim MR, Qazi QH, Andeerson VM, Valencia GB. A genetic male infant with female phenotype in camptomelic syndrome: A relationship to exposure to oral contraceptives during pregnancy. *Am J Obstet Gynecol.* 1995;172:1042-3

172.   Kjaer SK, *et al.* Case-control study of risk factors for cervical squamous-cell neoplasia in Denmark. 111. Role of oral contraceptive use. *Cancer Causes and Control.* 1993; 4(6):513-9, Ma

173.   Klebanoff SJ. Effects of spermicidal agent nonoxynol-9 on vaginal
        micro-flora. *Int Infect Dis.* 1992;165:19-25.

174.   Klein R, Raymond J, Dumble L. *RU-486; Misconceptions, Myths and
        Morals* Spinifex Press, Melbourne, Victoria, Aust. 1991

175.   Kohler U, Wuttke P. Results of a case-control study of the current
        effect of various factors of cervical cancer risk. 2. Contraceptive
        behaviour and the smoking factor. *Zentralblatt fur gynakologie.*
        1994;116(7): 405-9,. Ma

176.   Kolata Gina. Will the Lawyers Kill Off Norplant. *The New York Times.*
        28.5.95. pp.,1&5. Sect 3

177.   Kondo K, Tsuzuki H, Sasa M, Sumitomo M, Uyama T, Monden Y. A
        dose-response relationship between the frequency of p53 mutations
        and tobacco consumption in lung cancer patients. *J Surg Onco.*
        1996;61:1,20-6 Ma

178.   Kurman R, Wallach EE, Zacur HA. Letter *NEJM.* 1995;332:1300-1302

179.   Lamptey P, Klufio C, Smith SC, *et al.* Ortho vaginal tablets and Emko
        vaginal tablets in Accura,Ghana. *Contraception.* 1985;32:445-454.

180.   La Vecchia C. Reproductive factors, oral contraceptives, and breast
        cancer: The importance of unifying hypotheses. *Dev Oncol.* 1991;63:
        69-88,. Ma

181.   La Veechia, *et al.* Oral contraceptives and primary liver cancer. *Br J
        Cancer* 1989; 59: 460-461

182.   Lawson C. Stoke victim doggedly blinks trial testimomy. *The Ottawa
        Citizen.* April. 1997. E-mail. <a1a34216@bc.sympatico.ca>

183.   Lafferty FW, Spencer G E, Pearson O H. Effects of
        androgens,estrogens, and high calcium intakes on bone formation and
        resorption in osteoporosis. *Am J Med.* 1964; 36: 514-528

184.   Lancet. 1991; 337: 969-70

185.   Larriera A. Safe sex drive fails to stop herpes spread. *The Sydney Morning Herald*. (Aust) 8/9/95

186.   Law MR, Hackshaw AK. Environmental tobacco smoke. *Br Med Bull*. 1996;52:1,22-34

187.   Lawrence J. Three Pill studies showed increased risk of blood clots. *The Times*. 21.10.95

188.   Layde P M, Beral V. Further analyses of mortality in oral contracepetive users. *Lancet*. 1981;541- 546

189.   Lefevre T. To verify, please phone +33 1 47 901998, fax +33 1 47 338187 or e-mail tdd1001@ibm.net

190.   *Le Monde* 10.4.91, *Le Figaro* 9.4.91

191.   *Le Quotidien de Medecin Paris* 30.4.90.

192.   Leroy O, *et al*. Deep venous thrombosis and antibodies to cyproterone acetate. *Lancet*;1990;336:509

193.   Lewis MA, Spitzer WO, LAJ Heinemann, MacRae KD, Bruppacher R, Thorogood M. on behalf of Transnational Research Group on Oral Contraceptives and the Health of Young Women. Third generation oral contracepives and risk of myocardial infarction: an international case-control study. *BMJ*.1996;312:88-90

194.   Liberman UA, Weiss SR, Broll J, Minnie HW, *et al*. Effects of oral alendronate on bone mineral density and the incidence of fractures in postmenopausal osteoporosis. *NEJM*.1995;333:1437-1443.

195.   Llewellyn-Jones D. *Everywomen*. 2nd Edition 1978. Faber and Faber, London

196.   Lowe G, Rumley A,Woodward M, Reid E.(Letter). *Lancet*.1997;349:1623

197. Lowry S, Russell H, Hickey I, Atkinson R. Incessant ovulation and
      ovarian cancer.(letter) *Lancet.* 1991; 337:1544-5

198. Lund E. Oral contraceptives and breast cancer.a review with some
      comments on mathematical models.*Acta Oncologia.*1992;31(2):183-6,
      Ma

199. Lytle CD, Tondreau SC, Truscott W, Budacz AP, Kuester RK, Venegas
      L, Schmukler RE, Cyr WH. Filtration size of human immunodeficiency
      virus type 1 and surrogate viruses used to test barrier materials.
      *Applied and Enviromental Microbiology.*1992;58:2:747-749

200. Mackenzie Dr.F. Healthwise,*Australian Women's Weekly,* May 1991

201. *Macquarie Dictionary.* A. Delbridge (Ed) Kevin Weldon Production
      1982. Sydney. Aust.

202. Madden J.(Mrs.) B. Pharm MPS (letters) *Australian Journal of
      Pharmacy.*1995:76. April

203. Mann JR, *et al.* Transplacental carcinogenesis (adrenocortical
      carcinoma) associated with hydroxyprogesterone hexanoate. *Lancet.*
      1983;ii, 580.

204. *Martindale- the Extra Pharmacopoea.* 1982-1995 Roy. Pharm. Soc.
      G.B. 29th Edition

205. McClung MR. Current bone mineral density data on bisphosphates in
      postmenopausal osteoporosis.*Bone.*1996;19:5 (suppl)195S-198S.

206. McCrystal P. What kind of prescription? *Chemist & Druggist.* 1995;
      Feb 25:304

207. McPherson K. Third generation oral contraception and venous
      thromboembolism. (Editorial).*BMJ.* 1996;Vol.312#7023: *http://www.bmj.
      com/archive/7023e.htm*

208. McPherson K, Neil A, Vessey M.P, Doll R. Oral contraceptives and
      breast cancer.*Lancet.* 1983;ii:1414-5.

209.   McPherson K, Vessey M.P, Neil A, Doll R, Jones L, Roberts M. Early
        oral contraceptive use and breast cancer: Results of another case-
        control study. *Br J Cancer.* 1987;56:653-660

210.   Meade TW, Greenberg G, Thompson SG. Progestogens and
        cardiovascular reactions associated with oral contraceptives and a
        comparison of safety of 50- and 30-ug estrogen preparations. *BMJ.*
        1980;280:1157

211.   *Media Tracking Service.* Monday, August 21, 1995 No.177(Aust).

212.   Meirik O, Adami H-O, Christoffersen T, Lund E, Bergstrom R, Bergsjo
        P. Oral Contraceptive use and Breast Cancer in Young Women .
        Lancet. 1986;2; 650-654

213.   Meirik O, Farley T, Lund E, Adami H-O, Christoffersen T, Bergsjo P.
        Breast cancer and oral contraceptives: patterns of risk among parous
        and nulliparous women-further analysis of the Swedish-Norwegian
        material. *Contraception.* 1989;39(5):471-5,

214.   Meland MR, Flehinger BJ. Early incidence rates of precancerous
        cervical lesions in women using contraceptives. *Gynecol Oncol*
        1973;1:290-8

215.   *Mellon's Illustrated Medical Dictionary* 3rd Ed (1993) NewYork.

216.   Memorial Sloan-Kettering Cancer Center. Scientists Link Smoking, p53
        and bladder cancer. 1996 *http://.mskcc.org/document/cn950801.htm*

217.   *Merck Manual* 15th Ed. (1987), 16th Ed (1992) Robert Berkow (Ed)
        1987. Merck & Co., Inc. Rahwat, N.J. U.S.A.

218.   *Micromedex* , Inc (Computerised Clinical Information System) Vol
        84,Vol 85, Vol 86, Vol 92. Drug monographs.

219.   Miller DR, Rosenberg L, *et al.* Breast Cancer before age 45 and oral
        contraceptive use: new findings. *American Journal of Epidemiology.*
        1989;129(2):269-80, Ma

220. *MIMS on CD. V2* 1 Feb- 20 April 1997. MIMS Australia. 2 Chandos St, St. Leonards. N.S.W. Aust.

221. Mishell DR. Pharmacokinetics of depot medroxyprogesterone acetate contraception. *J Reprod Med.*1996;41:5 Suppl, 381-90 Ma

222. Modern Oral Contraceptives. Your questions answered. Schering Pty. Ltd 27-31 Doody St. Alexandria NSW

223. Moore P. Smoking in pregnancy may cause limb defects. *Lancet.*1997; 349:#9051

224. Morelli S. Lourdes: Clinic violated teaching. *Binghamton Press & Sun.* 1997 (March 28)

225. *Mosby's Medical, Nursing and Allied Health Dictionary* 3rd Edition 1990 N. Darlene Como (Ed)

226. Murphy S, Munday PE, *et al.* Anti-HIV substances for rape victims (letter)*JAMA.* 1989; 262:2090-209

227. Murphy S Munday PE, *et al.* Rape and subsequent seroconversion to HIV (letter) *BMJ.*1990;300:118

228. *National Alliance of Breast Cancer Organisations.* (NABCO).1989; Vol. 3 #4 *http://nysernet.org/bcic/*

229. *News Weekly* (Melbourne, Aust) Abortion Drug Further Discredited June 22nd 1991 p.10.

230. Nieman LK, Chrousos GP, Kellner C, Spitz IM, Nisula BC, Cutler GB, Merriam GR, Bardin CW, Loriaux DL. Successful Treatment of Cushings Syndrome with the Glucocorticoid Antagonist RU-486. *Journ Clin Endocrin Metabol.* 1985;61:536-540

231. NSW Cancer Incidence and Mortality. NSW Central Cancer Registry. Cancer Epidemiology Research Unit 1991 & 1996

232. Odeblad E.Prof. Regolazione Naturale Della Fertilita Femminile. 1988

233. Odeblad E. Prof. Paper presented at the Families of Australia Foundation International Conference in Sydney, Australia. 119-24 July, 1988

234. Olsen D. Pill policy will help victims of rape:hospital. *The Peoria Journal Star* (Illinios, USA). Monday , November 13, 1995.

235. Olsson H & ML, Moller TR, Ranstam J, Holm P. Oral contraceptive use and breast cancer in young women in Sweden. *Lancet.* 1985. March 30. 748-49.

236. Olsson H, Borg A, Ferno M, MollerT, Ranstam J. Early oral contraceptive use and breast in Southern Sweden. *Proc Annu Meet Am Soc Clin Oncol.* 1989:A367, Ma

237. Olsson H, Moller TR, Ranstam J. Early oral contraceptive use and breast cancer among premenopausal women: Final report from a study in Southern Sween. *Journal of the National Cancer Institute.* 1989;81(12):1000-4

238. Olsson H. Oral contraceptives and breast cancer. A review. *Acta Oncologica.* 1989;28(6):849-63, Ma

239. Olsson H, Ranstam MA, Baldetrop, Ewres SB, Ferno M, Killander D, Sigurdsson H. Proliferation and DNA ploidy in malignant tumours in relation to early oral contraception use and early abortions. *Cancer.* 1991;67(5) 1285-90,

240. Olsson H, Borg A, Ferno M, Moller TR, Ranstam J. Early oral contraceptive use and premenopausal breast cancer - a review of studies performed in Southern Sweden. *Cancer Detection and Prevention.* 1991;15(4):265-271

241. Olsson H, Borg A, Ferno M, Ranstam J, Sigurdsson H. Her-2/neu and INT2 Proto-oncogene amplification in malignant breast tumours in relation to reproductive factors and exposure to exogenous Hormones. *J Natl Cancer Inst.* 1991;83:1483-87

242. Olsson H, Jernstrom H, Alm P, Kreipe H, Ingvar C, *et al*. Proliferation of the breast epithelium in relationship to menstrual cycle phase, hormonal use, and reproductive factors. *Breast Cancer Research and Treatment.* 1996;40:187-196

243. Ory HW, *et al*. A Preliminary analysis of oral contraceptive use and risk of developing premalignant lesions of the uterine cervix. In: Garratini S, Berendes HW, Eds. *Pharmacology of steroid contraceptive drugs*. New York, Raven Press 1977 211-24.

244. *Osborn's Concise Law Dictionary* (6th Ed). J Burke (Ed) . Sweet & Marshall 1976

245. *Oxford Concise Medical Dictionary* 4th Ed 1994.

246. Painter K. Norplant gets a shot in the arm. *USA TODAY*. 22.8.95

247. Painter K. As perfect a Method as You Can Have. *USA Today* Dec 6, 1990 (cover story) in A Hidden Side of Norplant, by Kristine M Severyn, R.Ph., Ph.D. published by *Celebrate Life* July/August 1994

248. Palmer JR, Rosenberg L, Rao RS, Strom BL, *et al*. Oral contraceptive use and breast cancer risk among African-American women. *Cancer Causes & Control.*1995;6(4):321-31. Ma

249. Park TW, Fujiwara H, Wright TC. Molecular biology of cervical cancer and its precursors. *Cancer.*1995;76:10(Suppl),1902-13 Ma

250. Patel S. Current and potential future drug treatments for osteoporosis. *Ann Rheum Dis.*1996;55:10,700-14. Ma

251. Pater A, Bayatpour M, Pater MM. Oncogenic transformation by human papillomavirus type 16 deoxyribonucleic acid in the presence of progesterone or progestins from oral contraceptives. *Am J Obstet Gynecol.* 1990 Apr; 162:4,1099-103. Ma

252. Paul C. Depo-medroxyprogesterone (Depo-Provera) and risk of breast cancer. *BMJ.* 1989; 299: 759-62

253.   *Pearce's Medical and Nursing Dictionary and Encyclopedia.* 15th Ed. 1983

254.   Peritz E, Ramcharan S.The incidence of cervical cancer and duration of oral contraceptive use. *Am J Epidemiol.* 1977; 6: 462

255.   Perrault D, Eisenhauer EA, Pritchard KI, Panasci L, Norris B, Vandenberg T, Fisher B. Phase II study of the progesterone antagonist mifepristone in patients with untreated metatastic breast carcinoma: A National Cancer Institute of Canada Clinical Trials Group Study. *Journal of Clinical Oncology.*1996 (Oct); 14:2709-2712

256.   Persaud R. (letter).*Lancet.*1995;346:1431

257.   Pike MC, Henderson BE, Krailo MD, Duke A. Breast Cancer in young women and use of oral contraceptives: possible modifying effect of formulation and age at use.*Lancet.* 1983;2: 926-929

258.   Pike MC, Spicer DV, Dahmoush L, Press MF. Estrogens, progestogens, normal breast cell proliferation, and breast cancer risk. *Epidemiologic Reviews.*1993;15:1,17-35

259.   Poulter NR, Meirik O. Haemorrhagic stroke, overall stroke risk, and combined oral contraceptives: results of an international, multicentre, case-control study. *Lancet.*1996;348:#9026. *http://www.thelancet.com/ lancet/User/vol348no9026/articles/article2.html*

260.   Poulter NR, Meirik O. Ischaemic stroke and combined oral contracep-tives: results of an international, multicentre, case-control study. *Lancet.*1996;348:#9026. *http://www.thelancet.com/lancet/User/ vol348no9026/articles/article1.html*

261.   Powell L, Seymour R. Effects of depo-medroxyprogesterone acetate as a contraceptive agent. *Am J Obstet Gynecol.* 1971; 110:36.

262.   Powles TJ, Hardy JR, Ashley GM, Farrington GM, *et al.* A pilot trial to evaluate the acute toxicity and feasibility of tamoxifen for prevention of breast cancer *BrJCancer* (1989) 60;126-131

263. Priore GD, Robischon K, Phipps W. Letter. *NEJM.* 1995;332:1300-1302

264. Profumo R. *et. al.* Neonatal choreoathetosis following prenatal exposure to oral contraceptives. *Pediatrics.* 1990;86:648-9

265. Prudence with the Pill. Health warnings are meant to cause alarm. *The Times.* 21.10.95

266. Rabone D. Postcoital contraception - coping with the Morning After. *Current Therapeutics.* Jan.1990

267. Rahwan R. Prof. of Pharmacology & Toxicology. College Of Pharmacy, Ohio State University. *Chemical Contraceptives, Interceptives and Abortifacients,* 1995

268. Rahwan R. (letter), *Lancet* 1995;346:252

269. Ranstam J, Olsson H, Garne J-P, Aspegren K, Janzon L. Survival in breast cancer and age at start of oral contraceptive usage. *Anticancer Research.* 1991; 11:2043-6.

270. Ranstam JP. Oral contraceptives and breast cancer. *Diss Abstr Int(C)* 1992;53(4):705, Ma

271. Regelson W. Beyond Abortion: RU-486 and the Needs of the Crisis Constituency. *JAMA.* 1990; 264, #8,1027

272. Reubinoff BE, *et al.* Effect of low-dose estrogen oral contraceptives on weight, body composition, and fat distribution in young women. *Fertility and Sterility* 1995;63;(3) 516-520 Ma

273. Reuters - Hoechst gives away patent to RU-486 in Europe. Apr.4 1997 *http://www.reutershealth.com*

274. Reynolds C. School of Law, Flinders University of South Australia, Adelaide. Common law duties of prescribers. *Aust Prescriber.* 1996; 19(1):18-20

275.   Reynolds R.The 'Modified U' technique: a refined method of Norplant
       removal. *The Journal of Family Practice.•*, Vol. 40, No.2 (Feb), 1995

276.   Richard BW, Lasagna L. Drug regulation in the United States and the
       United Kingdom: the depo-provera story. *Ann Intern Med.* 1987; 106:
       886-891.

277.   Right To Life Of Greater Cincinnati *Newsletter,* April 1991.

278.   Roberts IF, West RJ. Teratogenesis and maternal progesterone. *Lancet.*
       1977; ii, 982.

279.   Robinson Assoc.Prof M, Benrimoj Prof. C, Kot T, Dight D, Parker J.
       CNS Medicines - Drug Information for Health Care Pharmacists.
       University of Queensland. 1992

280.   Rodriguez-Contreras R, *et al.* Oral contraceptives and cancer of the
       cervix uteri. Analysis of the strength of the association. *Revista de
       Sanidad e higiene Publica.* 1991;65(1): 25-38, Ma

281.   Rodriguez C, Tatham LM. Thun MJ, Calle EE, Heath CW Jrn. Smoking
       and fatal prostate cancer in a large cohort of adult men. *Amer Journ
       Epidem.* 1997;145: No.5. p.473

282.   Romieu I, *et al.* Oral contraceptives and breast cancer. Review and
       meta-analysis. *Cancer.* 1990;66(11): 2253-63, Ma

283.   Rookus M A, E van Leeuwen. Oral contraceptives and risk of breast
       cancer in women aged 20-54 years. *Lancet* 1994; 334; 884-851

284.   Rosenberg L. The risk of liver neoplasia in relation to combined oral
       contraceptive use. *Contraception.* 1991; 43:643-652 In *Micromedex* Vol
       84

285.   Rosenberg L, Palmer JR, Rao RS, Zauber AG, *et al.* Case-control study
       of oral contraceptive use and risk of breast cancer. *Amer J
       Epidemiol.* 1996;143:25-37

286. Rosing J. Tans G, Nicolaes GAF, Thomassen M, van Oerle R, van der Ploeg P, *et al.* Oral contraceptives and venous thrombosis: different sensitivities to activated protein C in women using second- and third-generation oral contraceptives. *Br J Haem.* 1997;97:233-238

287. Rosner B, Colditz GA, Willett WC. Reproductive risk factors in a prospective study of breast cancer: the Nurses' Health Study. *Am J Epidem.* 1994;139:819-35.

288. Rossing MA, Daling J.R., Weiss NS, Moore DE, Self SG. Ovarian tumors in a cohort of infertile women *N Eng J Med.* 1994; 331: 771-776

289. Rossing MA, Daling JR, Weiss NS. Letter. *N Eng J Med.* 1995; 332: 1300-1302

290. Rowe PM. Investigations into long-term contraceptives. *Lancet.* 1995;346:693

291. Rowe PM, IOM (Institute of Medicine -USA) report calls for research into new contraceptives. *Lancet.* 1996;347:1611

292. Rowe PM. Nonoxynol-9 fails to protect against HIV-1. *Lancet.* 1997; 349:#9058.

293. Rowland CW, in *News Weekly* 1993; Sept 11. Melbourne (Aust) B.A. Santamaria (Ed).

294. Rushton L, Jones DR. Oral contraceptive use and breast cancer risk: a meta-analysis of variations with age at diagnosis, parity and total duration of oral contraceptive use. *Br J Obst Gynae.* 99(3):239-46,1992 Ma

295. Sambrook PN. The treatment of postmenopausal osteoporosis. *N Eng J M.* 1995;333:1495-1496

296. Schlesselman JJ. Cancer of the breast and reproductive tract in relation to use of oral contraceptives. *Contraception.* 1989;40(1): 1-38

297. Schlesselman JJ. Net effect of oral contraceptive use on the risk of cancer in women in the United States. *Obstet Gynecol* 1995;85:5 Pt 1, 793-801 Ma

298. Schonhofer PS, *et al.* Brazil: misuse of misoprostol as an abortifacient may induce malformations. *Lancet.* 1991;337:1537-5

299. Schueler's *Home Medical Advisor Pro*. CD Version. 10460 Tropical Trail Merritt Island, Florida 32952. Ph. 4077790310. Fax. 4077770323

300. Schuurman AG, van den Brandt PA, Goldbohm RA. Exogenous hormone use and the risk of postmenopausal cancer: results from the Netherlands Cohort Study.*Cancer Causes and Control.*1995;6:416-424

301. *Science News Update* April 9, 1997. *http://www.ama-assn.org/sci-pubs/sci-news/1997/snr0409.htm#oc7194*

302. Shanner L. Informed consent and inadequate medical information. *Lancet* 1995;346:251

303. Shapiro S. Oral contraceptives - time to take stock. *N Eng J Med.*1986; 315;7;450-451

304. Shapiro S. (letter). *N Eng J Med.* 1995;332:1300-1302

305. Sharp D. Venous thrombosis and the modern pill.*Lancet.* 1996; 347:181

306. Shu XO, Brinton LA, Gao YT, Yuan JM. Population-based case-control study of ovarian cancer in Shanghai. *Cancer Res.* 1989 (Jul 1); 49:13, 3670-4 Ma

307. Shushan A, Paltiel O, Iscovich J, Elchalal U, Peretz T, Schenker JG. Human menopausal gonadotropin and the risk of epithelial ovarian cancer. *Fertility and Sterility.*1996;65:13-18

308. Sieghart M A. What is their Pill doing to my body? *The Times.* (London).21.10.95

309. *Sixty Minutes*, USA CBS TV April 9 1989. (Transcript)

310. Skegg DC, Noonan EA, Paul C, Spears GFS, Meirik O, Thomas DB. DMPA and breast Cancer. *JAMA.* 1995 :273:799-804

311. Smith R W. 'Safe' sex?. *Bridgetown Evening News*.(USA) 25.1.93

312. Somkuti SG, Sun J, Yowell CW, Fritz MA, Lessey BA. The effects of oral contraceptive pills on markers of endometrial receptivity. *Fertil Steril.* 1996;65:(3):484-488

313. Soussi T. The p53 tumour suppressor gene: a model for molecular epidemiology of human cancer. *Mol Med Today.* 1996;2:1,32-7. Ma

314. Sparrow M.J. Pregnancies in reliable pill takers. *New Zealand Med J.*1989;102:575-577

315. Spinnato JA. Mechanism of action of intrauterine contraceptive devices and its relation to informed consent. *Am J Obstet Gynecol.* 1997;176.503-6

316. Spiera H. Scleroderma After Silicone Augmentation Mammoplasty. *JAMA.* 1988;260:236-238

317. Spirtas R, Kaufman SC, Alexander N., Fertility drugs and ovarian cancer: red alert or red herring? *Fert Steril.* 1993; 59: 291-293

318. Spitzer WO, Lewis MA, Heinemann LAJ, Thorogood M, MacRae KD. Third generation oral contraceptives and risk of venous thrombo-embolic disorders: an international case-control study. *BMJ.* 1996;312: 83-8

319. Stadel BV, Schlesselman JJ. Oral contraceptives and breast cancer. *Lancet.* 1986;I:922-3

320. Stanford JL. Oral contraceptives and neoplasia of the ovary. *Contraception.* 1991;43:(6). p543

321.   Steadman M S, Probst JC, Jones WJ, Keisler DL. Norplant prescribing in family planning. *Journ Fam Practice.* 1996;42 (3):267-271.

322.   *Stedman's Medical Dictionary* 26th Ed 1995. Williams & Wilkins (Pub).

323.   Stryer L. *Biochemistry* 2nd Ed.,1980, W.H. Freeman & Co., San Francisco. USA

324.   Stubblefield PG. The effects on hemostasis of oral contraceptives containing desogestrel. *Am J Obstet Gynecol.* 1993;168:1047-52.

325.   Sweet M. The Contraceptive Revolution - still a bitter pill. *Sydney Morning Herald. (Aust).* March 13, 1995.

326.   Sweet M. Mystery as rarer types of cancer gain ground. *Sydney Morning Herald (Aust).* May 17, 1997, p.5

327.   Symons E-K, Pill safety row still unresolved. *The Sunday Telegraph* (Sydney, Australia) 1.10.95; p.181

328.   Taylor D. Spare the rod. *The Guardian* (U.K.) March 12, 1996, p11.

329.   Taylor S, Armour C. The debate is on: should men receive equal osteoporosis treatment? *Retail Pharmacy (Aust).* May 1997 p.18

330.   The writing group for the PEPI trial. Effects of hormone therapy on bone mineral density. Results from the postmenopausal estrogen/ progestin interventions (PEPI) trial. *JAMA.* 1996;276:1389-1396

331.   Thomas DB, Noonan EA. Breast cancer and depo-medroxyproges-terone acetate: a multinational study. WHO collaborative study of neoplasia and steriod contraceptices. *Lancet.* 1991;338:833-838

332.   Thomas DB, Ray RM, Pardthaisong T, Chutivongse, Koetsawang S, Silpisornkosol S, *et al.* Prostitution, condom use, and invasive squamous cell cervical cancer in Thailand. *Amer Journ Epidem.* 1996; 143:779-86

333. Thomas DB, Ray RM . Oral contraceptives and invasive adenocar-cinomas and adenosquamous carcinomas of the uterine cervix. *Am J Epid.*1996;144:281-289

334. Thomas Jr A G, LeMelle S. The Norplant system:where are we in 1995? *The Journal Of Family Practice*, 1995;40:No 2 Feb ,

335. Thomas SHL. Mortality from venous thromboembolism and myocar-dial infarction in young adults in England and Wales. *Lancet.* 1996;348: #9024. *http://www.thelancet.com/lancet/User/vol348no9024 /letters/ index.html#Mortalityfrom*

336. Tonti-Filippini N., RU-486: Dispelling Some Myths. *St.Vincents Bioethics Newsletter* Vol.8, No.2, 1990.

337. Toynbee P. The pill is still a girl's best friend. *The Independant.* 20.10.95.

338. Trisequens/Trisequens Forte Consumer product Information. Novo Nordisk Pharmaceuticals Pty Ltd. 22 Loyalty Rd, North Rocks NSW 2151

339. UBINIG. "The price of Norplant is TK.2000! You cannot remove it." Clients are refused removal in Norplant trial in Bangladesh. *Issues in Reproduction and Gen Engin.* 1991; 4: (1). 45-46

340. Ursin G, Peters R K, *et al.* Oral contraceptive use and adenocarcinoma of cervix. *Lancet.* 1994; 344; 1390-1394

341. Ursin G, Aragaki CC, Paganini-Hill A, *et al.* Oral contraceptives and premenopausal bilateral breast cancer: A case-control study. *Epidemiology.*1992; 3(5):414-9 Ma

342. *United States Pharmacopiel Dispensing Information* (USPDI) - Drug Information for Health Care Professionals. 12th ED. 1992;IB

343. Van der Vange, N. Ovarian activity in low dose oral contraceptives. *Contemporary Obstetrics and Gynaecology.*In: Chamberlain G, (Ed). *Butterworths*, London 1988;317- 326

344.   Van Voorhis BJ, Anderson DJ and Hill JA. The Effects of RU-486 on Immune Function and Steroid-Induced Immunosuppression In Vitro *Journ Clinical Endoc & Metab.*1989; 69: #6,1195-1199

345.   Vandenbroucke J P, Koster T, Briet E, Reistma PH, Bertina RM, Rosendaal FR. Increased risk of venous thrombosis in oral contraceptive users who are carriers of factor V Leiden mutation. *Lancet* 1994; 344: 1454-1457

346.   Vandenbroucke JP, Bloemenkamp KWM, Helmerhorst FM, Rosendaal FR. Mortality from venous thromboembolism and myocardial infarction in young women in the Netherlands. *Lancet.*1996;348:#9024.

347.   Vandebroucke JP, Helmerhorst FM. Risk of venous thrombosis with hormone-replacement therapy. *Lancet.*1996;348:#9033. *http://www. thelancet.com/lancet/Users/vol348no9033/editorial/commentary. html*

348.   Vandebroucke JP, Rosendaal FR. End of the line for "third-generation-pill" controversy? *Lancet.*1997;349:1113-1114.

349.   Vessey MP, Doll R, Sutton PM. Oral contraceptives and breast neoplasia: a retrospective study. *BMJ.* 1972:3:719-724

350.   Vessey MP, Doll R, Jones K. Oral contraceptives and breast cancer. Progress report of an epidemiology study. *Lancet.* 1975:1:941-944

351.   Vessey M.P, Doll R, Jones K, McPherson K,Yeates D. An epidemiological study of oral contraceptives and breast cancer. *BMJ.* 1979; 1:1757-8

352.   Vessy MP, McPherson K, Yeates D, Doll R. Oral contraceptive use and abortion before first term pregnancy in relation to breast cancer risk. *Br J Cancer.* 1982;45:327-331

353.   Vessey MP, McPherson K, Lawless M, Yeates D. Neoplasia of the Cervix uteri and contraception: A possible adverse effect of the pill. *Lancet,* Oct 22 1983; 930-934

354.   Vessey MP, Lawless M, Yeates D, McPherson K. Progestogen-only contraception. Findings in a large prospective study with special reference to effectiveness. *Br J Fam Planning.* 1985;10:117-121

355.   Voeller B, Nelson J, Day C.,Viral leakage risk differences in Latex condoms. *AIDS Research and Human Retroviruses.* 1994;10:701-710. Mary Ann Liebert, Inc., Publishers

356.   Wade ME, McCarthy PM, Harris GS, Danzer HC. *Am Obstet Gynecol.* (Letters). 1980; March 1:p.698

357.   Was ist da dran?, *Medical Tribune. Internationale Wochenzeitung - Ausgabe fur die Schweiz.* 1989;16,20. Translated by Ania Kurkowski B.Pharm.

358.   *Washington Post.* 22.4.1992 . Interview with C.M.Roland, Editor, Rubber Chemistry and Technology.

359.   Watt AH.Oral contraceptives and venous thromboembolism. *Lancet.* 1995;346:1430

360.   Weinstein AL, *et al.* Breast cancer risk and oral contraceptive use: results from a large case-control study. *Epidem.* 1991;2(5):353-8, Ma

361.   Weiner JJ, Evans WS. Uterine rupture in mid-trimester abortion: a complication of gemeprost vaginal pessaries and oxytocin-a case report. *BrJ Obstet Gynaecol.* 1990;97:1061-62

362.   Weisberg E. Oral contraceptives: fine tuning clinical use. *Patient Management.* 1988;6:19-35

363.   Weisberg E. OCs and community failure rate. *Current Therapeutics.* 1995 (Sept)

364.   Weisberg E, Fraser IS, Carrick SE, Wilde FM. Emergency contraception; General practioner knowledge, attitudes and practices in New South Wales. *Med Journal Aust.* 1995;162:136-138

365.　White M. The Pill: the Gap between Promise and Performance.1985., Published by *Responsible Society Research and Education Trust*, Wicken, Milton Keyes, Bucks, MK196BU, England.

366.　Whittelmore AS, Harris R, Itnyre J, and the Collaborative Ovarian Cancer Group (COCG). *Amer J Epidem*. 1992: 136:1184-1203.

367.　Whittlemore AS. The risk of ovarian cancer after treatment for infertility. *N Eng J Med.*1994;331;12;805-6.

368.　Wilkins L. Masculinization of female fetus due to use of orally given progestins. *JAMA*. 1960;172:1028-32

369.　Wiles J. Contraception: what's new, what works. *Australian Women's Weekly.*1997 (Feb) p.33

370.　Woodcock J, Hope J. Tragic girl given the Pill at 14. *Daily Mail* (UK). 1996; March 27: p.8.

371.　World Health Organisation, Task Force on Methods for the Determination of the Fertile Period, Special Program on Research, Development and Research Training in Human Reproduction, "A prospective Multi-centre Trial of Ovulation Method of Natural Family Planning. 1. The Teaching Phase". *Fertil Steril*. 1981;36:152.

372.　Wingo PA, Lee NC, *et al.* Age-specific differences in the relationship between oral contraceptive use and breast cancer. *Cancer*. 1993;71(4 Suppl): 1506-17,

373.　Women sue over Pill risks. *The Daily Telegraph-Mirror* (Sydney, Aust.). 13.4.95, p 22

374.　Ye Z, Thomas DB, Ray RM, and the WHO collaborative study of neoplasia and steroid contraceptives. Combined Oral Contraceptives and Risk of Cervical Cancer in situ, *International Journal of Epidemiology,* 1995;24:19-26,

375.   Zondervan KT, Carpenter LM, Painter R, Vessey MP. Oral
        contraceptives and cervical cancer — further findings from the Oxford
        Family Planning Association contraceptive study. *Br. J. Cancer.* 1996
        (May); 73:10, 1291-7

NB: The letters Ma at the end of some references denotes a MEDLINE abstract.

16. ACKNOWLEDGEMENTS.

Dr. Susan Moore Ph.D. English Literature, for tireless hours of editorial assistence. Her generosity is beyond repayment.

Drs Richard and Catherine Lennon, and Dr Kevin Hume (Sydney) for medical input, corrections and advice.

Prof. Tony Shannon, Dean, University of Technology - Sydney, Professor of Applied Mathematics, for statistical editing and assistance .

Mrs Mary Helen Wood, Mrs Anna Krohn, Mr Andrew Mullins, Dr A Foong and Melinda Reist, for directional and content advice with earlier drafts.

The library staff at St Vincent's Hospital Therapeutic Medicines Information Centre for their prompt supplying of research papers.

To Bo Kuhar, who unknowingly started me on this project, & Mrs.Judie Brown (USA), Brendan (UK) and Patrick (Ireland) for frequent faxes of relevant medical information.

To David Brandao, a bridge over troubled waters.

To Michael Conyngham, of Autralian Computer Almanac, for converting the MS into PageMaker format.

To Michael Penatta - for always coming through.

To Steve Hitchings - a vigilant typo spotter.

To Harry Z - he knows why.

To my team of barristers and lawyers, for their prudent advice and editing. To my Q.C. - his recommendations were invaluable.

To my children, for their forebearance whilst I spent many long nights and week-ends away from them , "on that stupid computer", preparing this book.

Finally, to my dear wife Jane, for her constant encouragement throughout a long, trying 24 months of research and writing, and for her editorial input.

Mea culpa - any errors are mine, and should not reflect poorly on the above thanked persons. The author would appreciate notification of any errors uncovered.

17. ERRATA TO FIRST EDITION.

Please note the five errors of fact.

p.11, Lines 32-33 should read: "They all contain a progesterone (levonorgestrel or medroxyprogesterone), but in a different drug delivery system and with different developmental histories.

p.100, Reference 389. It should read that the Billing's Method is 97% effective, not 99% effective.

p.179, Line 21 should read " A decrease in health (not *longevity*) is the price women will pay for the exclusion of this vital medical information."

p.203, Minulet contains gestodene, not desogestrel as the active progestogen.

p.243, Endnote 464. Delete "- referred to in the literature as ovulatory age-", which occurs midway through this entry.

18. ABOUT THE AUTHOR.

John Wilks has worked as a community pharmacist for more than fifteen years and has owned and managed his own pharmacy for ten years. During this time he has developed a strong interest in patient counselling and in the correct administration of drugs. He is the Director of the Drug Information Service of Western Sydney and was one of the first Australian community pharmacists to utilize Micromedex, a drug- information CD, as an adjunct to patient counselling.

He lectures part-time to graduate pharmacists at the University of Sydney, is a Director of API (Australian Pharmaceutical Industries) Health Care/Pharmacist Advice group and provides consultancy services to other community pharmacists interested in patient counselling. He has been a research investigator involved in a variety of projects linked both with the University of Sydney and pharmaceutical manufactures.

He has made numerous appearances on TV, radio and in the press on matters related to the correct community use of drugs and related health matters.

September, 1997